Obstetrics and Gynecology

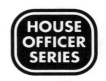

HOUSE OFFICER SERIES

Obstetrics and Gynecology

William F. Rayburn, M.D.

John W. Records Chair
Professor and Chief of Obstetrics
The University Hospital
Director, Section of Maternal-Fetal Medicine
Department of Obstetrics and Gynecology
The University of Oklahoma College of Medicine
Oklahoma City, Oklahoma

J. Christopher Carey, M.D.

Vice Chairman
Professor and Chief of Gynecology
The University Hospital
Department of Obstetrics and Gynecology
The University of Oklahoma College of Medicine
Oklahoma City, Oklahoma

Williams & Wilkins

BALTIMORE • PHILADELPHIA • HONG KONG
LONDON • MUNICH • SYDNEY • TOKYO

A WAVERLY COMPANY

Editor: Charles W. Mitchell
Managing Editor: Marjorie Kidd Keating
Production Coordinator: Kimberly S. Nawrozki and Anne Stewart-Seitz
Copy Editor: John J. Guardiano
Designer: Dan Pfisterer
Illustration Planner: Wayne Hubbel
Cover Designer: Wilma Rosenberger
Typesetter: Peirce Graphic Services, Inc.
Printer: Victor Graphics

Copyright © 1996 Williams & Wilkins
351 West Camden Street
Baltimore, Maryland 21201-2436 USA

Rose Tree Corporate Center
1400 North Providence Road
Building II, Suite 5025
Media, Pennsylvania 19063-2043 USA

Accurate indications, adverse reactions and dosage schedules for drugs are provided in this book, but it is possible that they may change. The reader is urged to review the package information data of the manufacturers of the medications mentioned.

Printed in the United States of America

First Edition, 1984
Second Edition, 1988

Library of Congress Cataloging-in-Publication Data

Rayburn, William F.
    Obstetrics and gynecology / William F. Rayburn, J. Christopher Carey.
        p.   cm.
    Includes index.
    ISBN 0-683-07181-5
    1. Gynecology—Outlines, syllabi, etc.   2. Obstetrics—Outlines, syllabi, etc.   I.
    Carey, J. Christopher.   II. Title.
RG112.R39 1995
618—dc20
                                                                        95-23109
                                                                            CIP

The publishers have made every effort to trace the copyright holders for borrowed material. If they have inadvertently overlooked any, they will be pleased to make the necessary arrangements at the first opportunity.

95 96 97 98 99
1 2 3 4 5 6 7 8 9 10

Preface

Every woman deserves optimal primary care before, during, and after her reproductive years. Good clinical judgment is essential in individualizing patient care, and current advances in medicine must be kept in proper perspective. This manual will serve as a quick reference for house officers who see patients with obstetric and gynecologic problems in the clinic, office, or emergency room. The scope of this manual is wide, covering most aspects of obstetric and gynecologic outpatient care. Descriptions of surgery are beyond the scope of this reference.

Guidelines used at The University of Oklahoma Health Sciences Center are presented in dealing with such problems. It must be remembered that this text describes one or two aspects of proper management; there may be other appropriate alternatives to good care. Information was gathered from a review of the current literature, American College of Obstetricians/Gynecologists Technical Bulletins, peer review literature, discussions with respected colleagues, and our own combined clinical impressions.

Approaches to common clinical conditions continue to evolve and change over time, as identified in our original obstetrics textbook 12 years ago (1984) and in the second edition 8 years ago (1988). Those familiar with these previous editions will recognize immediately that the organization of the present volume remains largely intact for obstetrics but incorporates new information about gynecology. Pertinent information is presented in the many tables highlighting the text. Clinical investigations continue to provide new information pertaining to disorders unique to the female patient.

Our hope for the book is to present this contemporary information in an easy-to-read manner with direct clinical application. We would like to thank Mary Long and Karen Johnston for their tireless hours in preparing the manuscript and Margaret Huffman for her thoughtful review of the manuscript.

William F. Rayburn, M.D.
J. Christopher Carey, M.D.

Contents

Obstetrics

Chapter 1

Prenatal Care

GESTATIONAL AGE DETERMINATION

Along with counseling the patient in preparing for pregnancy changes and childbirth, accurate dating of the pregnancy is essential for timing of a repeat cesarean section, assessment of fetal growth, decision making if pregnancy intervention is planned, timing of an amniocentesis (genetic, fetal lung maturity), assessment of multifetal gestation, avoiding iatrogenic premature delivery, and predicting neonatal survival if preterm delivery is anticipated. Accuracy in predicting the delivery date is improved by combining the methods described below and documenting these landmarks on the prenatal record.

Methods

Last Menstrual Period

If known with certainty, the date of the last menses is the most reliable clinical estimator of gestational age. However, dating is uncertain in 14–58% (average 40%) of all pregnancies. Menstrual dating requires a history of any contraceptive method (particularly oral contraceptives) and any menstrual irregularities.

Initial Positive Pregnancy Test

Methods for measuring human chorionic gonadotropin (hCG) and the earliest time for accurate measurements are listed in Table 1.1.

Initial Uterine Examination

Uterine size may be large-for-dates in the presence of a full bladder, trophoblastic disease, uterine fibroids, or twins.

Table 1.1
Pregnancy Tests to Detect hCG

Method	Detectable (+) results (weeks postconception)	Test sensitivity (mIU/mL)
Hemagglutination inhibition	3–4	750–3500
Enzyme-linked immunosorbent assay (ELISA)	2	25 (serum) 50 (urine)
Agglutination inhibition	2–3	100–200
Radioimmunoassay (RIA)		
Rapid, qualitative	2	20–40
24–48-hour, quantitative	1	2–4

Initial Fetal Heart Auscultation

With amplified Doppler auscultation, the fetal heart sounds should be heard by 12 weeks or sooner, depending on whether the uterus is pushed up out of the pelvis by a full bladder. Unamplified heart sounds are usually heard by 20 weeks in nonobese patients.

Initial Perception of Fetal Movement

A primigravid patient usually perceives light fetal movements by 19–20 weeks, whereas a multigravid patient often feels motion by 17–18 weeks. This parameter is often inexact.

Serial Uterine Fundal Height Examinations

An excellent correlation exists between fundal height measurement (in centimeters) from the upper symphysis to fundus and the gestational age (in weeks) between 18 and 30 weeks. This measurement is influenced by fetal position, differences between examiners, an empty or full bladder, or a patient's obesity.

Ultrasonography

Ultrasound examination should be performed to confirm pregnancy dating if the historical dates are in question, if obstetric intervention or elective delivery is to be required, or if a uterine size-date discrepancy exists. While abdominal scanning reliably detects the gestational sac at 6 weeks by menstrual dating, transvaginal scanning can identify the sac by 5 menstrual weeks. Fetal echoes should be seen by 7 weeks' gestation by abdominal scanning and before 6 weeks when vaginal scanning is used. Fetal heart activity may be viewed with abdominal scanning at 7 weeks by menstrual dating and at 6 weeks with transvaginal scanning. Measurement of fetal crown-rump length between 8 and 13 weeks can define gestational age to within 5 days in 95% of cases. The crown-rump length in centimeters plus 6.5 approximates the gestational age.

Beyond the 13th week, the average of gestational age predictions using biparietal diameter, head circumference, abdominal circumference, and femur length measurements is the best estimate of fetal age. These measurements can define gestational age to within 8 days before 20 weeks. However, this averaging method loses reliability if one measurement is incompatible with other measurements. Less frequently used parameters are outer orbital diameters, transcerebellar diameter, and foot length. The transcerebellar diameter in millimeters corresponds to the gestational age in weeks between 14 and 24 menstrual weeks.

Large variations ($\pm$ 3 weeks) in normal fetal measurements during the third trimester compromise the accuracy of late pregnancy ultrasonography in establishing gestational age. Nevertheless, the measurements do allow for estimation of fetal weight and assessment of fetal growth.

RECOMMENDATIONS TO PATIENTS

Symptoms during Pregnancy

Knowing that nausea and even vomiting are favorable signs, the patient may be able to handle these symptoms without medical intervention. Simple nausea is often treated expectantly with reassurance and diet manipulation. It is often helpful to avoid dehydration and hypoglycemia and to ingest frequent small feedings beginning upon awakening. Emotional factors undoubtedly contribute. Prenatal vitamins that contain vitamin B_6, antihistamines, or both may be helpful. Drug therapy is recommended to avoid maternal dehydration, weight loss, and electrolyte imbalance. Intravenous fluids (typically 1–3 liters of lactated Ringer's solution) on an outpatient basis often provide temporary relief. Phenothiazines, notably promethazine (Phenergan), and piperazine dihydrochloride (meclizine), are used commonly and without added risk of fetal anomalies. Less is known about the use of metoclopramide or H_2 blockers. If conservative therapy and antiemetic drugs are inadequate, enteral fluid and nutrient therapy (especially parenteral nutrient therapy) may be necessary at home or in the hospital.

Breast tenderness is another frequent symptom that occurs early in pregnancy, often before the first missed period. The degree of tenderness is variable and may be influenced by sexual stimulation and temperature changes, being worse during cold weather. The patient should wear a well-supporting, well-fitting bra, especially if she is physically active. The cup size of the bra is expected to increase by as much as two sizes during pregnancy. Nursing bras are available and may be worn later in pregnancy.

Profound fatigue can be expected, particularly during the first and last trimesters. Proper nutrition and daily rest with frequent naps are necessary during this period. In addition, a daily routine of exercise, such as walking, swimming, or bicycling, is recommended.

As additional weight is carried, the ligaments holding the pelvis together soften to allow fetal descent in anticipation of childbirth. For the most part, back and pelvic discomforts are normal, and lying on the side or a change in posture will usually give temporary relief. Persistent back pain should be sought, since this may suggest a urinary tract infection, premature labor, or a herniated disk.

Edema of the feet and legs is common, especially after standing or sitting for long periods. Support pantyhose may be worn while working and standing erect. Knee-hose should be avoided, because they further constrict the flow of blood returning from the lower extremities. It is important to note whether any rings become tight and difficult to remove if there is any swelling of the hands or face. Diuretics should rarely be given during pregnancy, because they decrease the blood volume and blood flow to the uterus and fetus.

Urinary frequency is one of the earliest signs of pregnancy. Going to the bathroom nearly twice as frequently is most noticeable during the first and last trimesters. Since the kidneys function best at night while the patient is lying on her side, she should expect to awaken several times to empty her bladder. Should she experience any burning or pain in the bladder area or the back, a urinary tract infection may be present which should be treated promptly.

The expanded blood volume during pregnancy often leads to nasal congestion, which can cause difficulty in breathing and sleeping, and can cause nausea. Decongestants and antihistamines are used frequently. Bleeding of the nose may occasionally accompany nasal congestion. This may be worse during winter because of dry air in heated buildings. Placing Vaseline on the inner aspect of each nostril before going to bed will help.

Changes occur during pregnancy in the stomach and intestines that will result in more efficient absorption of food. One of these changes is increased acid secretion by the stomach, and this can result in heartburn. If prone to heartburn, the patient should avoid smoking, drinking caffeinated beverages, and lying down after a meal. At night the entire head of the bed (not just the patient's head) should be elevated at least 3 inches. This can be done by placing a brick or other suitable object under the frame of the bed. Antacids, such as Tums, Maalox, and Mylanta, may be taken up to every 2 hours.

Many patients experience constipation during all stages of pregnancy. This is due in part to the iron content of vitamin pills, absorption of more fluids into the bloodstream, and compression of the bowel by the enlarging uterus. Constipation will be lessened by increasing fluid intake to three or more glasses of water or milk each day. We also recommend eating high-fiber foods, such as bran cereals and fresh fruit. Stool softeners are not recommended routinely, but cellulose powders (Metamucil) may be taken without harm.

Hemorrhoids may occur during pregnancy (and particularly after delivery) due to the softening of tissues, including the blood vessels, and to the increase in the circulating blood volume. These rarely require surgery and will usually subside after delivery. Preparation H, Anusol, or Tucks may be used without concern to decrease the swelling and relieve the pain. In addition, a cold compress will often help.

Although choice of clothing is a personal matter, those worn before pregnancy will become very tight and uncomfortable. It is important that garments be loose-fitting and comfortable. In addition, shoes should be comfortable, allowing for the modest swelling that is a normal symptom of pregnancy, and they should be of a style that provides stability, helping to prevent trips or falls.

An increase in vaginal discharge is an expected symptom of early and late pregnancy and does not require therapy. A speculum examination may be necessary to search for bacterial vaginosis, trichomoniasis, and other forms of infection, which may promote premature labor. Pregnancy can predispose to monilial infections, which may result in a further increase in the vaginal discharge, a change in its color or odor, a staining or crusting on undergarments, or itching of the labia. Should these symptoms occur, the physician should prescribe the appropriate therapy. Douching during pregnancy should be discouraged.

Precautions to Take during Pregnancy

A woman's prepregnancy body mass index (BMI) and her total weight gain during pregnancy are important determinants of newborn weight. Ranges of recommended weight gain during pregnancy according to the National Academy of Sciences are listed in Table 1.2. Nutritional advice during pregnancy includes a balanced daily diet containing approximately 35 calories for each kilogram of optimal body weight plus 300 calories. A proper diet is essential. We recommend fresh fruit, fresh vegetables, lean meats (chicken, fish), whole-grain breads and cereals, and low-fat dairy products. Intolerance to milk is common during pregnancy and may cause heartburn and induce cramping, diarrhea, and excess flatulence. It is acceptable to substitute cheese or yogurt or to add lactase (Lactaid) to the milk.

Most doctors prescribe prenatal vitamin supplements, but they are not essential during pregnancy as long as nutrition is adequate. Iron supplementation is necessary to maintain body stores and minimize the occurrence of iron deficiency anemia. Therefore, a prenatal vitamin supplement containing iron or an

Table 1.2
Recommended Weight Gain in Pregnancy

Patient's Original Weight	Pregnant BMI	Weight Gain Total (lb)	Rate (lb/weeks)
Underweight	<19.8	28–40	5.0
Normal weight	19.8–26.0	25–35	4.0
Overweight	26.1–29.0	15–25	2.6
Obese	>29.0	15	2.0

Adapted with permission from Nutrition during pregnancy. Washington, DC: National Academy Press, 1990.

iron tablet alone should be taken daily during pregnancy and lactation. Junk food and fast foods, though economical and convenient, should be discouraged as a regular part of the diet because they contain excess fat, salt, sugar, etc. A list of foods in any special diet (for example, a vegetarian diet) should be sought.

Sex need not be discontinued during pregnancy. The anticipation of a new family member may result in an increase in normal sexual desires. As pregnancy progresses, sexual activity becomes more difficult, more tiring, and sometimes uncomfortable. However, there is no reason to discontinue sexual activity, as it is generally believed not to pose any risk to the fetus or to result in an increased risk of premature labor or delivery. Orgasm will frequently cause uterine contractility, which may be uncomfortable but does no apparent harm. On the other hand, if the patient experiences any signs of an abnormal discharge or any recent vaginal bleeding, she should abstain from sexual activity until after she has been examined. In addition, a history of a "weak" or incompetent cervix, premature labor, or an untreated genitourinary infection should be sought. The mucus in the cervix during a normal pregnancy forms an effective plug such that the ejaculate remains in the vagina and does not gain access to the uterus.

The patient should refrain from using very hot water while bathing. Sitting in a sauna bath or hot tub with water temperatures higher than 110°F should be avoided or at least not continued for more than 10 minutes. The water is too hot if it reddens the skin. It is common to become very lightheaded, particularly late in pregnancy, and especially when changing positions from lying down to standing, sitting to standing, and getting out of the bathtub.

Pregnancy induces changes in the gums and teeth, and dental care is encouraged during pregnancy. Major procedures that require much manipulation or surgery should be discussed beforehand. Most dentists are very cautious about performing any dental procedure during the first and last few months of pregnancy. Dentists provide protective aprons that shield the fetus from any x-ray exposure.

During pregnancy, women can continue to exercise and derive health benefits even from mild-to-moderate exercise routines. Exercise in the supine position should be avoided after the first trimester. Non-weightbearing exercises such as cycling or swimming will minimize the risk of injury and facilitate the continuation of exercise during pregnancy. Any type of exercise involving the potential for even mild abdominal trauma or loss of balance should be avoided. Exercise during pregnancy requires an additional 300 calories/day, adequate hydration, appropriate clothing, and optimal environmental surroundings. While maternal fitness and a sense of well-being may be enhanced by exercise, no level of exercise during pregnancy has been conclusively demonstrated to be beneficial in improving perinatal outcome.

During the initial prenatal visit, time should be allotted to discuss the recurrence of any pregnancy complications. General risk figures are relatively encouraging and often helpful for patient education. The data are usually derived from large groups of heterogeneous pregnancies and may be subject to methodological bias. The risk of recurrence is less if no contributing factor (twins, anemia, hypertension, etc.) is present in any subsequent pregnancy. The etiology of complications is also often obscure and likely to remain so. An honest appraisal of the chances of success in any future pregnancy is necessary for the patient's support. Table 1.3 indicates recurrence risk figures for some of the most severe complications.

Only 6% of births in the United States involve women aged 35 or older. Those with an advanced maternal age often have postponed beginning a family until their education has been completed and a career has been started. Although most of such pregnancies are successful, there appears to be a greater risk of

Table 1.3
Recurrence Risks for Common Pregnancy Complications

Previous Complication	Recurrence Risk (%)	
Hydatidiform mole	1.3–2.9%	
Recurrent miscarriage	20%–30%	
Ectopic pregnancy	50%	for involuntary infertility
	35%–40%	for successful pregnancy
	10%–15%	for recurrent ectopic
Mild preeclampsia	2.0%	for severe preeclampsia
	29.0%	for mild preeclampsia
Severe preeclampsia	7.5%	for severe preeclampsia
	30.0%	for mild preeclampsia
Preterm labor × 1	15%	
× 2	30%	
Gestational diabetes	20%–30%	

spontaneous abortion, and the stillbirth rate doubles by the late 30s and increases to threefold to fourfold by the mid-40s. Chromosomal abnormalities, especially trisomies 13, 18, and 21, and sex chromosome aneuploidies increase logarithmically with maternal age starting in the 30s. Genetic counseling should therefore be offered to any expectant mother who is 35 or older. Bleeding from a placenta previa or abruptio placentae is also thought to be more common in late gestation of older patients. Hypertension, preeclampsia, and diabetes are not only more frequent, but also seem to carry a greater risk, resulting in more frequent fetal demise. There also appear to be more abnormal labor patterns and a higher incidence of cesarean section.

Travel late in pregnancy should be discussed. As a general rule, we discourage long trips within the last month, particularly within the last 2 weeks of pregnancy or when a complication has occurred. If there are situations that require travel late in pregnancy, we encourage a vaginal examination before leaving to determine the dilation of the cervix. It is also wise for the patient to have the name of a competent obstetrician in the community to be visited. If travel is by automobile, a stop is recommended at least every 2 hours. During this travel break, it is necessary to ambulate and to empty the bladder. It is safe to fly during pregnancy, and there is no increased risk of abortion or anomalies to the fetus.

Vaginal bleeding at any time during pregnancy should be sought. It is not uncommon for slight spotting to occur after sex or a pelvic examination. However, this should be reported if it persists.

Uterine contractions within 2 months before the due date are common but should be reported. Irregular contractions occurring less frequently than every 8 minutes are particularly common and likely to be Braxton-Hicks contractions. The physician should be notified if these persist as frequently as every 5 minutes after rest and hydration.

Approximately 1% of all pregnant women are exposed to abdominal x-rays during the first trimester. Radiation exposures usually result in doses much lower than 5 rads. A dose of about 10 rads is the lowest amount associated with structural embryonic or fetal defects. Should x-rays be necessary (such as a dental, chest, or abdominal film), the uterus should be shielded, which renders these necessary x-rays quite safe. On occasion, a patient will report that an x-ray was performed very early in pregnancy when pregnancy was unsuspected. Any added risk to the fetus is highly unlikely, and there is no indication for a therapeutic abortion. After fertilization, radiation effects are likely to be "all or none" during tubal transport, and the embryo after implantation may be more resistant.

Fevers of 100°F or greater should also be reported. This may be due to a flu-like illness but may also represent a more serious infection such as pyelonephritis or pneumonia. The actual harm to the fetus from high fevers cannot be clearly determined but a targeted ultrasound scan and a maternal serum alpha-fetoprotein test are recommended with first-trimester exposure.

Blood pressure changes can be monitored in the clinic and at home. For patients with a prior history of high blood pressure or kidney disease, we frequently ask that they purchase a blood pressure cuff and stethoscope at their local drug or department store. By monitoring blood pressure levels at home as well as in the clinic, we have a better idea of the degree of the problem and can better counsel the patient. Severe, continuous headaches are uncommon during pregnancy and should be reported.

Severe or persistent abdominal pain or cramping are associated with an abruptio placentae or premature labor. These pains are often sharp and well-localized. On the other hand, it is common to have occasional abdominal cramps that are related to Braxton-Hicks uterine contractions. A sudden escape of fluid from the vagina indicates either a loss of urine or a rupture of the membranes.

A decrease in fetal movement is a common patient concern. Fetal movement charts are available for patients who have a pregnancy complication or notice a decrease in fetal movement. The patient is asked to keep a daily record of the fetus's activity during at least one convenient hour while lying on her side. Documented fetal inactivity suggests compromise and requires more objective evaluation.

Preparing for Childbirth and Infant Care

Specific information about childbirth classes should be available in any prenatal clinic. We strongly encourage our patients to prepare for labor by attending these classes even if a repeat cesarean section will be undertaken. If there are any concerns about delivery, discuss these with the patient and any other doctor who is likely to perform the delivery. Also discuss what to expect during labor and delivery, and what may be used for analgesia. Discuss with her the possibility or probability of needing a cesarean delivery or bilateral tubal ligation.

Cesarean section classes are usually available if the patient has an interest in learning more about the surgery. A prior cesarean section does not necessarily compel a repeat cesarean section. Every effort can be made to allow a vaginal birth experience if the patient and her spouse desire.

Information should be provided about options available during the course of labor and after delivery. These options include an intravenous line to be maintained throughout labor, electronic fetal heart monitoring, vaginal preparation, sibling visitation, 24-hour rooming-in, early hospital discharge, and nurse visits to the home. A labor-delivery-recovery room or "birthing room" may decrease the admission-to-delivery interval, allow more freedom of movement, increase rooming-in time, and decrease hospital costs.

State laws require that each infant receive an application of silver nitrate, erythromycin, or tetracycline to the eyes to guard against gonorrhea. If desired, a circumcision is performed in the first few days after the baby boy is delivered. We encourage that you seek the patient's thoughts on circumcision before labor. Information about the pros and cons of circumcision should be available from the clinic. Although the complication rate is very low, a circumcision is cosmetic and not medically necessary.

We also recommend that a pediatrician or family physician be chosen before delivery. It is not necessary for that doctor to attend the delivery or see the baby shortly after delivery. The baby's first visit should be scheduled 2 to 4 weeks after delivery.

Baby furniture such as a crib and dresser should be purchased before delivery. There are many products available, and parents may wish to discuss these items with a physician or nurse during the antepartum visits. It is a law in many states that the baby leave the hospital in a safety-approved car seat.

We are often surprised that many patients have not chosen a baby's name before birth. This can be an anxiety-provoking situation, and we encourage selection before birth.

OUTPATIENT LABORATORY TESTS

It is essential for the physician who assumes responsibility for prenatal care to be familiar with normal physiologic and pathologic changes. The intervals for routine tests and procedures, as recommended by the American College of Obstetricians and Gynecologists, are summarized in Table 1.4. Indications for special tests are shown in Table 1.5.

DRUG EFFECTS ON THE FETUS

With the increased awareness of drug effects on the unborn infant, there is a general reluctance among patients to take drugs during pregnancy. Despite this trend, the average pregnant patient takes two drugs, besides iron or vitamin supplements, before labor. This number of drugs actually increases rather than decreases as gestation progresses, and approximately one-half of these drugs are over-the-counter preparations (aspirin, acetaminophen, decongestants). The initial prenatal examination should include a history of any prescribed or nonprescription drugs taken at conception, during the first trimester, or currently.

Most drugs have no apparent structural effect on the fetus. Drugs or chemicals account for no more than 1% of all major

Table 1.4
Recommended Intervals for Routine and Indicated Prenatal Tests

Time	Assessment
Initial (as early as possible)	Hemoglobin or hematocrit
	Urinalysis, including microscopic examination and infection screen
	Blood group and Rh type
	Antibody screen
	Rubella antibody titer
	Syphilis screen
	Cervical cytology
	Hepatitis B virus screen
8–18 weeks	Ultrasound
	Amniocentesis
	Chorionic villus sampling
16–18 weeks	Maternal serum alpha-fetoprotein
26–28 weeks	Diabetes screening
	Repeat hemoglobin or hematocrit
28 weeks	Repeat antibody test for unsensitized Rh-negative patients
32–36 weeks	Ultrasound
	Testing for sexually transmitted disease
	Repeat hemoglobin or hematocrit

Table 1.5
Indications for Special Tests during Pregnancy

Special Test	Indications
Gonorrhea culture	Prior venereal infection, vaginitis, drug abuser, adolescent; may be required routinely in certain states
Clean-catch urine for culture	Patients with consecutive positive Testurias, symptoms strongly suggestive of urinary tract infection, or prior history of renal disease
Herpes culture	Vulvar lesion, prior infection, recent exposure
HIV antibody	Patients at increased risk of exposure to the AIDS virus, i.e., intravenous drug abusers, prostitutes, hemophiliacs, and gravidas whose sexual partners may be at increased risk because of the above factors or homosexual activity. Informed consent should be obtained prior to testing because of the potential adverse psychosocial implications of a positive result
Shielded chest x-ray	Positive tuberculin skin test, significant past or present respiratory or cardiac illness
Ultrasound	Uncertain menstrual dates, uterine size disparity, prior cesarean section, medical or obstetric complications, poor obstetric history
1-hour post 50 g glucola glucose determinations (before 24th week)	Family history of diabetes, prior macrosomic fetus, prior poor obstetric history, persistent glycosuria, suspected polyhydramnios, maternal age 35 or older, obesity, recurrent moniliasis, or prior anomalous infant
Hemoglobin A_{lc}	Maternal diabetes or prior macrosomic infant
Rubella titer (later in pregnancy)	If prior titer was 1:8–1:16, or suspected exposure to rubella if titer less than 1:16
Paternal blood typing	Rh-negative mother-to-be, uncertainty of father-to-be's Rh status

malformations, while multifactorial or unknown causes are implicated in two-thirds of all human malformations. Teratogenic effects include not only obvious malformations or abortions, but also altered fetal growth, carcinogenesis, functional deficits, or mutagenesis. Therefore, no drug can be considered absolutely safe to use during pregnancy.

Our limited knowledge about specific drugs is gathered from case reports, epidemiologic studies, or animal studies in which different experimental animal species and strains are typically exposed to high drug doses during early fetal development. The few drugs with known teratogenic effects include anticonvulsants, warfarin (Coumadin), alcohol, folic acid antagonists (methotrexate, aminopterin), diethylstilbestrol, androgens, and thalidomide (Table 1.6). Except for phenytoin, those drugs with known teratogenic effects are unnecessary during pregnancy. Suspected teratogenic drugs include alkylating agents, nicotine, sulfonylureas, isotretinoin (13-*cis*-retinoic acid), valproic acid, and benzodiazepines.

General Recommendations

The overall incidence of birth defects in the general population is 2–4%. Most drugs pose no obvious threat to the fetus, but added risks are related to the dose, duration, any drug metabolites, and gestational age at the time of exposure. The genotype of the mother and fetus and the effect from any other drugs must also be considered.

Accurate dating of gestational age is necessary when a patient expresses concern about drug exposure during early pregnancy. The drug or chemical may have been taken before implantation or after organogenesis. Unless absolutely necessary, all drugs should be avoided during the first trimester.

An amniocentesis to screen for drug or metabolite levels is not recommended. A maternal serum alpha-fetoprotein (MSAFP) level between 15 and 18 weeks may be helpful, especially when a drug has been taken which is thought to be associated with an increased risk of open neural tube defects, such as valproic acid or carbamazepine. Ultrasonography is useful for dating a gestation, searching for major malformations, and assessing fetal growth. Reassuring findings are not a guarantee of a "normal" fetus, however.

The risks and benefits must be considered when prescribed medications are necessary to treat any underlying medical or ob-

Table 1.6
Drugs with Known or Suspected Teratogenic Effects

Drug	Teratogenic Effect(s)
Known teratogens	
Anticonvulsants (phenytoin, trimethadione)	Facial dysmorphogenesis, mild mental retardation, growth retardation, cardiac defects
Anticoagulants (warfarin and congeners)	Nasal hypoplasia, epiphyseal stippling, optic atrophy, mental retardation
Alcohol	Fetal alcohol syndrome—growth retardation, mild mental retardation, increase in anomalies
Folic acid antagonists (methotrexate, aminopterin)	Abortion, multiple malformations
Hormones Diethylstilbestrol and congeners	Vaginal adenosis, carcinogenesis, cervical and uterine anomalies, epididymal abnormalities
Androgens	Masculinization of female fetus
Methyl mercury	CNS damage, growth retardation
Thalidomide	Phocomelia
Valproic acid	Open neural tube defects
Isotretinoin 13-*cis*-retinoic acid	Hydrocephalus, cardiac defects, ear and hearing defects
Suspected teratogens	
Alkylating agents	Abortion, anomalies
Lithium carbonate	Ebstein's anomaly (?)
Nicotine	Growth delay
Sulfonylureas	Anomalies (?)
Carbamazepine	Open neural tube defects

stetric complication. As a general rule, perinatal outcomes are more favorable with the appropriate selection of a drug (or drugs) to treat an underlying medical disorder. Even though the lowest effective doses are desired, total serum concentrations of such prescription drugs as phenobarbital, phenytoin, or digoxin decrease during pregnancy. Therefore, increased doses of these medications are required to maintain adequate therapeutic levels.

Specific Drugs

Mild Analgesics

No conclusive evidence exists that aspirin causes fetal malformations in humans. Salicylates may inhibit prostaglandin synthesis and reduce platelet aggregation. Gestation and labor may be prolonged if large doses have been taken. Prolonged bleeding time, even with small doses, may last for 5–7 days, and blood loss at delivery may be increased.

Salicylates cross the placenta freely, and premature closure of the ductus arteriosus is theoretically possible. This event may cause pulmonary arterial hypertension and cardiopulmonary complications in the newborn. Other potential fetal or neonatal problems include increased bleeding time and jaundice from competition with bilirubin and albumin binding.

Because of these potentially harmful effects in the third trimester, it is preferable to avoid aspirin and to substitute acetaminophen if necessary. Acetaminophen has similar analgesic and antipyretic properties, which may result from prostaglandin synthetase inhibition or direct hypothalamic stimulation. To the best of our knowledge, no consistent information has revealed any detrimental effect of acetaminophen on the fetus when used in the recommended doses.

Decongestants and Antihistamines

Physiologic nasal congestion, upper respiratory viral infections, and allergic symptoms are common during pregnancy and frequently require decongestant and antihistamine therapy. Pseudoephedrine-containing decongestants have not been shown to be teratogenic in human fetuses. Patients with hypertension, however, should avoid or minimize the use of these medicines during pregnancy.

Compared with a group of pregnant patients who took no drugs, no increased incidence of congenital anomalies has been reported in patients using such antihistamines as brompheniramine, chlorpheniramine, and meclizine. Antihistamines and decongestants are excreted in breast milk, but neonatal effects are not significant in the usual dosages.

Antacids

Over-the-counter antacid preparations contain either aluminum hydroxide, calcium carbonate, sodium bicarbonate, or magnesium hydroxide. Antacid use is most common in late pregnancy for relief of heartburn from gastric hyperacidity. It is considered safe, unless high doses are ingested chronically.

Adverse effects from antacid use include constipation and

impaired absorption of such drugs as tetracyclines, cephalosporins, and chlorpromazine. Although absorbed calcium or magnesium from within these preparations may cross the placenta or be excreted in breast milk, effects on the fetus or neonate are not considered to be significant.

Penicillins

Penicillins are commonly prescribed during pregnancy for treatment of urinary tract or upper respiratory infections. To achieve serum drug concentrations similar to those in the nonpregnant state, large or more frequent dosages may be necessary. Many clinical studies have failed to show adverse effects of penicillins on the developing fetus. Penicillins may therefore be considered safe to use in nonallergic patients. Most antibiotics will appear in breast milk and may cause diarrhea and candidiasis in the nursing infant with prolonged exposure.

Antiemetics

If the patient is unresponsive to conservative therapy, such as frequent, small, dry meals, phenothiazine medications have been prescribed. Products such as promethazine (Phenergan) are not associated with an increased risk of fetal anomalies. Phenothiazines may cause drowsiness, disorientation, hypotension, and extrapyramidal signs and are not currently approved by the Food and Drug Administration for routine use during pregnancy.

Caffeine

Caffeine and its metabolites cross the placenta without apparent difficulty and are detected in the serum and urine of newborn infants. Caffeine also crosses into the breast milk, and withdrawal of moderate or continual doses may explain jitteriness, wakefulness, or irritability in a sensitive infant.

Documentation is lacking about human malformations attributable to caffeine ingestion in normally consumed amounts. An association between excess caffeine intake (800 mg or more each day; six or more 6-ounce cups of coffee) and increased fetal loss have been reported. Large, well-controlled epidemiologic studies have failed to show any obvious effects from excess caffeine on the developing fetus, however. Decaffeinated beverages may be substituted, although this is not absolutely necessary.

Oral Contraceptives

When taken during early pregnancy, oral contraceptives may increase maternal nausea and vomiting and promote cholestatic jaundice. A review of the literature shows that most studies have failed to reveal an increased incidence of congenital anomalies, spontaneous abortion, and chromosomal abnormalities in pregnancies delivering at term.

A combination of anomalies involving the vertebrae, anus, cardia, trachea, esophagus, and limbs ("VACTERL" syndrome) has been associated with sex steroid exposure during early gestation. On the other hand, several reports have failed to confirm this teratogenicity, especially cardiac defects. Masculinization of the female fetus is theoretically possible from prolonged exposure to androgen-like progestins. However, this finding has been reported in only 0.3% of all exposed female fetuses.

In our experience, the patient will discontinue oral contraceptive use soon after discovering the pregnancy. An abortion is to be discouraged, and the patient should be reassured that the risk of a malformation is no greater than the usual 2–4% incidence.

Cigarette Smoking

Approximately one-third of women are smokers at the time they conceive. Carbon monoxide has an affinity for adult hemoglobin 200 times greater than that of oxygen, and an even higher affinity for fetal hemoglobin, resulting in a decrease in oxygen carrying capacity. Nicotine's action on the adrenal gland results in increased levels of circulatory norepinephrine, epinephrine, and acetylcholine, which lead to a decrease in uteroplacental perfusion. Nicotine crosses the placenta and increases blood pressure in the fetus. It may also affect the fetal gastrointestinal, genital, urinary, and central nervous systems and decrease breathing.

Smoking is also associated with reproductive health problems such as lower overall fecundity, ovulatory and tubal disorders, increased perinatal mortality, bleeding complications of pregnancy, decreased mean birth weight (by 220 g or 5 oz), and higher incidences of small-for-gestational-age babies, low-birthweight babies, and preterm deliveries. The goal of the provider is to help a woman to stop (or at least reduce) smoking, refrain from smoking during pregnancy, and avoid relapse after delivery through intensive smoking cessation programs. The package inserts of the nicotine gum and transdermal patches suggest that pregnant women not use these therapies.

Alcohol

Jones and Smith reported in 1973 a constellation of abnormalities described as the "fetal alcohol syndrome." Nearly all of these infants were born to daily heavy alcohol drinkers. Studies show that a daily intake of greater than 2.2 g of ethyl alcohol per kilogram (5 ounces or six hard drinks) significantly increases the frequency of central nervous system dysfunction, growth deficiencies, and facial abnormalities. Mental retardation is a common manifestation. Microcephaly, hydrocephaly, and incomplete development of the cerebral cortex have also been described. It is uncertain whether heavy alcohol use affects early fetal loss.

No absolute safe level of consumption has been determined, so all pregnant women should be cautioned to reduce alcohol intake to the barest minimum and encouraged to eat properly. It is unknown whether light or moderate drinking causes any added risk of malformation or abortion. Concentrations in breast milk are not significant with light or moderate consumption, but infant lethargy and prolonged sleeping may occur when the mother consumes excessive amounts.

Nutritional Supplements

All women of childbearing age in the United States who are capable of becoming pregnant should consume 0.4 mg folic acid per day for the purpose of reducing their risk of having a pregnancy affected with spina bifida or other open neural tube defects (NTDs). Prenatal vitamins contain 0.8 mg or 1 mg of folic acid. Foods with high folate content, such as green, leafy vegetables or breakfast cereals and bread fortified with folic acid, may be consumed instead. Because the benefit of folic acid in preventing first occurrences of NTDs has not been established, obstetricians should continue to offer maternal serum alpha-fetoprotein screening routinely.

Nutritional factors have been implicated in the etiology of hypertensive disease in pregnancy. The role of calcium in the development of hypertension has been proposed in recent epidemiologic and experimental data. Preliminary evidence of the effect of a large daily dose of calcium (1 g) in normal pregnant women reveals a significantly lower diastolic blood pressure in the third trimester. This pattern is in contrast to that seen in similar patients who received either no treatment or a 2-g daily dose and was seen despite there being no changes in blood levels of calcium, magnesium, phosphorus, and proteins.

The fluoride content in most water supplies is usually sufficient. Despite this, prenatal fluoride tablets (1 mg daily) have been recommended for pregnant women. Preliminary evidence suggests that the enamel of teeth exposed prenatally to fluoride is resistant to caries. This is especially true of the surface enamel observed on electron microscopy.

Aspartame, a synthetic sweetener found in diet drinks, contains phenylalanine and aspartic acid. There is no cause for concern about its use during pregnancy. Another sweetener, saccharin, also has not been associated with an increased risk of malformations.

Antibiotics

The most commonly prescribed medications during pregnancy are antibiotics. There has not been any reported increased risk of malformations specifically or overall with first trimester exposure. A short-term course of antibiotics is also not thought to adversely affect the fetus. Ampicillin remains the most commonly prescribed antibiotic, but first and second generation cephalosporins are also considered safe. Less is known about other β-lactam antibiotics (synthetic penicillin, third generation cephalosporins). Erythromycin crosses the placenta negligibly, and therefore would not be effective in treating the fetus. Although metronidazole is not associated with an increased risk of malformations, its use during pregnancy should include folate supplementation and be limited to the second and third trimesters.

Nitrofurantoin is useful for treating urinary tract infections, and, although rarely, is associated with hemolysis. Fetal hyperbilirubinemia is not known to be a concern. Sulfonamides are bacteriostatic agents that interfere with folate synthesis and may cause kernicterus. Use of these during pregnancy should be avoided. Staining of deciduous teeth (enamel hypoplasia) associated with prenatal tetracycline exposure is not reported to result during the first trimester; instead, this finding is associated with the development of adult teeth, which does not begin until the second half of pregnancy. Little has been reported on the use of quinolones during pregnancy, but skeletal dysplasias have not been documented.

Acne Preparations

Acne is a common dermatologic problem during pregnancy. Most acne products are topical preparations that contain benzoyl peroxide, colloidal sulfur, salicylic acid, or antibiotics. These creams, liquids, or gels are absorbed in small amounts and cause no direct harm to the fetus.

Recalcitrant cystic acne is sometimes treated with retinoic acid (vitamin A_1 acid). Oral isotretinoin (Accutane), which contains 13-*cis*-retinoic acid, is contraindicated during pregnancy because of teratogenicity in humans, rats, and rabbits. Case reports of major central nervous system defects in human fetuses and newborns have described microcephaly, hydrocephalus, and abnormalities of the external ear (micropinna, small or absent external auditory canals).

Psychotropic Medications

A common drug safety inquiry concerns the use of psychotropic medications before and during pregnancy. The lowest effective dose is desired. Common side effects and symptoms of toxicity are often confused with pregnancy-induced physiologic changes such as drowsiness, hypotension, nausea, anxiety, headache, increased maternal heart rate, constipation, cholestasis, and fatigue. The risk of fetal anomalies is not thought to be greater than usual, although exposed central nervous system cells continue to divide rapidly throughout fetal development. It is unknown whether intrauterine exposure to those drugs leads to any subtle impairments of behavior and cognitive learning.

Chlorpromazine (300–800 mg daily) is the antipsychotic drug used most commonly, but extrapyramidal, hypotensive, and sedative effects are less with molindone (50–100 mg daily). The plasma half-lives of these drugs are long, often permitting only once daily dosing. All of these compounds undergo hepatic metabolism, which varies significantly between individuals but is not affected by pregnancy alone. For acute psychotic reactions, haloperidol (1–5 mg orally or intramuscularly) is to be repeated hourly until the desired effect is achieved.

Pregnant patients requesting sedative-hypnotic or anxiolytic drugs would best be managed with counseling and behavioral modifications. The antihistamines diphenhydramine (25–50 mg orally at bedtime) for sedation and hydroxyzine (25–100 mg orally every 4 hours) for anxiety are likely safer than the benzodiazepines. None of the benzodiazepines is to be clearly preferred, but lorazepam has a shorter half-life and no active metabolites, unlike alprazolam, chlordiazepoxide, and diazepam.

It is unclear which antidepressant (tricyclics, trazodone, fluoxetine) provides the least risk to the fetus. Serotonin reuptake inhibitors (Zoloft, Prozac) are better tolerated than the tricyclic antidepressants. Any association between lithium and Ebstein's anomaly in the fetus is rare, but fetal echocardiograms continue to be requested. An association between lithium and premature delivery is preliminary and requires confirmation.

MATERNAL SERUM TESTING

Alpha-fetoprotein (AFP) is a fetal-specific α-globulin that is synthesized within the fetal yolk sac, gastrointestinal tract, and liver. During the first half of pregnancy, the concentration of AFP is 100 times greater in the fetal serum than in the amniotic fluid. Fetal and amniotic fluid concentrations peak at 14 weeks, then decline significantly until term. Maternal serum alpha-fetoprotein (MSAFP) values are 1000 times less than those in the fetal serum before 20 weeks, and they gradually increase during gestation.

Elevated MSAFP

The major clinical application of AFP testing is for the detection of fetal open neural tube defects (prevalence in the U.S. 1–2/1000 births). Couples with an affected first degree relative should be offered an ultrasound-directed amniocentesis for the evaluation of amniotic fluid AFP. However, this approach will detect only approximately 10% of all affected infants with neural tube defects.

It has become routine for most American obstetricians to offer MSAFP screening to gravidas with a negative family history. It is important that the patient understand that such screening is voluntary, and that further testing would be required if abnormal screening results occur. Routine screening is appropriate on a select patient population at risk for neural tube defects or malformations: poor obstetric history, diabetes (either controlled by diet alone or insulin-dependent), distant family member who has an open neural tube defect, or seizure disorder requiring valproic acid or carbamazepine therapy.

An initial MSAFP sample is obtained at 15–18 weeks. A normal value, 0.5–2.0 multiples of the median, rules out an open neural tube defect with a probability of about 80–90%. Between 3 and 7% of American women's initial AFP will be elevated. If the value is greater than 2.0 but less than 3.0 multiples of the median (MOM) and the gestational age is less than 18 weeks, a repeat sample should be obtained. Approximately half of the repeat values will be normal, and in these cases no further testing is required. The remaining patients and those gravidas whose initial MSAFP value is more than 3.0 MOM or whose gestational age is more than 18 weeks should be encouraged to have amniotic fluid AFP and acetylcholinesterase measurements.

Causes of falsely elevated MSAFP values include more advanced gestational age, twins, threatened abortion, fetal death, maternal hepatitis, and Rh disease. Acetylcholinesterase determination using gel electrophoresis is less influenced by fetal blood, thereby eliminating most false-positive amniotic fluid AFP values. The absence of acetylcholinesterase strongly suggests the absence of an open neural tube defect. Patients with elevated MSAFP values in whom no genetic defect is found appear to have approximately a 40% risk of delivering a low-birth-weight infant either due to intrauterine growth retardation or premature labor. A repeat ultrasound examination is therefore recommended at 28–32 weeks to assess fetal growth.

Down Syndrome Screening

Approximately 9% of routinely screened patients will have an abnormally low MSAFP serum level, defined as less than 0.4 multiples of the median. Low MSAFP values can be used in conjunction with maternal age to predict risks for Down syndrome. An amniocentesis is recommended (rather than repeating the MSAFP test) when the risk approaches that for a 35-year-old woman, that is, 1 in 270. To increase the sensitivity of MSAFP as a screening tool for Down syndrome, many investigators have recommended the addition of two other serum markers—unconjugated estriol and/or human chorionic gonadotropin (hCG). Women with a Down syndrome fetus are more likely to have a low MSAFP value along with low serum unconjugated estriol levels and elevated serum hCG levels.

Women who are less than 35 years of age and who are between 15 and 18 weeks of gestation by menstrual dating should be offered serum screening to assess Down syndrome risk. At this time, multiple serum marker testing in women over the age of 35 cannot be recommended for routine screening as an equivalent alternative to prenatal cytogenic diagnosis. However, it may be offered as an option for those women who do not accept the risk of amniocentesis or who wish to have this additional information prior to making a decision about having an amniocentesis. Screening should be voluntary and based on informed consent.

Based on the data available, a specific multiple biochemical marker protocol other than MSAFP alone cannot be exclusively recommended at this time. The specific combination of tests and the particular assays that are performed will yield a Down syndrome detection rate of 20–25% with MSAFP alone and at least 55–60% with MSAFP, hCG, and unconjugated estriol.

Reporting should include information about (*a*) the patient's age-related risk, (*b*) the patient's risk as adjusted by the laboratory results, and (*c*) an indication of the patient's adjusted risk relative to a specific cutoff level (e.g., greater or less than that of a 35-year-old woman). All patients who have a risk higher than the selected cutoff should have ultrasonography performed to confirm gestational age. Revision of gestational age should be based on biparietal diameter and not femur length measurement, because the femurs are shortened in some fetuses with Down syndrome.

ANTEPARTUM RH IMMUNE GLOBULIN

The availability of $Rh_O(D)$ immune globulin has provided a means to virtually eliminate fetal erythroblastosis from anti-D antigen sensitization. While certain cases result from omission or administration of inadequate doses of $Rh_O(D)$ immune globulin at delivery, most Rh isoimmunization occurs from the omission of globulin therapy at the time of elective or spontaneous abortion, ectopic pregnancy, amniocentesis, antepartum uterine bleeding, and fetal-maternal hemorrhage.

All Rh-negative unsensitized pregnant patients are eligible for antepartum $Rh_O(D)$ immune globulin unless the father is known to be D-negative. Indications for and dose of antepartum $Rh_O(D)$ immune globulin are shown in Table 1.7. The dose is determined by gestational age and can be calculated by Kleihauer-Betke testing after the first 12 weeks.

Table 1.7
Indications and Doses of Antepartum Rh$_o$(D) Immune Globulin for Rh-negative, Unsensitized Women

Indications	Dose

Gestational age at or before 12 weeks:
    Abortion, spontaneous or induced
    Ectopic pregnancy
    Chorionic villus sampling
	50 μg[a] to protect against 5 mL transfused whole blood

Gestational age after 12 weeks:
    Abortion, spontaneous or induced
    Ectopic pregnancy
    Amniocentesis
    Persistent vaginal bleeding
    Stillbirth
    Fetal-maternal hemorrhage
    Abnormal trauma
	300 μg (minimum)[b] to protect against 30 mL transfused whole blood

Transfusion
    Red cells, whole blood,
        platelets or granulocytes
	300 μg (minimum)[b]

[a] Microdose brands include MICRhoGAM and Mini-Gamulin Rh.
[b] Regular dose brands include RhoGam, Gamulin Rh, and HypRho-D.

We no longer perform D testing during maternal blood typing, since it is not cost-effective. Only 1% of Rh-negative people are D-positive, and there is no harm in administering the globulin to a D-positive mother. If the cord blood at delivery is D-positive, D testing should be done on the mother.

Since 1–2% of Rh-negative women will become sensitized in their current pregnancy before delivery, Rh$_O$(D) immune globulin is administered routinely at approximately 28 weeks to all Rh-negative unsensitized patients. An indirect Coombs' test is not performed thereafter, and another injection is not given routinely for the remainder of the antepartum period.

The administration of a standard 300 μg vial of Rh immune globulin reduces the incidence of such sensitization to 1/1000. The 300-μg dose may cause a mildly positive Rh titer (1:4), but it is less than one-tenth of the dose required to cause significant harm to the fetus. Causes of failures of Rh$_O$(D) immune globulin include antenatal sensitization, inadequate dose, misinterpretation of maternal Rh type, previous Rh$_O$(D)-positive transfusion, failure of administration when indicated, immunization to cross-reacting antigen, and delay in administration.

The half-life of $Rh_O(D)$ immune globulin is 23 days. A repeat injection at 28 weeks and after delivery (for Rh-positive infants) is recommended for those Rh-negative women who undergo a genetic amniocentesis. This additional globulin should maintain an adequate level of antibody to prevent enhancement. If the last injection was administered 4 or more weeks previously, there is no contraindication to administering the product again.

Even though this IgG antibody will cross the placenta, it will not cause any appreciable hemolysis. There is no risk of transmission of viral disease, including HIV and hepatitis B, although a false-positive hepatitis serology is possible. Severe anaphylactic reaction or serum sickness is exceedingly rare. After the delivery of the Rh-positive infant, Rh immune globulin (300 μg) should be administered intramuscularly despite a weakly positive direct Coombs' titer of cord blood.

AMNIOCENTESIS BEFORE REPEAT CESAREAN SECTION

The accessibility of ultrasound and amniocentesis has provided a means to determine gestational age more accurately and to document fetal pulmonary maturity. Given the current level of obstetric technology, iatrogenic prematurity after an elective delivery should be rare.

The need for accurate gestational dating cannot be overemphasized. The following factors are necessary to define a reliable gestational age: (*a*) the patient is initially seen during the first half of pregnancy; (*b*) the date of her last menses is known; (*c*) uterine size is consistent with gestational age between the 18th and 30th gestational weeks; and (*d*) an ultrasound examination for gestational dating is performed before the 26th week.

Inaccurate Gestation Dating

An amniocentesis for fetal lung maturity testing should be performed when estimation of gestational age appears inaccurate. The amniocentesis should be undertaken between the presumed 37th and 38th completed weeks for nonemergent conditions. All amniocenteses should be preceded by or performed during real-time ultrasonographic visualization. Any "bloody tap" or transplacental insertion of the needle requires fetal heart rate monitoring and the administration of Rh immune globulin to any Rh-negative, unsensitized patient.

An amniocentesis does not need to be performed if: (*a*) the procedure appears to be technically difficult because of reduced amniotic fluid volume; (*b*) biparietal diameter measurement is more than 92 mm; (*c*) placenta is consistently grade 3; or (*d*) free-floating particulate matter in the amniotic fluid is strongly suggestive of fetal lung maturity. A safe alternative is to wait to perform the surgery until labor begins if concern remains about the accuracy of dating, ultrasound findings, or technical difficulties with an amniocentesis.

Accurate Gestation Dating

With accurate dating or once fetal lung tests indicate maturity, an elective repeat cesarean section is performed between the 38th and 39th completed gestational weeks, before the onset of labor. If estimation of gestational age is accurate, an amniocentesis is not routinely recommended. Confirmation of the ultrasound findings described above is also reassuring. The advantages in not routinely performing an amniocentesis include cost considerations and avoiding an invasive procedure which may cause fetal injury or placental bleeding.

Suggested Readings

American Academy of Pediatrics, American College of Obstetricians and Gynecologists. Guidelines for perinatal care. 3rd ed. Elk Grove Village, Illinois: AAP; Washington, DC: ACOG, 1992.

American College of Obstetricians and Gynecologists. Alpha-fetoprotein. ACOG Technical Bulletin 154. Washington, DC: ACOG, 1991.

American College of Obstetricians and Gynecologists. Antenatal diagnosis of genetic disorders. ACOG Technical Bulletin 108. Washington, DC: ACOG, 1987.

American College of Obstetricians and Gynecologists. Folic acid for prevention of recurrent neural tube defects. ACOG Committee Opinion 120. Washington, DC: ACOG, 1993.

Haddow JE, Palomaki GE, Knight GJ, Williams J, Pulkkinen A, Canick JA, et al. Prenatal screening for Down's syndrome with the use of maternal serum markers. N Engl J Med 1992;327:588–593.

Institute of Medicine, Subcommittee on Nutritional Status and Weight Gain during Pregnancy. Nutrition during pregnancy. Washington, DC: National Academy Press, 1990.

Jack BW, Culpepper L. Preconception care: risk reduction and health promotion in preparation for pregnancy. JAMA 1990;264:1147–1149.

Mehta L, Young ID. Recurrence risks for common complications of pregancy—a review. Obstet Gynecol Surv 1987;42:218–223.

Chapter 2

Medical Disorders During Pregnancy

GESTATIONAL DIABETES

A woman is more likely to develop glucose intolerance during pregnancy because of counterinsulin hormones and enzymes produced primarily by the placenta. One to six percent of all women in the United States will have documented glucose intolerance during pregnancy. When diabetes is diagnosed, the following conditions are more common: (*a*) fetal loss (incidence up to 2 or 3 times greater than in the general population); (*b*) fetal macrosomia and its attendant complications (even when fasting glucose concentrations are normal); (*c*) deterioration of glucose metabolism resulting in the need for insulin (in approximately 20–50% of gestational diabetics); (*d*) increased risk of operative or mechanical deliveries because of increased fetal size; and (*e*) later development of type II diabetes (within 20 years in 20% of gestational diabetics).

Diagnosis

In the past, obstetricians tended to screen selectively for gestational diabetes in the presence of historical or clinical risk factors (family history of diabetes, previous macrosomic infant, poor obstetric history, persistent glycosuria). Several studies have indicated, however, that the incidence of gestational diabetes is the same whether or not risk factors are present. Therefore, the National Institute of Health, the American Diabetes Association, and the American College of Obstetricians and Gynecologists recommend that all pregnant patients be screened for diabetes.

Screening for gestational diabetes is routine at 24–28 weeks gestation and earlier in the presence of risk factors. A serum glucose determination of 140 mg/dL 1 hour after a 50-mg glucose challenge requires more definitive evaluation by a 3-hour glucose tolerance test (GTT). Using a 100-mg glucose load, a 3-hour GTT requires fasting blood as well as a sampling at 1-hour, 2-hour, and 3-hour intervals. Any two values greater than the expected levels (fasting, 105 mg/dL or more; 1-hour, 190 mg/dL or more; 2-hour, 165 mg/dL or more; 3-hour, 145 mg/dL or more) are diagnostic of gestational onset glucose intolerance (Class A diabetes).

Management

Adequate control of the mother's glucose levels by dietary manipulation and blood glucose monitoring is necessary to decrease the increased risk of perinatal morbidity, primarily from fetal macrosomia and its attendant medical and metabolic complications. Most patients will be treated sufficiently with a daily caloric intake according to current weight in relation to ideal body weight (less than 80%: 35–40 calories/kg of body weight; 80–120%: 30 calories/kg; 120–150%: 24 calories/kg; more than 150%: 12–15 calories/kg). Approximately 40–50% of the typical 2000–2500 calories/day intake should be foods containing complex carbohydrates. One hundred grams of protein are also essential each day. Sweets, junk food, and greasy fried foods should be avoided.

More frequent clinic visits are recommended (usually every 2 weeks until 36 weeks, and weekly thereafter) and glucose monitoring should be performed periodically. Fasting and 2-hour postprandial glucose determinations are recommended during the more frequent examinations. The patient should be instructed to avoid eating after midnight and to have her "fasting" blood drawn when seen initially in the clinic, then to eat a "regular" meal at the cafeteria or brought from home before returning in 2 hours for a postprandial glucose determination. A fasting serum glucose level less than 100 mg/dL and a 2-hour postprandial value less than 120 mg/dL are desired. Capillary blood glucose determinations by the patient using a reflectance photometer are more convenient and cost-effective but tend to be slightly higher than plasma levels. Therefore, a fasting capillary glucose level less than 115 mg/dL (plasma less than 100 mg/dL) and two-hour postprandial level less than 140 mg/dL (plasma less than 120 mg/dL) are desirable.

If either glucose value exceeds recommended levels, it is necessary to get a more detailed history of the patient's diet, consult a dietitian, and consider insulin therapy. Gestational-onset diabetic women are eligible for insulin therapy if the diet is inadequate. The initial daily dose of Humulin insulin (0.5 U/kg/day in the first trimester, 0.6 U/kg/day in the second trimester, and 0.7 U/kg/day in third trimester) should be started as early in gestation as possible to reduce the risk of the fetus's becoming large-for-gestational-age. Once insulin is begun, principles of management are the same as those for already insulin-dependent women. An empiric algorithm divides the estimated daily insulin requirements into thirds, with two-thirds being given before breakfast (two-thirds as NPH, one-third as regular). and one-third before the evening meal (split evenly between NPH and regular).

Gestational age should be determined accurately. Ultrasonography is quite helpful and may also be used during the last weeks of pregnancy to search for signs of a large-for-gestational-age fetus or polyhydramnios.

Pregnancies of Class A diabetic patients may be described as being either uncomplicated or complicated (i.e., coexistent hypertension or history of previous stillbirth). Uncomplicated Class A pregnancies are at low risk for antepartum stillbirth and may be followed until labor occurs spontaneously.

The need for antepartum fetal testing in uncomplicated Class A pregnancies is not firmly established. Fetal movement charting often provides a useful method for monitoring and is recommended beginning at approximately the 34th gestational week. Many authorities advocate nonstress testing beginning at approximately the 36th gestational week.

Complicated Class A pregnancies are at increased risk for antepartum stillbirth, so fetal movement charting and nonstress testing should be initiated at 32 weeks' gestation or earlier, depending on the patient's previous obstetric history. Gestation is not usually allowed to advance beyond the estimated date of confinement.

Fetal pulmonary maturity may be delayed in Class A patients, so an amniocentesis for pulmonary maturity testing is often performed before most elective deliveries. The physician who will care for the infant should also be notified well before the anticipated delivery, because there is a significantly greater risk of neonatal complications even in patients with well-controlled

Class A diabetes. Some women with low mean glucose values may still deliver macrosomic infants.

INSULIN-DEPENDENT DIABETES

Fifty years ago, maternal mortality among insulin-dependent diabetics was 50% and perinatal mortality was nearly 100%. Maternal mortality is now rare, and perinatal mortality is related to a certain extent to the duration of maternal diabetes and any evidence of vascular disease. Current management techniques of type I (insulin-dependent) diabetic patients have made perinatal survival less dependent on the diabetes class. With the exception of Class H patients, perinatal mortality is less than 5% in most tertiary centers. These improvements have resulted from the meticulous execution of comprehensive protocols for the management of pregnant diabetics. Table 2.1 lists the current classification of diabetes during pregnancy. The duration of diabetes is related to end organ derangement.

Strict maternal glucose control is often difficult during pregnancy. Hypoglycemia is common in the first and third trimesters, while hyperglycemic tendencies are frequent in the second and third trimesters. Ketoacidosis occurs in pregnant patients at glucose levels much less elevated than in nonpregnant patients. Urinary tract and surgical infections are also common. Hypertensive disorders occur relatively frequently, especially in the more advanced classes. Cesarean section rates are high, often 50% at tertiary centers. Progression of proliferative retinopathy occurs in 30–50% of Class R patients.

Table 2.1
Classification of Diabetes during Pregnancy

Class	Description
A	Gestational onset diabetes
A-1	Adequate control by diet alone
A-2	Requires insulin
B	Overt diabetes, onset after age 20 or duration 10 years or less
C	Overt diabetes, onset at age 10–19 or duration 10–19 years
D	Overt diabetes, duration more than 20 years or onset before age 10, or benign retinopathy
F	Nephropathy (proteinuria, uremia)
R	Proliferative retinopathy (retinitis proliferans)
H	Arteriosclerotic heart disease

Although the etiology of antepartum stillbirth in diabetic pregnancy is not firmly established, the application of various antepartum fetal testing modalities has decreased the stillbirth rate. Fifty to seventy percent of perinatal deaths result from congenital anomalies which are found in approximately 6–8% of diabetic pregnancies. Because increased placental transfer of glucose, amino acids, and free fatty acids results in fetal hyperinsulinemia, adipose deposition is promoted and infants of diabetic mothers experience higher rates of macrosomia and attendant birth trauma. Neonatal hypoglycemia and hypocalcemia are common. Lung maturation is delayed in some infants, causing hyaline membrane disease and transient tachypnea to be more common than in infants delivered of mothers without diabetes.

Cautious glucose control appears to reduce the incidence of maternal complications. Normoglycemia at conception and in the first trimester decreases the incidence of congenital abnormalities and spontaneous abortions. While the relationship between neonatal complications and maternal glucose control is not firmly established, all investigators believe that attempts should be made to achieve the best possible control at all times.

Clinic Visits and Hospitalizations

At the initial prenatal visit, many patients with insulin-dependent diabetes, regardless of the duration or age at onset, require control of blood glucose, patient education, baseline renal function tests, electrocardiogram, and ophthalmologic examination. Hospitalization may be avoided if patient knowledge about pregnancy expectations is adequate and glucose control is already strict. If there is evidence of renal, retinal, or cardiovascular compromise, the option of pregnancy termination should be discussed in early gestation.

The patient should visit the clinic every 1 or 2 weeks, depending on the compliance in home blood glucose monitoring and the level of her glucose control. Beyond the 30th week, the patient should be seen in the clinic on a weekly basis, and hospitalization is necessary for inadequate glucose control or any worrisome obstetric or other medical complication.

Control of Serum Glucose

A fair correlation exists between mean daily capillary glucose values over 4 weeks and the subsequent glycosylated hemoglobin

(Hb A_{Ic}) level. We recommend that a Hb A_{Ic} value be determined (*a*) at the initial visit, (*b*) when there is a question of control, (*c*) when the patient is seen initially after maternal transport, or (*d*) after delivery of a large-for-gestational-age infant. A markedly elevated Hb A_{Ic} value before 14 weeks' gestation is associated with a 22% incidence of major congenital malformations, compared with 5% or less if the value is within the normal range. A maternal serum alpha-fetoprotein value should be determined between 15 and 18 weeks.

To avoid ketosis and to decrease the risk of perinatal mortality, strict control of glucose levels is desirable by adjustments of insulin dose and redistribution of caloric intake. Most patients can learn how to determine and record blood sugar results in a cost-effective manner at home using a reflectance meter (Accucheck, Dextrometer, Glucometer), either loaned from the clinic or purchased (approximately $100–$200). We recommend that blood sugar determinations be made at least four times daily (usually to include levels for fasting, two hours postprandial, and bedtime).

Control of glucose levels should be as strict as possible. Ideally, a fasting capillary glucose value should be less than 115 mg/dL, a 2-hour postprandial glucose determination less than 140 mg/dL, and before meals less than 110 mg/dL.

The patient's diet should be the same as that described for the Class A diabetic. In addition, a readjustment of caloric intake throughout the day may be necessary to control the blood glucose levels more adequately.

Attempts to maintain strict glucose control should begin before conception. There is no role for oral hypoglycemic agents during pregnancy. Biosynthetic, recombinant DNA human insulin (Humulin) is less immunogenic, requires a lower dose, and acts more rapidly than bovine or porcine insulin. Most diabetics are accustomed to using the rapid-acting (regular; peak effect 2–6 hours, duration 14–28 hours) insulin preparations.

Care of the pregnant diabetic patient requires an understanding of anticipated insulin therapy changes. Regardless of metabolic control and duration of diabetes, average daily insulin requirements are expected to increase approximately twofold during pregnancy. The degree of increase is related only to maternal weight at the initial visit and weight gain during weeks 20–29 and is inversely related to the duration of diabetes. The period during which insulin doses are most likely to decrease would be during early gestation, because of inadequate caloric intake from nausea, and in the third trimester, when placental insufficiency is most likely.

Unacceptably high glucose levels require use of a sliding scale of intravenous regular insulin such as the following, in which the listed doses are given every 4 hours: for glucose levels of 125–149 mg/dL, 2 units insulin; 150–174 mg/dL, 4 units; 175–199 mg/dL, 6 units; 200–224 mg/dL, 8 units; 225–249 mg/dL, 10 units; and 250 mg/dL or higher, 12 units.

Daily self-monitoring of fasting postprandial glucose values should be done using reflectance glucometers. Insulin is usually administered on two or three occasions each day using a mixture of regular and NPH U-100 Humulin insulins. Experience with subcutaneous insulin infusion during pregnancy has been limited to those with "brittle" diabetes requiring more than three daily doses. Portable or implantable intravenous or subcutaneous insulin pumps have been used when strict or fair glucose control has not been achieved despite diligent efforts.

Frequent episodes of hypoglycemia (less than 60 mg/dL) or hyperglycemia (greater than 200 mg/dL) should be avoided, even though no relationship exists between maternal hypoglycemia and damage to the fetus. Although rarely necessary, the patient's family should be instructed on the use and administration of intramuscular glucagon (using 1-mg kits) and buccal glucose tablets to treat a hypoglycemia reaction, which occurs most often at night. We recommend a 0.5-mg dose of glucagon, then the ingestion of juice, rather than administering a full dose, to minimize any profound adrenergic response. Ketonuria is seen occasionally in fasting states (early morning clinic) but is not necessarily worrisome if serum glucose levels are appropriate and ketonuria is absent later in the day.

Diabetic ketoacidosis is associated with intrauterine fetal demise. However, it is uncommon in pregnancies in which glucose is strictly monitored. Fluid and metabolic derangements should be corrected as soon as possible by frequent evaluation of the clinical and laboratory status. Baseline serum glucose, ketones, potassium, sodium, blood urea nitrogen (BUN), creatinine, and HCO_3 levels should be determined. Bicarbonate therapy (1 ampule, 44 mEq) is to be started in the presence of a pH less than 7.1, shock, or coma. A bolus of regular insulin at 0.15 units/kg body weight should be followed by a constant insulin infusion at 0.15 units/kg body weight/hour (5–10 units are mixed with 100 mL normal saline). The maintenance dose may be doubled if the serum glucose value has not fallen to 200 mg/dL during the first 2 hours. A 5% glucose solution should be used once the glucose level is normalized and once the pH returns to normal. A sliding-scale insulin regimen should be continued until a liquid diet is tolerated. Long-acting insulin may be added the next morning.

Fetal Surveillance

Maternal serum alpha-fetoprotein (MSAFP) levels should be drawn between the 15th and 18th weeks to screen for any elevation from open neural tube defects. Ultrasound examination for fetal age and growth assessments are usually done on the initial visit and at 4–6-week intervals.

The risk of intrauterine fetal demise increases as gestation proceeds beyond 30 weeks. The etiology of fetal death is often unclear; however, patients with preeclampsia, uteroplacental vascular lesions, and maternal hyperglycemia are at increased risk. The patient should be instructed on charting fetal movement beginning at the 29th gestational week. Weekly nonstress tests, contraction stress tests, or biophysical profiles should be initiated between the 28th and 32nd gestational weeks and increased to twice weekly by the 34th gestational week. Testing should begin earlier and be undertaken more frequently in the presence of cardiovascular disease, poor glucose control, or poor obstetric history.

Hospitalization of the diabetic before delivery is not routine, provided that excellent metabolic control and adequate fetoplacental testing can be accomplished on an outpatient basis. Pregnancy may be allowed to continue until the 38th week, when most authorities recommend that an amniocentesis for fetal lung maturity testing be performed. The lung maturity screen should include a determination of the lecithin/sphingomyelin (L/S) ratio and phosphatidylglycerol (PG). An L/S ratio of 3 alone, or an L/S ratio of 2–3 with a positive PG, strongly suggests fetal lung maturity with a very minimal risk of subsequent development of hyaline membrane disease. Induction should be undertaken if lung maturity is present, the fetus is in a vertex presentation, the estimated fetal weight is less than 4000 g, and the Bishop score is favorable. If the cervix is unfavorable, it is permissible either to ripen the cervix or to delay delivery until the anticipated due date, provided that the metabolic and fetoplacental status remains stable. If the estimated fetal weight is more than 4000 g or if the fetus is in a breech presentation, the option of cesarean delivery should be offered to reduce the risk of birth trauma.

Hospitalization may be required when there is evidence of worsening end organ damage (proliferative retinopathy, neuropathy), hypertension, inadequate glucose control, poor patient compliance, or abnormal fetoplacental function tests. Every attempt should be made to optimize glucose control. In addition to daily fetal movement charting, the frequency of fetoplacental testing should be increased. An amniocentesis may be performed before the 38th week. The decision to deliver is usually dependent on the worsening of any of the above conditions or the presence of fetal lung maturity. Cesarean section is often necessary because the cervix remains unfavorable; however, the use of cervical ripening agents is gaining wider acceptance.

The pediatric staff must be notified of any impending delivery, since these infants often require intravenous glucose therapy and may need respiratory support. Metabolic complications include hyperbilirubinemia, hypoglycemia, hypocalcemia, and poor feeding. The reported incidence of major malformations in infants born to diabetics is 8% (most notably cardiac and neural tube defects). Perinatal mortality (approximately half of which are stillbirths) at most perinatal regional centers is less than 5%.

Insulin Requirements during and after Delivery

Before Labor

Despite close antepartum glucose monitoring, maternal hypoglycemia or hyperglycemia may occur during labor and delivery, and neonatal glucose control may be significantly compromised. Before the anticipated day of delivery, the usual evening dose of insulin is given. The patient is kept NPO after midnight, and insulin on the day of delivery is given intravenously. Before induction of labor or cesarean section, a serum glucose level is determined and an intravenous line is begun. A D_5W (5% dextrose) drip is run at 150 mL/hour (7.5 mg/hour).

Intrapartum

The desired goal is to maintain a serum glucose level within the 60–120 mg/dL range, determined every 1–3 hours. Insulin is given intravenously with capillary glucose levels being determined with a bedside glucometer. Thirty units of regular insulin are drawn into a 50 mL syringe, and mixed with 50 mL of normal saline (0.6 units insulin/mL). The insulin may adhere to the syringe, so 1 mL of the patient's blood should be drawn into the syringe and the contents mixed well.

A constant-rate pump is used to begin infusing the insulin at 2 mL/hour (1.2 units/hour) in a "piggyback" manner. Insulin requirements during labor are often negligible. The average patient requires 1.2 units insulin per hour (range 0–2 units/hour). Oxytocin may be infused through the same vein using another line.

Postpartum

Placental hormones are metabolized and eliminated rapidly after delivery, and insulin requirements decrease dramatically. In our experience, prepregnancy insulin requirements are usually reached within 4–7 days after delivery, and dose requirements are approximately one-half to one-third those necessary for adequate control late in pregnancy.

If delivery was vaginal, insulin infusion should continue until the patient is transferred from the recovery area. In the first few days after delivery, strict glucose control is not necessary, and we strive for glucose values less than 200 mg/dL. Regular insulin may be administered by a sliding-scale regimen based on blood glucometer results obtained every 4–6 hours. For example, 5 units regular insulin may be administered subcutaneously for a glucose level of 200–249 mg/dL, 10 units for 250–200 mg/dL, and 15 units for 300 mg/dL or higher.

After cesarean section, insulin infusion may be continued through the first day or until oral intake is tolerated, with bedside glucose monitoring every 2–4 hours. Minimal or no insulin is usually necessary. Insulin requirements do not appear to be affected greatly by the patient's mode of delivery or whether breast-feeding is undertaken. NPH or Lente is usually begun around the 4th postpartum day after 1 full day of eating solid foods.

If the patient is a Class A-2 diabetic, insulin is usually unnecessary before discharge. Patient instructions should include an emphasis on proper nutrition, physician notification of excess fatigue, and continued glucose monitoring (fasting and postprandial two or three times weekly). A 75-gram 2-hour glucose tolerance test is recommended at the 6-week postpartum visit.

OBESITY

There is disagreement about the proper definition of obesity in pregnancy, although various authors have suggested pregnancy weights greater than 175 pounds or at least 40% (usually 100 pounds or more) above ideal body weight. Obese women are at increased risk for hypertension, gestational diabetes, urinary tract infection, and episiotomy or wound infections. Pregnancy dating is often limited because of irregular menstrual cycles and difficulties with uterine height examinations.

In most studies, maternal mortality rates are increased, largely from thromboembolic, infectious, or anesthetic complications. Fetal macrosomia is also more common. Although perinatal mortality is usually not increased and low-birth-weight infants are uncommon, an optimal pregnancy outcome is associated with a weight gain of at least 15 pounds for these mothers.

Antepartum Management

1. Nutritional counseling at first visit and follow-up visits
2. Screening urine culture
3. Ultrasound examination at approximately 20 weeks to confirm pregnancy dating
4. Diabetes screen initially, and at 24–28 weeks
5. Frequent blood pressure monitoring, using a large cuff if arm circumference is 35 cm or more
6. Prophylactic rest at least 1 hour each day in the third trimester
7. Pulmonary function tests followed by an anesthesia consult in early third trimester if the patient is morbidly obese and any suggestion of pulmonary compromise exists
8. Discuss tubal ligation if chance of cesarean delivery

Intrapartum and Postpartum Management

1. Prophylactic heparin (5000 units subcutaneously every 12 hours) during labor and until fully ambulatory
2. Notify anesthesia staff of patient's presence in labor and delivery
3. Careful monitoring for preeclampsia, using a large blood pressure cuff
4. Careful attention to the progress of labor
5. Anticipation of fetal shoulder dystocia because of possible macrosomia

6. Meticulous hemostasis during episiotomy repair
7. If cesarean section is required: (*a*) prophylactic antibiotics, (*b*) Smead-Jones closure if vertical incision, and (*c*) continuous suction drain (such as a Jackson-Pratt) in subcutaneous space
8. Early ambulation
9. Continued nutritional counseling in the postpartum period

CHRONIC HYPERTENSION

Approximately 2% of all pregnant patients will have chronic hypertension, which is defined as any interval of sustained elevation of the blood pressure (140/90 mm Hg or greater) before pregnancy or before the 20th week of the present pregnancy. These patients are frequently obese and may have been on antihypertensive medication. A search for end organ damage such as renal or cardiac disease is necessary, since either may affect the prognosis of the mother and fetus.

Antepartum Management

The preliminary outpatient investigation (inpatient if blood pressure is elevated) should include: (*a*) a 24-hour urine study for protein and creatinine clearance, (*b*) serum electrolyte levels, (*c*) urinalysis and urine culture, (*d*) ultrasound examination, (*e*) electrocardiogram, (*f*) trial of medications if normotensive, and (*g*) patient instruction on self blood pressure monitoring. Return clinic visits should be a minimum of every 3 weeks until 20 weeks' gestation, every 2 weeks until 32 weeks, and every week after 32 weeks. The patient should be encouraged to record blood pressure levels at home and to share these results with her physician. Bed rest is encouraged for one or more hours each afternoon.

Methyldopa (Aldomet) is the drug of choice (up to 1 g four times daily) because it poses minimal risk to the fetus and there has been extensive experience with its use during pregnancy. The safest second-line antihypertensive is a disputed matter. Many women with chronic hypertension have been treated with β_1-adrenergic blockers throughout pregnancy (labetalol, atenolol, metoprolol), and no adverse fetal effects have been demonstrated with these drugs. A comparison of atenolol and the calcium channel blocker nifedipine reported no differences between the two. Oral nifedipine is rapid-acting and has been used without complications; however, there have been no long-term trials of calcium channel antagonists in pregnancy.

Fetal heart rate testing is usually begun between the 32nd and 34th gestational weeks if medications are used or if the hypertension worsens. Serial ultrasound examinations to assess fetal growth and placental morphology are recommended early in pregnancy and usually no more frequently than every 3 weeks. Daily fetal movement charting should begin during the early third trimester.

Hospitalization is indicated for a persistent elevation of systolic-diastolic values 30/15 mm Hg above previous levels, or if there are signs of superimposed preeclampsia or a suspicion of acute fetal compromise (e.g., oligohydramnios, abnormal fetal heart rate (FHR) pattern).

Consider delivery as soon as fetal lung maturity is attained, or by 40 weeks if fetal growth has been normal and maternal blood pressure has been well-controlled. If delivery is anticipated before 34 weeks, glucocorticoids may be given to enhance fetal lung maturity if the mother's condition is stable and blood pressure values are no more than 160/105 mm Hg.

Intrapartum Management

If superimposed preeclampsia develops, delivery is indicated and intravenous magnesium sulfate is begun for seizure prophylaxis. Continuous electronic FHR monitoring is recommended.

Epidural anesthesia is permissible, as long as the blood pressure is not greater than 160/105 mm Hg and an experienced anesthesiologist is available. Bearing-down efforts by the mother should be avoided, and outlet or low forceps delivery may be necessary to shorten the second stage of labor.

PREGNANCY-INDUCED HYPERTENSION

Next to anemia, hypertension is the most common medical complication during pregnancy. Pregnancy-induced hypertension is more common than chronic hypertension during pregnancy and affects up to 10% of all pregnancies. Hypertension during pregnancy is defined as any elevated blood pressure of 140/90 mm Hg or greater, or any elevation of the systolic/diastolic values of more than 30/15 mm Hg on two occasions 6 hours apart.

Pregnancy-induced hypertension is often fluctuant and has an onset beyond the first 20 weeks. Differentiating between pregnancy-induced hypertension and mild preeclampsia is often difficult, but preeclampsia should be suspected if there is a weight gain of 2 pounds or more per week or persistent proteinuria of greater than 300 mg but less than 5 g/24 hours. In either circumstance, end organ damage is not usually extensive enough to cause liver dysfunction, central nervous system involvement, coagulopathies, or pulmonary edema.

Surveillance Techniques

The following measures are recommended in monitoring the mother and fetus during the third trimester. If blood pressure values remain elevated, hospitalization is necessary.

Maternal

1. Check for headaches, blurred vision, abdominal pain, chest pain, respiratory symptoms, brisk deep tendon reflexes, and clonus
2. Instruct patient on home blood pressure monitoring
3. Weigh daily
4. Dipstick test for proteinuria daily
5. High protein diet (100 g daily) if proteinuria is present
6. Salt substitute, no diuretic therapy
7. Complete blood count and peripheral blood smear (burr cells, schistocytes, polychromasia) on admission and as indicated
8. Liver function study (SGOT) on admission and as indicated
9. Coagulation study (especially platelets) on admission and as indicated
10. Renal function testing (24-hour urine study for protein and creatinine clearance) on admission and as indicated

Fetal

1. Daily fetal movement charting
2. Antepartum FHR testing or biophysical profile
3. Ultrasound scan for fetal growth assessment every 3 weeks
4. Consider umbilical Doppler flow studies

Therapy in Hospital

1. Bed rest in lateral decubitus position with bathroom privileges
2. If hyperreflexia or clonus are present, or BP is greater than

160/105 mm Hg, begin intravenous magnesium sulfate while monitoring urine output

3. Intermittent boluses of intravenous labetalol 20 mg if BP is greater than 160/105 mm Hg
4. Pregnancy intervention if there is evidence of fetal lung maturity, fetal distress, deteriorating maternal end organ function, or worsening, persistently-elevated BP values
5. Discharge home only if the reliable patient can remain sedentary, is asymptomatic with no laboratory abnormalities, can monitor her urine protein output and blood pressure daily, and lives nearby so that she can be seen semi-weekly in clinic. A home monitoring program is appealing but remains investigational.

SEVERE PREECLAMPSIA OR ECLAMPSIA

Severe preeclampsia or eclampsia is an extension of pregnancy-induced hypertension or mild preeclampsia. Hospitalization is required for immediate attention to the mother and fetus. Under these circumstances, there is a greater likelihood of placental abruption, fetal distress, and fetal demise, along with end organ changes in the mother such as renal failure, liver failure, cerebrovascular accident, heart failure, consumptive coagulopathy, and thrombocytopenia. The primary goals of therapy include stabilizing the maternal blood pressure, correcting any accompanying medical complications, and delivering the fetus in the near future.

General Recommendations

1. Admit to labor floor for close monitoring
2. Strict bed rest in a lateral position and quiet environment
3. Seizure precautions (side rails up, tongue blade available, oral airway unobstructed)
4. Foley catheter drainage for output measurement
5. External monitoring of fetal heart rate and any spontaneous uterine activity
6. Notify pediatricians of patient's status

Surveillance Techniques

The frequency of the following surveillance techniques is dependent on the patient's clinical status.

1. Intake and output: hourly measure of urine volume, specific gravity, and quantitative protein
2. Blood pressure, respirations, pulse hourly
3. Deep tendon reflexes (patellar-depressed or brisk), clonus
4. Bedside ultrasound examination and nonstress test
5. Immediate laboratory tests:
   a. Blood type and screen for possible whole blood administration
   b. Complete blood count with peripheral blood smear
   c. Urinalysis
   d. Serum electrolytes, BUN, creatinine, uric acid
   e. Platelets and fibrinogen
   f. SGOT
   g. 24-hour urine collection for protein and creatinine clearance determinations
6. Frequent laboratory tests
   a. SGOT
   b. Platelet count
   c. 24-hour urine collection for protein and creatinine clearance determinations

Therapy

1. Intravenous magnesium sulfate with a 4–6 g loading dose and 1–3 g/hour maintenance dose
2. Intermittent intravenous labetalol 20 mg to lower blood pressure to within a 140–155/90–105 mm Hg range. Persistently elevated blood pressure levels may be lowered using continuous intravenous labetalol hydralazine (40 mg in 500 mL D_5W), carefully titrated according to present recordings. A reduction in placental blood flow is possible with an abrupt decrease in blood pressure.
3. Nasal oxygen 5–7 liters/minute if eclampsia is present
4. Delivery once maternal condition is stable
   a. Induction of labor if there is cephalic presentation and cervix is favorable; fetal monitoring and maternal observation for excess vaginal bleeding or uterine tenderness
   b. Cesarean section if cervix is unfavorable (especially if time permits a trial of cervical ripening which has failed), fetal distress is suspected without imminent vaginal delivery, or other obstetric conditions (twins, breech, placenta previa, infant anticipated to weigh less than 1500 g).

5. Plasma expanders such as albumin or Plasmanate may be used to increase a low central hemodynamic pressure reading
6. Same parameters to be monitored postpartum with continued intravenous magnesium sulfate for next 12–24 hours. Intravenous labetalol as necessary. Avoid excess intravenous sodium and fluid overload (D_5 ½ NS (5% dextrose, 0.45% NaCl) at less than 200 mL/hour).
7. Consider a Swan-Ganz catheter placement in the presence of renal failure, pulmonary edema, heart failure, or persistently high blood pressure values despite parenteral antihypertensive medications

CARDIAC DISEASE

Cardiac disease is found in 1–3% of all pregnant women. Improvements in antibiotic prophylaxis for rheumatic fever and surgical correction of congenital lesions have reduced the number of childbearing women with rheumatic heart disease and increased those with corrected congenital defects. Intravascular volume, heart rate, stroke volume, and cardiac output increase beginning early in pregnancy and reach a peak at approximately 28–30 weeks. These changes remain relatively stable and decrease slightly near term. The increases are further magnified during labor and the immediate postpartum period.

As a result of these physiologic alterations, there is a marked increase in cardiac work, and the pregnant cardiac patient is thus subjected to significant stress in the antepartum and peripartum periods. Her prognosis depends on the functional capacity of her heart, the presence or absence of other diseases complicating the pregnancy (such as hypertension, infection, etc.), the quality of her medical care, and the resources available in her family and community.

Historical and Clinical Findings

Symptoms such as fatigue and mild dyspnea and physical findings such as a systolic murmur, third heart sound, and edema may be signs of cardiac disease in nonpregnant women but are usually normal physiologic alterations during pregnancy. Further evaluation for cardiac disease is warranted if any of the following symptoms or physical findings are present: dyspnea severe enough to limit activity, progressive orthopnea, paroxysmal nocturnal dyspnea, hemoptysis, syncope immediately following activity, chest pain with an anginal pattern associated with physical activity or emotional stress, a greater than III/VI systolic murmur (diastolic, prediastolic, or continuous), unequivocal cardiac enlargement, severe arrhythmia, cyanosis, or clubbing.

The New York Heart Association Classification in Table 2.2 may be used to classify cardiac patients during pregnancy. The prognosis for the pregnancy outcome can be assessed to a certain extent using this classification. If medication is required to maintain a lower classification, the prognosis is somewhat worse.

General Recommendations

The initial history and physical examination of a person with worrisome heart disease should include a baseline ECG, echocardiogram, and a cardiology consult. In general, the treatment of most serious cardiac disorders in pregnancy should follow the same principles as in the nonpregnant patient (Table 2.3). The patient should be seen weekly or biweekly in the obstetric clinic. If the heart condition is a congenital structural defect, a fetal echocardiogram is recommended at mid-gestation.

Infections may predispose to cardiac failure. Patients should be instructed to report to their physician any signs of infection and to avoid individuals with respiratory infections. Antibiotic prophylaxis against rheumatic fever (either a monthly injection

Table 2.2
New York Heart Association Classification

Class 1	Patients have no limitations of physical activity. Ordinary physical activity does not cause undue fatigue, palpitations, dyspnea, or anginal pain
Class 2	Patients have slight limitation of physical activity. Ordinary physical activity results in fatigue, palpitations, dyspnea, or anginal pain.
Class 3	Patients have marked limitations of physical activity. Less than ordinary activity causes fatigue, palpitations, dyspnea, or anginal pain.
Class 4	Patients are unable to carry on any physical activity without discomfort. Symptoms of cardiac insufficiency or anginal syndrome may be present even at rest. When physical activity is undertaken discomfort increases.

Table 2.3
Cardiac Drugs Utilized during Pregnancy

Drug	Primary Use	Loading Dose	Maintenance Dose
Digoxin	Paroxysmal supraventricular tachyarrhythmia; rate control in atrial fibrillation	0.75–1.25 mg intravenously in 0.25-mg increments at 4-6-hr intervals 1.25–2.0 mg orally in increments at 4-6-hr intervals	0.25–0.50 mg daily, orally
Propranolol	Atrial and ventricular premature beats; reentrant ventricular and supraventricular tachyarrhythmia; rate control in atrial flutter and fibrillation	0.05mg–0.15 mg/kg intravenously by slow infusion; no more than 0.15 mg/kg should be administered in a 6-hr period	40–160 mg daily in 3–4 divided doses, orally
Phenytoin	Supraventricular and ventricular arrhythmia due to digitalis toxicity	100 mg intravenously every 5 min until arrhythmia controlled or adverse effects occur; total dose should not exceed 1000 mg/24 hr 1000 mg orally in divided doses over 24 hr	500 mg orally in divided dose
Verapamil	Paroxysmal supraventricular tachyarrhythmia; rate control in atrial flutter or fibrillation	5–10 mg intravenously over 2–3 min; may be repeated in 30 min if arrhythmia persists	80–120 mg 3–4 times daily, orally

of benzathine penicillin G (Bicillin) 1,200,000 units, or penicillin G 200,000 units orally two times daily) should be used in the rare patient with well-documented rheumatic heart disease.

Many patients are on warfarin (Coumadin) therapy after valve replacement. This drug should be avoided during pregnancy because of its teratogenic risk and the increased incidence of fetal and neonatal deaths from hemorrhage in the later trimesters. Heparin should be used instead, with 5000–8000 units administered subcutaneously every 6–8 hours on an outpatient basis, or intravenously using an anticoagulation dose when hospitalized.

For Class 1 and Class 2 patients, management is usually on an outpatient basis. Patients should rest several times daily to reduce cardiac work and should be hospitalized if there is any sign of heart failure or significant arrhythmia. Patients should have continuous ECG monitoring and oximetry during delivery if significant abnormalities are detected on the outpatient ECG or if symptoms of ischemia occur during labor.

Because of the substantially increased risk of maternal mortality, Class 4 patients should be counseled against becoming pregnant. Extensive bed rest is necessary. A Swan-Ganz catheter and continuous ECG monitoring are required during any labor and at delivery. Determination of the pulmonary capillary wedge pressure is the most useful parameter for evaluating cardiac function in pregnant eclampsia. Pressures at 5–12 mm Hg are usually associated with failing heart functions, as wedge pressures normally range from 13–17 mm Hg. Higher values (especially above 20 mm Hg) indicate ventricular overdistension, and values of 5 mm Hg or less indicate inadequate vascular volume.

Cardiac failure should be treated aggressively with rest, oxygen, rotating tourniquets, digoxin (0.5 mg intravenously over 10 minutes followed by 0.25 mg intravenously every 2–4 hours up to 2 mg as needed), and morphine (10–15 mg intravenously every 2–4 hours). Significant maternal tachycardia should be treated with propranolol (0.2–05 mg intravenously every 3 minutes until the rate is below 110 bpm), digoxin (as above), or cardioversion (25–100 watt-seconds).

The American Heart Association recommends that in pregnant patients with valvular heart disease antibiotics be administered before a cesarean section or urethral catheterization is performed, or during a complicated vaginal delivery. Antibiotics are not required in most patients with heart disease for pelvic examination, dilation and curettage of the uterus, or uncomplicated vaginal delivery, however. The recommended drug regimen for bacterial endocarditis prophylaxis is shown in Table 2.4.

Beta-agonists for the treatment of premature labor are contraindicated in patients with significant cardiac disease. Magnesium sulfate may be used cautiously, since cardiotoxicity is possible with high doses.

A cesarean section should be performed only for obstetric indications. Cardiac surgery such as a commissurotomy is reserved for those patients who are unresponsive to medical management and is performed preferably during the second trimester. Adequate oxygenation and mild hypothermia are desired during the procedure. Electronic fetal monitoring may be helpful, since the fetal heart rate is influenced by the maternal blood pressure and oxygenation.

Specific Disorders

Mitral Stenosis

Because the physiologic changes of pregnancy serve to aggravate the underlying pathophysiology of cardiac disorders, patients with mitral stenosis are at relatively high risk for developing congestive failure, atrial fibrillation, and supraventricular tachycardia. One in four will develop symptoms of cardiac decompensation during pregnancy. Initial therapy consists of bed rest. If this does not suffice, judicious use of digoxin and diuretics may be required. Epidural anesthesia during labor and delivery may re-

Table 2.4
Drug Regimen for Bacterial Endocarditis Prophylaxis

Aqueous penicillin (2 million units) or ampicillin (1 g) i.v. or i.m. **plus** either gentamicin (2.5 mg/kg i.m. or i.v.) or streptomycin (1 g i.m.) 0.5–1 hour before the procedure.

If gentamicin is used, repeat the dose of penicillin or ampicillin and gentamicin every 8 hours for 2 additional doses

If streptomycin is used, give penicillin or ampicillin with streptomycin every 12 hours for 2 additional doses after the procedure

If the patient is allergic to penicillin, vancomycin (1 g i.v. infused over 30 minutes) about 1 hour before the procedure, and gentamicin or streptomycin as above can be used. The same dose of these agents may be repeated in 8–12 hours for 2 more doses

---

lieve anxiety and pain, reduce cardiac afterload, and improve cardiac function.

Mitral Insufficiency

Congestive changes with mitral insufficiency tend to occur at a later age than with mitral stenosis. Most women of childbearing age with this disorder are asymptomatic and tolerate pregnancy without difficulty. If congestive changes are present, acute deterioration and atrial fibrillation may occur and should be treated as outlined for patients with mitral stenosis. Regional anesthesia is recommended.

Aortic Stenosis

High maternal and fetal mortality rates have been reported in the past in patients with aortic stenosis. Pregnant women with this lesion rarely develop congestive failure, but angina often occurs more frequently. Patients have difficulty maintaining cardiac output in the face of acute increases in afterload or decreases in preload. Therefore, hypertension, fluid overload, and hypotension due to blood loss or regional anesthesia must be avoided.

Aortic Insufficiency

Most patients with this lesion tolerate pregnancy without difficulty. However, congestive failure occasionally occurs, requiring rest, digoxin, and diuretics. Regional anesthesia is recommended for labor and delivery.

Pulmonary and Tricuspid Lesions

These lesions are rare and usually well-tolerated during pregnancy. However, patients with symptomatic pulmonary stenosis are at substantially increased risk and should undergo corrective surgery prior to attempting pregnancy.

Periportal Cardiomyopathy

This idiopathic primary congestive cardiomyopathy is present within the first 5 postpartum months. Moderate respiratory distress is accompanied by mild to severe heart failure. Cardiomegaly, a protodiastolic gallop, and an abnormal electrocardiogram are present. Complications include digitalis toxicity, thromboembolism, arrhythmias, and bronchopneumonia. The prognosis is guarded, and the incidence of recurrence is high with any subsequent pregnancy.

Atrial Septal Defect, Ventricular Septal Defect, Patent Ductus Arteriosus

Patients with these lesions usually tolerate pregnancy without substantial deterioration unless right to left shunting and pulmonary hypertension are present. Bacterial endocarditis prophylaxis is required for VSD and PDA, but not for ASD.

Mitral Valve Prolapse

Patients with mitral valve prolapse alone usually do well during pregnancy. The prevalence of arrhythmias is higher, and 20% require propranolol to control this problem. The need for prophylactic antibiotics for an uncomplicated labor and delivery is controversial.

Idiopathic Hypertrophic Subaortic Stenosis

The hemodynamic changes associated with pregnancy often result in a decrease in outflow obstruction and improvement in symptoms. However, situations predisposing to catecholamine release (pain and anxiety, hypotension due to blood loss or regional anesthesia) may aggravate symptoms during labor and should be avoided.

Coarctation of the Aorta

Patients with this disorder may be separated into complicated or uncomplicated categories on the basis of the presence or absence of associated cardiac valvular lesions. Patients with uncomplicated coarctation usually do well during pregnancy. However, gravidas with complicated coarctation are at higher risk due to potential rupture of associated intracranial aneurysms and/or aortic dissection. Therapy for the latter group consists of control of hypertension, rest, and beta-blockers as prophylaxis against dissection.

Marfan's Syndrome

Patients with Marfan's syndrome who have an aortic arch greater than 4.0 cm in diameter or who have cardiac decompensation are at high risk for sustaining a ruptured aortic aneurysm or further cardiac deterioration. Pregnancy is contraindicated in such women. Gravidas with an aortic arch diameter less than 4.0 cm and no cardiac decompensation are at relatively low risk. They should rest frequently, and beta-blockers may be considered to reduce pulse pressure.

Pulmonary Hypertension, Eisenmenger's Syndrome

Pregnancy is contraindicated in these cases because maternal mortality is 30–50%.

THROMBOEMBOLIC DISEASE

The physiologic changes of pregnancy increase the chances that a pregnant woman may experience Virchow's classic triad of factors predisposing to thrombosis: alteration in the composition of the blood, venous stasis, and vessel wall injury. During the antepartum period, the prevalence of deep vein thrombophlebitis remains similar to that found in nonpregnant women but increases by fourfold to sixfold during labor, delivery, and the postpartum period. Additionally, pulmonary embolism occurs at a rate of 0.5–1.2 per 1000 deliveries. Respiratory and cardiovascular compromise as a result of this medical complication are common causes of maternal mortality, especially in the postpartum cesarean patient.

The diagnosis of thrombophlebitis is often obscured due to musculoskeletal pain and edema, common in normal pregnancy. Doppler flow studies, impedance plethysmography, and limited venography may be diagnostic. Once the diagnosis is established, anticoagulant therapy has been demonstrated to decrease the probability of pulmonary embolus and result in decreased mortality. Because of the potential teratogenic and late fetal complications associated with warfarin therapy, heparin is the preferred anticoagulant during the antepartum period. It may be administered as a 70 U/kg intravenous bolus followed by an infusion of 300–400 U/kg/24 hours, or as a 5000 U bolus followed by a maintenance dose of approximately 1000 U/hour. The maintenance infusion should be titrated to achieve a partial thromboplastin time (PTT) of 50–75 seconds. Intravenous therapy should be continued for 7–10 days. In the postpartum period, warfarin therapy may be initiated and continued for three months. In the antepartum period, a moderate dose of subcutaneous heparin (approximately 10,000 U every 12 hours or 7,000 U three times a day, adjusted to maintain a therapeutic PTT level) may be administered for three months, followed by a subcutaneous dose 5000 U two times a day for the remainder of the pregnancy.

Unfortunately, laboratory studies used in the diagnosis of pulmonary embolism (Table 2.5) are often insensitive and nonspecific. If clinical suspicion of a pulmonary embolus is high and certain diagnostic tests are delayed or inconclusive, intravenous heparin therapy should be initiated in the dosage outlined above. Once the diagnosis is confirmed, long-term therapy should be utilized according to the above guidelines for a minimum of 3–6 months. If emboli recur after adequate anticoagulation, vena cava ligation should be considered.

Women who have experienced a thromboembolic event before pregnancy appear to have a 12% recurrence risk. This observation has led us to administer a minidose of subcutaneous heparin, 5,000 U every 12 hours during the first trimester, 7,500 U during the second trimester, and 10,000 U during the third trimester and until the patients are fully ambulatory postpartum. Some investigators have recommended that this practice be extended to other high-risk groups, including women with advanced maternal age, high parity, obesity, immobility, diabetes, hypertension, cardiac disease, or severe varicose veins.

DRUG ABUSE

It would appear that 10% is a minimal reasonable estimate of the prevalence of urine toxicologic evidence of substance abuse in the general pregnancy population in the United States. Although the risk of fetal malformation with inadvertent use in early gestation is unknown, no benefit from continued use is possible, and premature delivery is more likely. Furthermore, the effect of these drugs (which readily cross the placenta) on fetal neurobehavioral development cannot be assessed with certainty.

Cocaine use has gained nationwide attention and is a commonly abused substance of most pregnant drug addicts. Observations have suggested that cocaine use is related to a significantly higher rate of spontaneous abortion, growth retardation, stillbirth, and malformation. Infants and children exposed in utero to cocaine are also more likely to show depressed interactive behavior and poor organizational response to environmental stimuli.

Table 2.5
Tests Used to Diagnose Pulmonary Embolism

Test	Findings Suggestive of Pulmonary Embolus	Aids to Differential Diagnosis	Therapeutic Implications
Arterial blood gases	Low pO_2 and low or normal pCO_2 are nearly constant findings	Normal pO_2 nearly always excludes PE	Guide to oxygen therapy and prognosis
Chest x-ray	Enlargement of main pulmonary artery and right ventricle, lung infiltrate, pleural effusion, elevated diaphragm, or asymmetry of vasculature	To rule out pneumonia and congestive heart failure (may be secondary)	Presence of acute right ventricular enlargement indicates life-threatening embolism
ECG	Right axis shift and right ventricular strain	To rule out acute myocardial infarction or ischemia	Detection and treatment of arrhythmia
Ventilation/perfusion scan (V/Q)	Areas of oligemia (areas of the lung with a decreased concentration of radioactivity on perfusion studies with unmatched areas on ventilation)	Equivocal scan can be caused by pneumonia, atelectasis, or other pulmonary lesions	Extent of V/Q mismatch serves as a guide to severity
Pulmonary angiogram	Filling defects distally	Normal angiogram excludes large emboli, cutoffs of pulmonary arteries, areas of decreased perfusion	Most accurate guide to assess

Each patient should be questioned about substance abuse at her first prenatal visit. Abstinence and prenatal care are associated with improved perinatal outcomes. Abortion is not recommended for drug exposure alone. Tests of amniotic fluid to assess fetal involvement are not available. Periodic urine toxicology screening is a motivational tool to encourage abstinence but may be threatening to the patient and limited by the rapid clearance of most substances in 48–72 hours. Listed below are general recommendations for assessing the mother and fetus and for management of drug dependency.

Baseline Laboratory Studies

1. Complete blood count with indices
2. Blood smear
3. Urine culture (minimum of two during pregnancy)
4. Tuberculin skin test
5. Total protein and A/G ratio
6. Liver function profile
7. Rubella titer
8. Serologic test for syphilis (RPR, VDRL, etc.)
9. Gonorrhea and chlamydia culture (cervical) at initial visit and repeat at 36 weeks
10. HB_sAg (hepatitis B surface antigen)
11. Pap smear
12. Blood type, Rh, and irregular antibody screen
13. Ultrasound scan
14. Herpes culture (if positive history)
15. Sickle cell screen (if patient is anemic and African-American)
16. Serum HIV antibody titer

Nutrition

1. Diet consultation
2. Ingestion of fresh fruit, fresh vegetables, lean meats, dairy products
3. Prevent deficiency states
4. Prenatal vitamins
5. Frequent complete blood counts
6. Diet recall with each visit
7. Assess dental hygiene
8. Encourage smoking cessation

Infection

1. Examine for and treat any sexually transmitted disease
2. Screen for hepatitis B
3. Watch for and treat any other illness
4. Examine urine for infection
5. Search for preexisting bacterial endocarditis

Psychosocial

1. Establish contact with social services for care before and after delivery and for infant placement (if necessary)
2. Watch for suicidal depression (hospitalize without delay)

Drug Management

1. Watch for multiple drug use (including alcohol, marijuana, and tobacco); may need to perform urine drug screens intermittently
2. Supportive withdrawal: minor tranquilizers, sedatives, and amphetamines
3. Maintenance therapy for narcotic abuse: gradual detoxification with oral methadone, usually beginning with approximately 40 mg daily; decrease methadone dose (by 2 mg/week) with caution and attempt to achieve 20 mg/day or less by delivery to minimize any neonatal withdrawal

Fetal Assessment

1. Maternal serum alpha-fetoprotein screening offered at 15–18 weeks
2. No tests of amniotic fluid to assess fetal effects from drugs, nor a karyotype analysis, are recommended
3. Serial ultrasound examinations to search for intrauterine growth retardation (IUGR) and microcephaly
4. Perform fetal biophysical tests in third trimester if fetal compromise is suspected
5. Notify pediatrician before labor and delivery
6. Use of naloxone (Narcan) is contraindicated in newborns of drug-addicted mothers, since it may initiate an immediate withdrawal syndrome; support any respiratory depression with mechanical ventilation

7. Effects from specific abused drugs on the mother and fetus are listed in Table 2.6

Postpartum

1. Continue above recommendations
2. Drug analysis of meconium and newborn hair may identify neonates who may be at risk for developing long-term sequelae
3. Become familiar with state laws regarding urine testing during pregnancy, testing of newborns, and reporting results to child protection agencies

SEIZURE DISORDERS

Seizure disorders are found in approximately 1 in 100 pregnant women. Several years were required to recognize the teratogenic potential of most anticonvulsant medications because of the compounding effects of metabolic changes, seizure-related hypoxia, and genetic factors. Current therapeutic practice requires prescribing a minimal number of medications, selecting those with the least teratogenic potential, and using the lowest dose compatible with maternal seizure control.

An understanding of both the type of seizure disorder and any medications taken is necessary. Table 2.7 lists drug therapy for specific seizure disorders. Most patients requiring long-term drug therapy have grand mal or tonic-clonic seizures. The risk to an unborn child of developing epilepsy is 2–3%, or 5 times greater than in the general population. A patient should be discouraged from becoming pregnant if the seizures are difficult to control, causing her to be incapable of responsible parenting. The risk of a seizure disorder's worsening during the pregnancy is 50%, of being unaltered is 5%, and of improving is 45%. The risk of its worsening is greater, however, if seizures have occurred recently.

Petit mal seizures are rare in adults. Whether patients with petit mal or psychomotor seizure disorders should continue their medications during pregnancy is unclear. Consultation with a neurologist is recommended.

Antenatal Care

An attempt should be made to withdraw anticonvulsants over several months before pregnancy if the patient has been seizure-free

Table 2.6
Effects from Specific Abused Drugs

Drug Groups	Maternal Signs and Symptoms of Overdose	Maternal Withdrawal Symptoms	Fetal/Neonatal Effects
Alcohol	Unusual behavior; mostly depressant with stupor, loss of memory, hypotension	Agitation, tremors	Fetal alcohol syndrome (FAS): microcephaly, mental retardation, facial dysmorphia, failure to thrive
Marijuana	Pupils normal but conjunctivae inflamed	None	None known; meconium during labor(?)
CNS sedatives (barbiturates, chlordiazepoxide, alprazolam, diazepam, flurazepam, methaqualone)	Pupils fixed, BP decreased, respiration depressed, reflexes hypoactive, drowsiness, coma, lateral nystagmus, slurred speech, delirium, convulsions	Tremulousness, insomnia, chronic blink reflex, agitation, toxic psychosis	Decreased heart variability; sedation or respiratory depression (mild if present)
CNS stimulants (cocaine, antiobesity drugs, amphetamines)	Pupils dilated and reactive, respirations shallow, BP increased, reflexes hyperactive	Muscle aches, abdominal pain, hunger, prolonged sleep, suicidal	Hyperactivity with increased kicks, spontaneous abortion, premature labor, fetal demise, placental abruption, IUGR, SIDS, neuro-behavioral impairments; limb reduction defects (?), genitourinary malformations (?)

Hallucinogens (LSD, phencyclidine)	Pupils dilated, BP elevated, heart rate increased, reflexes hyperactive, face flushed, euphoria, anxiety, inappropriate affect, illusions, hallucinations	No withdrawal symptoms	No known fetal effects; behavior problems, facial abnormalities(?)
Narcotics (codeine, heroin, meperidine, morphine, opium)	Pupils constricted, respirations and BP decreased, reflexes hypoactive, sensorium obtunded	Flu-like syndrome, agitation, dilated pupils, abdominal pain	Intrauterine withdrawal with increased fetal activity, neonatal withdrawal, increased rates of IUGR and intrauterine fetal demise
Solvents (fumes from glue, gasoline, paint thinner, cleaning solutions)	Euphoria, toxicity to liver and kidneys	Agitation	"Fetal Solvent Syndrome" (similar to FAS)

Table 2.7
Drug Therapy for Specific Seizure Disorders during Pregnancy

Seizure Disorder	Primary Drug	Secondary Drug
Grand mal (tonic-clonic)	phenobarbital	carbamazepine phenytoin primidone
Psychomotor	primidone	phenytoin phenobarbital carbamazepine
Petit mal (absence)	ethosuximide	clonazepam
Status epilepticus	diazepam followed by phenytoin	phenytoin phenobarbital paraldehyde thiopental

for several years and has a normal electroencephalogram. Listed in Table 2.8 are adverse maternal and fetal effects from anticonvulsant use. If a combination of anticonvulsants has been taken before conception, an attempt should be made to see if the generalized (tonic-clonic) seizures can be controlled with one agent, preferably phenobarbital or carbamazepine. However, the patient should be maintained on as many medications as necessary to control the seizures, since a seizure with hypoxia is a greater concern than any drug-induced teratogenicity.

A preferred second-line drug is uncertain, but phenytoin (Dilantin) is most commonly used. Current estimates are that 7–10% of exposed children will show low intelligence quotients, low birth weight, midfacial hypoplasia, nail hypoplasia, hirsutism, hypotonicity, and mild developmental delays, whereas only 3% will show major anomalies like cleft lip/palate or heart disease when phenytoin is used alone. These figures increase when other drugs are taken in combination.

Valproic acid and carbamazepine (Tegretol) carry a reported 1% teratogenic risk of open neural tube defects. Despite reports of its safety, carbamazepine may be associated with a greater risk of minor craniofacial abnormalities, digital hypoplasia, and developmental delays. If the patient is first seen during pregnancy and seizures are well-controlled on her current regimen, the medications should not be withdrawn, as this may precipitate status epilepticus.

The patient should be advised that the risk of fetal anomalies

Table 2.8
Adverse Maternal and Fetal Effects from Anticonvulsant Use

Maternal	Fetal/Neonatal
Phenobarbital Drowsiness (transient), ataxia, respiratory depression, sleep abnormalities, hypotension, withdrawal	Possible low-level teratogenicity, neonatal depression, coagulopathy, hemorrhage
Carbamazepine (Tegretol) Diplopia, drowsiness, leukopenia, transient blurred vision, rash, disturbance of equilibrium	Open neural tube defect
Phenytoin (Dilantin) Cardiovascular collapse after rapid i.v. injection, ataxia, nystagmus, GI upset, increased incidence of seizures, behavioral changes	Probable teratogenicity (including nonspecific cardiac), neonatal coagulopathy, hypocalcemia, tetany
Valproic acid GI upset, sedation, ataxia, loss of coordination, hepatotoxicity, thrombocytopenia	Open neural tube defect
Diazepam (Valium) Depressed respiration, bradycardia, hypotension, cardiovascular collapse, paradoxical hyperexcitability, withdrawal	Possible low-level teratogenicity, decreased FHR variability, neonatal depression, withdrawal, impaired thermoregulation

is increased twofold to threefold (8% overall) when taking anticonvulsants, and there is some increased risk of mental retardation with certain agents. Excessive weight gain and sudden fluid retention may increase the risk of seizures. We routinely offer a targeted ultrasound scan and maternal serum alpha-fetoprotein (MSAFP) screening at 15–18 weeks and a fetal echocardiogram at 20–24 weeks because of the slightly higher risk of an open neural tube defect and nonspecific cardiac defects with the use of these medications.

Patients should be advised that there is a 50% risk that a seizure disorder will worsen during pregnancy and that this risk is even higher if she has had frequent seizures recently. The most common precipitant of seizures is noncompliance with drug therapy; other causes include fever, substance abuse, sedative drug withdrawal, and a metabolic or structural abnormality. Serum drug levels should be measured monthly during pregnancy, with adjustments in dosages to attain a total serum level in a low-normal therapeutic range (Table 2.9).

Anticonvulsants antagonize folic acid and vitamin K. Pregnant epileptics receiving phenytoin, phenobarbital, or carbamazepine should be given oral folic acid (4 mg daily before conception and 1 mg daily beyond the first 2 months of pregnancy; an 800-μg or 1-mg dose is found in standard prenatal vitamin preparations). The use of anticonvulsants during pregnancy is associated with a vitamin D–dependent bleeding disorder in the newborn. Biochemical abnormalities of vitamin K–dependent factors are much more common than is clinical bleeding. Studies have shown that administration of vitamin K (at least 10 mg/day) to the mother during the last month of pregnancy decreases the deficiency of vitamin K in newborns exposed to anticonvulsants.

Status epilepticus should be treated vigorously. Diazepam (Valium) 10 mg should be administered intravenously over 1–3 minutes after the patient's airway is opened and free exchange of air takes place. Phenytoin (Dilantin) 200–500 mg is then given intravenously depending on anticonvulsant blood levels.

Intrapartum/Postpartum Management

The pediatric staff should be notified of any impending delivery. Evidence of fetal malformations or neonatal depression and withdrawal should be sought. Coagulation studies of the cord blood should routinely be performed, and the infant should be given 1 mg of vitamin K intramuscularly shortly after birth.

Intravenous anticonvulsant therapy using phenytoin (500 mg intravenously over 30 minutes every 12 hours) or magnesium

Table 2.9
Daily Dosages of Specific Anticonvulsants to Maintain Therapeutic Serum Levels

Drug	Adult Daily Dosage (mg)	Therapeutic Level (μg/mL)
Phenobarbital	90–120	15–40
Phenytoin (Dilantin)	300–500	10–20
Carbamazepine (Tegretol)	800–1200	4–16

sulfate (1–2 g/hour) should be administered if the patient is to take nothing by mouth during active labor or cesarean delivery. Phenytoin should not be mixed in a dextrose-containing solution, because intravenous crystallization may occur.

Breast-feeding is permissible if no infant signs of depression are evident. Anticonvulsant drug doses should be decreased after delivery according to serum drug levels.

THYROID DISEASE

Hyperthyroidism

Next to diabetes, untreated or previously treated hyperthyroidism is the most common endocrine disorder encountered during pregnancy. The diagnosis of hyperthyroidism is often difficult, as signs and symptoms of thyroid hyperfunction are similar to certain normal patient complaints during pregnancy, and thyroid tests are altered by pregnancy-induced changes in the serum proteins. However, therapy is necessary to avoid maternal and fetal complications. If untreated, stillbirth rates are increased to 8–15%, and premature delivery may occur in up to one-fourth of affected patients.

Drug therapy of hyperthyroidism is the primary form of treatment during pregnancy. A subtotal thyroidectomy is best reserved for patients for whom medical management has been ineffective because of poor compliance, severe disease, or the need for excessive antithyroid medication. Medications are intended to decrease the amount of circulating thyroid hormones (antithyroid drugs) and to relieve severely bothersome maternal symptoms (β-adrenergic antagonists). The two principal antithyroid preparations, propylthiouracil (PTU) and methimazole (Tapazole), are thiourea derivatives that prevent the iodination of tyrosine by inhibiting the oxidation of iodide to iodine. They are equally effective and both are safe, but PTU is preferred over methimazole because placental transfer is less rapid. If either drug has been taken for 6 months, it may be gradually withdrawn before pregnancy. Most relapses occur within 3–6 months after discontinuation.

The response of hyperthyroidism to therapy is governed by the need to deplete thyroid stores. A 7–8-week period is the median time during pregnancy to normalize the free thyroxine (T_4) index. An adjustment of daily doses is dependent on relief of patient symptoms and circulatory levels of free T_4, which should be maintained within an upper-normal or slightly elevated range.

Daily doses exceeding 300 mg (usually 50–100 mg two or three times a day) should be avoided because of the greater potential of fetal thyroid effects. No increased risk of malformations (3%) is present, and overt hypothyroidism in the neonate is rare. Goiter formation in the fetus may be present in up to 10% of all infants and is dependent on the dose and duration of in utero exposure. Neonatal hypothyroidism lasts only a few days, but long-term intellectual development has not been compared to their siblings. Presumably, insignificant amount of PTU reach suckling infants, with no change in the infants' serum T_3, T_4, thyroid-stimulating hormone (TSH), or resin T_3 uptake levels.

Maternal symptoms relating to enhanced sympathomimetic activity such as tremors, tachycardia, and palpitations are seen with hyperthyroidism. A beta-blocker such a propranolol may be used when symptoms are severe. However, its beta-blocking action may also cause a loss of beat-to-beat variability, bradycardia, hypoglycemia, and transient respiratory depression in the newborn, and it should be discontinued, if possible, shortly before delivery to minimize peripartum drug effects.

Thyroid storm occurs rarely during pregnancy, most commonly in patients with no history of thyroid disease. It is characterized by a high fever (103°F or more), tachycardia, nausea and vomiting, or central nervous system involvement and is usually precipitated by infection, ketoacidosis, or surgery. Therapy for the pregnant patient with thyroid storm includes the following: copious intravenous fluids, propranolol (40 mg orally every 6 hours or 1–2 mg intravenously slowly until pulse rate less than 100 bpm), propylthiouracil (300 mg orally every 6 hours), hydrocortisone (100 mg intravenously every 8 hours), sodium iodine (1 g intravenously), and hypothermia induction.

Thyroid function should be monitored carefully in the first few postpartum months, since severe and unpredictable alterations may occur. The IgG immunoglobulin, LATS (long-acting thyroid stimulator), can cross the placenta easily in a small number of mothers with Graves' disease and remain within the newborn's circulation.

Hypothyroidism

Hypothyroidism is found most commonly after a subtotal thyroidectomy. Affected patients have symptoms similar to normal complaints during pregnancy, which include fatigability and cold intolerance. Most thyroidectomy or postirradiated patients are on thyroid replacement therapy at conception. This medication should be continued during pregnancy, since documented hypothyroidism may be associated with an increased risk of an unfavorable perinatal outcome and thyroid hormone reserves will become further depleted.

Symptoms of hypothyroidism overlap with those from pregnancy-induced physiologic changes. Low free T_4 levels and elevated TSH levels have been reported to be associated with an increased risk of infertility and recurrent pregnancy losses. It is recommended that thyroid supplementation be continued during pregnancy if laboratory evidence exists and patient symptoms persist.

Levothyroxine (Synthroid) is the first-line therapy, because it is T_4 only and is the most physiologic replacement. Thyroid supplements do not cross the placental barrier in appreciable amounts and should not affect the autonomous fetal thyroid-pituitary function. The usual nonpregnant daily dose of 0.1–0.2 mg may need to be increased slightly during pregnancy. The only major complication is overdose. Serum T_4 levels may be falsely higher when receiving maintenance therapy, and the dose of levothyroxine should be such that the TSH level is less than 10 mU/mL. Thyroid function should be monitored carefully in the first few postpartum months, since severe and unpredictable alterations may occur.

COLLAGEN VASCULAR DISORDERS

Systemic lupus erythematosus and rheumatoid arthritis are the most common collagen vascular disorders and perhaps those most amenable to therapy. Although many women experience reexacerbations after delivery, few cases actually develop de novo during pregnancy. Lupus nephritis is a particularly dangerous complication, however, and may be difficult to differentiate from preeclampsia.

Systemic corticosteroids are seldom indicated for the treatment of rheumatoid arthritis, but they form the mainstay of drug therapy for systemic lupus. Women who receive the medication are thought to have fewer exacerbations and less perinatal mortality than those without this drug therapy. These medicines are prescribed in the lowest doses to minimize symptoms and prevent recurrence. A daily dose of 20–40 mg of prednisone may be utilized for flare-ups with nonmajor organ involvement. The daily dose should be increased in the puerperium or if major organ involvement (nephritis, central nervous system, vasculitis) is present. The medication should be taken in the morning, and preferably on alternating days. Prenatal vitamins should be continued, because calcium and vitamin D should be supplemented. Signs of gestational diabetes and hypertension should be sought.

Salicylates form the first line of drug therapy for rheumatoid arthritis and may be helpful in controlling minor symptoms in patients with systemic lupus. These agents exert their therapeutic benefit by blocking prostaglandin synthetase activity through the inhibition of cyclooxygenase. Enteric-coated acetylsalicylate is the preferred preparation, in daily doses of 650–1300 mg every 4–6 hours. While there have been occasional reports suggesting an increased risk of fetal malformations, the overwhelming body of evidence has demonstrated no teratogenic effect. The length of gestation may be longer, the incidence of postdatism higher, and the duration of labor more prolonged for mothers who have been treated with salicylates because of the prostaglandin inhibitory properties. Premature closure of the ductus arteriosus and pulmonary hypertension in the newborn are unlikely but should be sought. Neonatal platelet dysfunction and an increased frequency of intracranial hemorrhage have been associated with maternal salicylate ingestion.

Less is known about other nonsteroidal antiinflammatory drugs (NSAIDs). What has been found with indomethacin is similar to what has been reported on full-dose aspirin. The lack of knowledge about immunosuppressive medications, penicillamine, and gold during pregnancy would warrant that they be avoided except in life-threatening situations.

ASTHMA

Asthma is one of the most common medical disorders, with a reported prevalence of 2% during pregnancy. Many drugs are available for the control of asthma, and therapy during pregnancy differs little from that in the nonpregnant adult. Patients with asthma, except those with mild and infrequent episodes of bronchospasm, should be continuously treated with appropriate medications. Much emphasis has been placed on maintenance therapy using a combination of inhaled corticosteroids (beclomethasone, triamcinolone, flunisolide) with beta-agonists. Systemic absorption is minimal, and any increased fetal risk from these drugs is negligible or nonexistent with standard dosing. Objective measurement of airflow using peak flow meters is useful and is essential in evaluating the response to maintenance therapy.

If intermittent therapy is acceptable, many patients can be treated solely with β_2–adrenergic agonists (albuterol, terbutaline, or metaproterenol) through metered-dose inhalers (MDI) or nebulizers. During short periods of wheezing, 2–4 puffs can be followed by 1–2 puffs every 10–20 minutes. Thereafter, 2 puffs every 4 hours can be taken until wheezing stops.

If inhalation therapy does not suffice, oral theophylline preparations may be continued or begun, although their value is being questioned. The most common preparation of these phosphodiesterase inhibitors is theophylline in a dose of 200–400 mg orally two times a day. Theophylline clearance is often increased during late pregnancy. For optimal effects, the dose should be adjusted to reverse wheezing and maintain therapeutic serum levels in the range of 10–20 mg/mL. Theophylline inhibits the force but not the frequency of uterine contractions, and its use is associated with the theoretic risk of prolonging gestation or labor. It may also accelerate fetal pulmonary maturity because of its phosphodiesterase-inhibiting properties.

If these women still experience respiratory symptoms, oral β-adrenergic agents should be prescribed. Several preparations are available, but terbutaline, using a dose of 2.5–5 mg orally two or three times a day, is standard. These agents exert their bronchodilating effect by stimulating β_2 receptors in bronchial smooth muscles, leading to an increased production of cyclic AMP (adenosine 3',5'-cyclic monophosphate). Because these drugs may also inhibit labor, there is a theoretic risk of prolonging gestation.

Orally-administered corticosteroids may be started for patients who remain refractory to the above mentioned therapeutic regimens. Varying doses of 40–60 mg of prednisone in a single daily dose are recommended, with clinical improvement usually being noted within 6 hours. The dosage is tapered over 5 to 14 days in most circumstances, and inhaled corticosteroids can be substituted in dosages of 2 puffs spaced apart 5–10 minutes four times daily. Those few patients continuing to receive oral corticosteroids should be given intravenous hydrocortisone (100 mg every 6 hours) during labor, delivery, and immediately postpartum.

Little or none of antiasthmatic medications appears in breast milk. Inhaled bronchodilators have minimal systemic absorption and are therefore probably not secreted in breast milk.

GASTROESOPHAGEAL REFLUX

Estimates of the incidence of gastroesophageal reflux (or "heartburn") during pregnancy range from 10–80% in select populations. Although heartburn is not more frequent in multiparous than nulliparous women, a tendency exists for symptoms to recur in women who experienced heartburn in a prior pregnancy. Mild esophagitis is common, but more severe complications are rare. Medications may be helpful if symptoms persist despite lifestyle changes and avoidance of certain foods (fatty, onions, garlic, caffeine, chocolate).

Antacids are usually successful in making heartburn more tolerable but do not usually provide complete relief. Although there are few data concerning fetal effects, antacids taken in doses not to exceed the manufacturer's recommendations are considered to be safe during pregnancy. No antacid is clearly preferred, although most obstetricians prefer the calcium-containing products. Tablets are more convenient than liquid antacids and may be more effective, since salivation is necessary during chewing.

Cimetidine (Tagamet) was the first histamine$_2$-receptor antagonist to be introduced as an antisecretory drug for peptic ulcer disease and GER. Given possible antiandrogenic effects of cimetidine, ranitidine (Zantac) or famotidine (Pepcid) should probably be preferred over cimetidine. Each crosses the human placenta by passive diffusion relatively slowly compared with other drugs. There are few published reports of antagonists being taken early in pregnancy, but there have been no adverse fetal effects noted.

INFLAMMATORY BOWEL DISEASE AND PERSISTENT DIARRHEA

Neither ulcerative colitis nor Crohn's disease is associated with infertility, and neither appears to worsen during pregnancy. Therapy begins with prenatal vitamins (vitamin B_{12}, iron, folate, vitamin E, magnesium) and modification of the diet to avoid lactulose, some fruits, and vegetables. Because there is an increased requirement during pregnancy, calcium intake may need to be supplemented with calcium tablets (e.g., Os-Cal 500 mg, 1 or 2 tablets two times daily).

Sulfasalazine is frequently used alone or in combination with corticosteroids for the treatment of inflammatory bowel disease. This medication is split by bacteria to form 5-aminosalicylate and sulfapyridine. The body of evidence suggests that prolonged therapy for the prevention of recurrences is of little benefit. Toxic maternal side effects include headache, nausea, vomiting, and abdominal pain. Sulfasalazine inhibits folate absorption in the small bowel, so folate supplementation in a prenatal vitamin is required during pregnancy. No teratogenic effect or jaundice has been attributed to use of this medication. Sulfasalazine is also secreted in breast milk, with concentrations approaching 30% of those of the simultaneous maternal serum. No adverse neonatal effects have been reported with its use.

Corticosteroids are usually employed for those patients who fail to respond to the above measures. They exert their beneficial effect by accumulating in the inflamed bowel tissue and exerting a dose-related inhibition of the inflammatory response. However, evidence on the efficacy of corticosteroids for preventing recurrences in quiescent ulcerative colitis has yielded conflicting results. Corticosteroids may be administered either orally, or as retention enemas if there is distal colitis. Prednisone in a dose of 40 mg is utilized initially. A single dose is preferable, and most patients experience a therapeutic response in 1–2 weeks. The dosage is then generally reduced to allow for 4–8 weeks of total therapy.

Nonspecific antidiarrheals are unnecessary with most bouts of acute diarrhea. These drugs are also not a substitute for treatment of the underlying illness. Bulk-forming agents (e.g., Metamucil, Konsyl) and absorbents (e.g., Kaopectate) are safe. Opioids or opioidlike compounds (codeine, Lomotil, loperamide) should best be avoided during pregnancy. Little or no experience has been reported with 6-mercaptopurine, azathioprine, and 5-aminosalicylate (mesalamine) during pregnancy.

MIGRAINE HEADACHES

Migraine headaches are common among women of childbearing age. Unilateral and throbbing discomfort is accompanied by nausea and visual, cognitive, motor, or psychic disturbances. Most investigators have noted a decrease in the frequency of migraines during pregnancy, especially beyond the first trimester. Recovery is enhanced by removing any provoking factors and resting in a quiet, dark, noise-free environment.

Ergot alkaloids administered at the earliest indication of an attack form the cornerstone of drug therapy in nonpregnant individuals. Most clinicians recommend that these agents be avoided during pregnancy due to their vasoconstricting effects. Ergot alkaloids are also relatively contraindicated in the breast-feeding mother due to associated neonatal vomiting, diarrhea, and blood pressure disturbances.

Simple analgesics such as acetaminophen with or without codeine are generally utilized for acute therapy during pregnancy. Prostaglandin synthetase inhibiting drugs (aspirin, indomethacin) and opioids are not encouraged for maintenance therapy during pregnancy. Published experience is limited on prophylactic therapy for recurrent headaches during pregnancy. Propranolol in doses of 20 mg orally two times a day may be used if analgesics are unsuccessful, particularly if blood pressure levels are elevated. Despite very limited experience, tricyclic antidepressants such as amitriptyline are occasionally prescribed in low doses before sleep, especially when coexisting depression is suspected.

No reports are available on the use of combinations of analgesics, sedatives, caffeine, or sympathomimetic amines (such as Midrin or Fiorinal) during pregnancy. Little is known also about the safety of monoamine oxidase (MAO) inhibitors, calcium channel antagonists, methysergide, and prednisone as prophylactic therapy for migraine or cluster headaches during pregnancy.

Suggested Readings

Bag S, Behari M, Ahuja GK, Karmarkar KG. Pregnancy and epilepsy. J Neurol 1989;236:311–313.

Clark, SL. Management of asthma during pregnancy. National Asthma Education Program Working Group in Asthma and Pregnancy. National Institutes of Health, National Heart, Lung, and Blood Institute. Obstet Gynecol 1993;82:1036–1040.

Davis LE, Lucas MJ, Hankins GDV, Roark ML, Cunningham FG. Thyrotoxicosis complicating pregnancy. Am J Obstet Gynecol 1989;160:63–70.

Landon MB, Gabbe SG. Diabetes mellitus and pregnancy. Obstet Gynecol Clin North Am 1992;19:633–654.

Maccato ML. Pneumonia and pulmonary tuberculosis in pregnancy. Obstet Gynecol Clin North Am 1989;16:417–430.

Metzger BE. Summary and recommendations of the Third International Workshop-Conference on Gestational Diabetes Mellitus. Diabetes 1991;40(2 Suppl):197–201.

Rosa FW. Spina bifida in infants of women treated with carbamazepine during pregnancy. N Engl J Med 1991;324:674–677.

Scialli AR. Fetal protection policies in the United States. Semin Perinatol 1993;17:50–57.

Slutsker L. Risks associated with cocaine use during pregnancy. Obstet Gynecol 1992;79:778–789.

Sorokin JJ, Levine SM. Pregnancy and inflammatory bowel disease: a review of the literature. Obstet Gynecol 1983;62:247–252.

Zuspan FP, Rayburn WF. Blood pressure self-monitoring during pregnancy: practical considerations. Am J Obstet Gynecol 1991;164:2–6.

Chapter 3

Antepartum Obstetric Complications

FIRST TRIMESTER BLEEDING

Approximately one-fourth of all pregnant patients will have some vaginal bleeding in early pregnancy. Along with a threatened or incomplete abortion, other causes include incorrect menstrual dating, a lesion of the cervix, an ectopic pregnancy, a missed abortion, and trophoblastic disease. A systematic examination is necessary to search for any abdominal tenderness, internal cervical ostium dilation, uterine enlargement, or an adnexal mass.

A proposed management plan is shown in Figure 3.1. The prognosis is favorable if fetal motion is seen sonographically beyond 6 weeks' gestation. In addition, serial quantitative serum human chorionic gonadotropin (hCG) testing will identify abnormal pregnancies, ectopic pregnancy, or those destined to abort in 85% of cases if a rate of increase less than 66% is noted within 2 days. Serum progesterone levels are also predictive of unsuccessful pregnancy. Viable pregnancies are very rarely associated with serum progesterone levels of less than 5 ng/mL. Most viable intrauterine pregnancies are associated with serum progesterone levels greater than 25 ng/mL, and most unsuccessful pregnancies have values less than 15 ng/mL.

ABNORMAL PAP SMEAR

A Pap smear should be obtained routinely during the pelvic examination at the initial prenatal visit. An endocervical brush can be safely used and may increase the yield of any abnormalities, compared with the use of cotton-tipped swabs. Pregnancy may contribute to an increased incidence of abnormal Pap smears be-

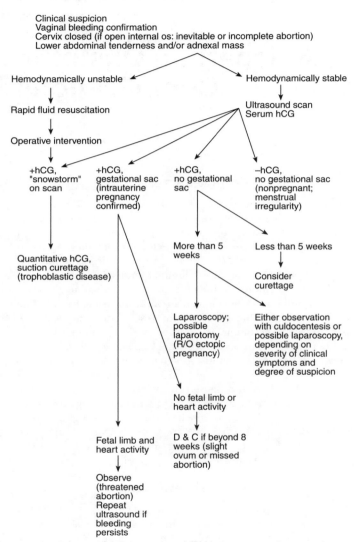

Figure 3.1.   Proposed management for first trimester bleeding.

cause of cervical eversion. However, a worsening of abnormal cytologic findings is not thought to occur, and many Pap smear abnormalities improve after delivery. Carcinoma in situ of the cervix is found in 1 in every 761 pregnant women, while invasive cervical carcinoma occurs in 1 in 2200 pregnancies.

All pregnant women with squamous cell intraepithelial lesions should undergo colposcopy. The hyperemic, redundant vagina occasionally obscures adequate visualization of the squamous-columnar junction. Although a cervical biopsy is associated with bleeding, a histologic diagnosis is usually necessary unless colposcopic expertise is available. If invasive disease is excluded, the need for further diagnostic or therapeutic intervention is delayed until after delivery. There is little indication for antepartum therapy for squamous cell intraepithelial dysplasia. Although term infants are delivered in 80% of pregnancies after conization and fetal salvage approaches 90%, the physician should be hesitant to perform conization unless an invasive lesion is indicated by cytologic or colposcopic evaluation and immediate therapeutic action is anticipated. Noninvasive lesions can be followed up with a repeat colposcopic evaluation during the third trimester, although the need for this repeat procedure may be questioned if an invasive lesion has been excluded.

If the diagnosis of an invasive lesion is established, therapeutic delays of up to 16 weeks are not associated with an adverse maternal prognosis with a low-volume, early-stage disease. Consideration of surgical versus radiation therapy is related to the extent of disease and actually differs little from the evaluation of a nonpregnant woman. There appears to be little benefit in a pretreatment induced abortion before radiation therapy. While serum tumor markers may aid in the evaluation and follow-up for squamous cancers, their use during pregnancy remains to be defined.

TRAUMA IN PREGNANCY

Trauma complicates approximately 1 in 12 pregnancies. It is the leading cause of death in women of reproductive age and accounts for 20% of nonobstetric maternal deaths. The most common cause of fetal death in major trauma is death of the mother, so stabilization of the mother takes immediate precedence over fetal welfare. Rapid assessment of maternal status includes assessing the level of consciousness, respiratory status, and cardiovascular status while the patient is placed in a left lateral tilt to displace the uterus off of the vena cava. Two or more large-bore intravenous lines, a Foley catheter, and oxygen should be given. An oxygen saturation of greater than 90% is necessary, and a pulse oximeter is usually preferable to arterial blood gases. The fetus should be monitored early in trauma assessment, because uterine hypoperfusion precedes maternal shock. However, no intervention for fetal indications should be considered if the mother is hemodynamically unstable.

Blood abdominal trauma is perhaps the most common type of trauma during pregnancy. It involves falls, automobile accidents, or spousal abuse. Abruptio placentae occurs early if it happens. In one study, no abruptions occurred when fewer than one contraction occurred every 10 minutes during a 4-hour period, while abruptions occurred in 20% of cases in which contractions occurred more often than every 10 minutes in the same period. The latest recommendation from the American College of Obstetricians and Gynecologists (ACOG) Committee on Maternal-Fetal Medicine is to monitor for 2–6 hours if no contractions, bleeding, or uterine tenderness are observed. Ultrasound scanning allows direct visualization of the fetal heart and rapid determination of gestational age. A normal-appearing placenta on ultrasound does not exclude a placental abruption.

A detailed secondary survey of the patient should be done to search for additional signs of trauma such as lacerations or contusions. A pelvic examination may help to diagnose pelvic bony fractures. Resuscitation and monitoring of the patient should not be interrupted if the patient is taken to radiology. Tetanus toxoid should be given if not current (within 10 years) or if the status of the vaccination is unknown. Peritoneal lavage (1 liter warm lactated Ringer's solution) has shown to be a safe and sensitive method of diagnosing intraabdominal hemorrhage in the presence of signs suggestive of intraperitoneal hemorrhage, altered sensorium, unexplained shock, major thoracic injuries, or multiple orthopaedic injuries. If the lavage is positive (grossly bloody fluid, red blood cell count greater than 100,000 cells/mm^3, white blood cell count greater than 175 cells/mm^3, amylase level greater than 175 units/dL) then a laparotomy is required. If the lavage is negative (red blood count less than 50,000 cells/mm^3, white blood count less than 100 cells/mm^3, amylase less than 75 units/dL), then the patient may merely be observed. If lavage results are intermediate, a repeat lavage or a laparotomy should be considered.

Penetrating abdominal trauma most commonly involves gunshot wounds or stab wounds. A bullet with sufficient energy can cause a "cone-shaped" injury proportional to the diameter of the bullet. A bullet that penetrates the uterus usually stays there if it is a low-powered bullet such as those from many handguns or small caliber rimfire rifles. Fetal injury or death occurs in two-thirds of cases in which the uterus is penetrated. A stab injury is limited to the width and breadth of penetration of the penetrating object. If it can be clearly shown that there is no penetration of the peritoneal cavity or retroperitoneal space, cleansing and closure of the wound may be all that is necessary. An upper abdominal injury usually penetrates multiple loops of bowel which have been displaced upward by the uterus. Hepatic or splenic injury is more common than in nonpregnant women.

Head trauma is seen with assaults or automobile accidents. In the presence of a minor injury, there is no history of severe impact, loss of consciousness, or skull fracture. In such cases, treatment for minor lacerations or abrasions is sufficient. Neurologic checks should be done every two hours to evaluate the level of consciousness and reactivity of the pupils. If severe injury is suspected, the first step after stabilization is to notify the neurosurgery service.

Many trauma cases can be prevented. A patient should be counseled that lap-shoulder restraints offer better protection to the fetus than lap restraints alone. The extreme flexion of the body that occurs with a lap seat belt in a sudden deceleration increases the risk of placental abruption. Identification of patients at risk for spousal abuse may prevent a case of maternal trauma by offering counseling, shelters, or legal intervention. Spousal abuse should be suspected when there is a pattern of injuries hidden by clothing or if injuries about the face and head are associated with "defense" injuries of varying ages on the forearms or hands.

ADNEXAL MASS

Current practice requires exploration and histologic evaluation of any adnexal mass (particularly with a complex ultrasound evaluation) greater than 5 cm if it persists into the second trimester. The risk of ovarian malignancy in this circumstance ranges from 2.2% to 8%. The most common coexisting adnexal abnormality includes benign cystic teratomas and mucinous cystadenomas or serous cystadenomas. Rapid histologic diagnosis is imperative.

Conservative surgery should be considered for an apparent stage I ovarian malignancy or tumors of borderline malignant potential when preservation of fertility is of prime concern. At a minimum, peritoneal cytologic tests and careful visual examination and palpation of the mesenteric surfaces, pelvic gutters, subdiaphragmatic spaces, omentum, and retroperitoneal areas should be performed and recorded. If any doubt exists intraoperatively, a lesser procedure should be performed, with the realization that a second, more definitive procedure may be necessary.

RH ISOIMMUNIZATION

In the last two decades the widespread use of anti-D immune globulin (RhoGAM) has diminished remarkably the incidence of Rh isoimmunization. It remains a potentially serious complication of pregnancy, and a successful perinatal outcome requires careful planning during the antepartum, intrapartum, and neonatal periods. Along with a knowledge of the maternal serum antibody titer to the specific erythrocyte antigen, the gestational age and the father's blood type and Rh antigen status must be determined. There is no need for further evaluation if the father is known to be negative for that particular antigen. Most cases involve sensitization (formation of IgG antibodies) to the D, C, d, c, E and Kell blood groups. Hemolytic disease associated with certain less common and atypical antigens may be variable in severity (Table 3.1).

The level of maternal antibody titer is usually predictive of the severity of fetal disease in the first sensitized pregnancy. The titer is of less prognostic value in subsequent pregnancies. In utero transfusion or preterm delivery are becoming less common and should not be performed on the basis of an antibody titer alone. Instead, an amniotic fluid delta OD_{450} analysis is more predictive of fetal status and a fetal hematocrit determined by cordocentesis (percutaneous umbilical blood sampling) is even more so. A cordocentesis allows for direct evaluation of fetal hematologic status and eliminates certain cases with falsely elevated delta OD_{450} results caused by old blood or meconium in the amniotic fluid.

Delivery should be planned carefully. Standard means of fetal surveillance testing are recommended. Particular attention

Table 3.1
Examples of Antibodies Causing Hemolytic Disease

Blood Group	Antigens	Severity of Hemolytic Disease
Rh	c, C, E	Mild to severe
	C, e	Mild to moderate
Lewis	Le	Not a proven cause
I	I	Not a proven cause
Kell	K, k	Mild to severe
Duffy	Fy^a	Mild to severe
	Fy^b	Not a proven cause
Kidd	Jk^a, Jk^b	Mild to severe
MNSs	M, S, s	Mild to severe
	N	Mild
Lutheran	Lu^a, Lu^b	Mild
Diego	Di^a, Di^b	Mild to severe
Xg	Xg^a	Mild
P	P, P$_1$, p^k, (Tj^a)	Mild to severe

should be placed on any decrease in fetal activity. Lung maturation is neither delayed nor accelerated in the isoimmunized pregnancy. Communication with blood bank and neonatal personnel is required to support the severely ill premature fetus and to prevent long-term neonatal complications.

Management of Atypical Antibody Screen

If the patient's antibody titer is below the "critical titer" established by that particular laboratory (usually 1:16 or less), it should be repeated at 20 weeks and then monthly. Provided that the titer remains below this critical level, no intervention is necessary, and delivery at term can be anticipated.

An eligible patient with an antibody titer above the critical titer should have an amniocentesis or cordocentesis performed beyond 22 weeks. Real-time ultrasonography is a necessary adjunct for evaluating fetal status. Signs of congestive heart failure would include placental thickening (more than 5 cm), enlarged liver, and diminished body motion. Ultrasonography is also helpful in guiding a 22-gauge needle for either the amniocentesis or the cordocentesis.

In more severely affected patients, many experts currently

recommend that a cordocentesis be used rather than an amniocentesis in the second trimester to assess the fetus. This is particularly important if the father is heterozygotic for the offending
antigen, since determination that the fetus is negative for that
antigen may obviate further invasive evaluation. The fetal hematocrit, antigen status, and direct Coombs' test result can be determined at the time of the initial blood sampling. Transfusion is
indicated at that time if the hematocrit is less than 30%. If the
hematocrit is greater than 30% and the relevant antigen is found
to be present in the fetal blood, the timing of future diagnostic
procedures depends on the patient's history, serial ultrasound
findings, and hematocrit at the time of last sample.

If an amniocentesis is performed, results of the delta OD_{450}
(indirectly measuring bilirubin concentration from hemolysis)
are plotted on the Liley curve shown in Figure 3.2.

The management outlined in Figure 3.3 is dependent on
whether the delta OD_{450} value remains within zone 1, 2, or 3 on
the Liley curve. Fortunately the need for in utero transfusion is
rare. Before delivery of a severely affected infant, O-negative
blood or blood compatible with the mother's should be available
for possible exchange transfusion by the pediatricians. A direct
Coombs' test, hemoglobin, serum bilirubin, and blood type will
need to be determined on the newborn infant.

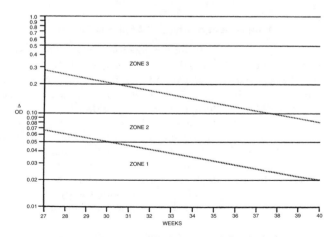

Figure 3.2.   Liley curve (27–40 weeks' gestation).

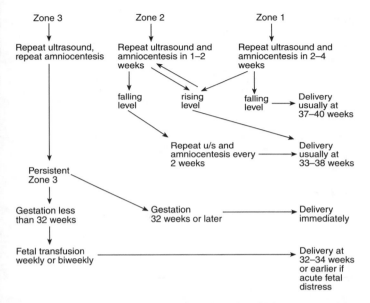

Figure 3.3. Evaluation after OD_{450} result of amniotic fluid at 22–26 weeks.

PRETERM LABOR

Approximately 7–10% of pregnant patients in the United States deliver prematurely. These premature infants account for 75% of all perinatal mortality. While the cause of preterm labor is unknown in more than 50% of cases, it is important for the obstetrician to be aware of conditions associated with premature labor (Table 3.2). A 20–50% recurrence risk is associated with prior premature labor or delivery.

Most current preterm-birth prevention programs have as an initial goal the detection of early signs and symptoms of preterm labor, so that more patients may be candidates for tocolytic therapy and the potential efficacy of tocolysis can be improved. Unfortunately, the benefit of various preterm prevention programs is unclear. There are no biochemical tests currently proven to predict preterm labor, although results are promising in the use of positive cervicovaginal fetal fibronectin in preterm labor patients with intact membranes. For selected very-high-risk patients, such as those with multiple gestations or previous recur-

Table 3.2
Conditions Associated with the Onset of Premature Labor

Maternal	*Uterine*
Acute severe systemic illness	Polyhydramnios
Chronic severe systemic illness	Foreign body (IUD)
Pyelonephritis, urinary tract infection	Trauma, surgical manipulation
Chronic hypertension	Cervical incompetence
Hyperthyroidism	Uterine anomalies
Hyperadrenalism	Amniocentesis
Previous history of premature labor	Chorioamnionitis
Fever or disseminated infection	Prior cone biopsy
Inadequate nutrition	Diethylstilbestrol exposure
Maternal age under 18 or over 35	
Excess smoking	*Fetoplacental*
Severe dehydration	Fetal death
Abdominal trauma	Placenta previa
	Abruptio placentae
	Fetal anomalies
	Multifetal gestation
	Ruptured membranes
	Fetal growth retardation

rent preterm labor and deliveries, some physicians elect to advise bed rest or at least increased rest, cessation of coitus, and pharmacologic treatment, but the efficacy of these approaches is not proven.

While tocolytic drugs have been designed to decrease the incidence of side effects, these medications may cause alterations in maternal metabolism. To prevent serious complications, the obstetrician must be aware of the proper selection criteria and safeguards required with the use of these agents.

Before beginning drug therapy to inhibit uterine contractions, true labor must be accurately diagnosed and any accompanying obstetric or medical disorders should be sought. The diagnosis of preterm labor is difficult. Proposed criteria for selecting patients for tocolytic therapy are outlined below, and recommended pretherapy screening tests are listed in Table 3.3.

(*a*) Clinical diagnosis
- Gestational age between 20 and 36 weeks
- Estimated fetal weight less than 2500 g (especially 1500 g or less)

Table 3.3
Tests before Beginning Tocolytic Therapy

Cervical cultures for gonorrhea, Group B beta-hemolytic streptococci, and chlamydia

Clean catch midstream or catheterized urine specimen for urinalysis and culture

Confirmation of the presence or absence of ruptured membranes

Ultrasound examination for biparietal diameter/abdominal circumference/ femur length, fetal presentation, twins, amniotic fluid volume, fetal anomaly, abnormal uterine contour, placental location, estimated fetal weight, site for possible amniocentesis

Baseline fetal heart rate tracing

Complete blood count with differential

Serum electrolytes

Electrocardiogram (if maternal cardiac disease)

- Uterine contractions every 10 minutes or less, lasting 30 seconds or more, for at least a 30-minute period
- Cervical dilation of 4 cm or less

(b) No remarkable antepartum complication or contraindication (Table 3.4)

No group of tocolytic drugs has been definitely shown to be helpful in prolonging gestation. Side effects from these drugs in the mother and fetus must be recognized, and patient education is necessary. Careful monitoring of the fetal heart rate (FHR) and uterine activity is paramount. When an undesired effect from a specific drug is manifested, or when intravenous therapy is required for more than 48 hours, the drug may be continued, discontinued, reduced in dosage, or a second drug used in combination. These decisions should be made by the clinician on the basis of an evaluation of the seriousness of the side effects, the probability of premature delivery, and the potential consequences of premature delivery at that gestational age.

Drug Therapy

Magnesium Sulfate

Magnesium sulfate is frequently used as the first-line drug in inhibiting premature uterine contractions, using doses which are approximately twice those used for seizure prophylaxis in preeclamptic patients. This drug may also be used in combination with

Table 3.4
Contraindications to Tocolytic Therapy

Absolute	
Fetal death	Severe cardiac disease
Fetal congenital abnormality incompatible with life	Severe preeclampsia
	Active vaginal bleeding
Life-threatening maternal illness	Unexplained uterine bleeding
	Intraamniotic infection

Relative	
Documented fetal pulmonary maturity	Placenta previa with minimal bleeding
Diabetes (beta-agonists)	
Mild cardiac disease	Abruptio placentae (suspected)
Pulmonary disease	Preterm ruptured membranes
Hypertension	Vascular headaches

β-adrenergic agents, so that uterine contractions may be inhibited more effectively, or when unwanted side effects from β-adrenergic therapy require small doses to be administered.

A 40-g dose of magnesium sulfate is mixed in 1 liter of 5% dextrose in water or 0.45% normal saline. The loading dose is usually 4–6 g in 100 mL over 20 minutes, followed by maintenance therapy of 2–4 g/hour intravenously. Signs of hypermagnesemia (hyporeflexia, depressed respiratory rate) should be sought periodically. After successful intravenous therapy, oral beta-agonists may be initiated. Oral magnesium gluconate in a dose of 1 mg every 4 hours may be employed if there is any contraindication, failure, or intolerable side effects for oral beta-agonist therapy.

Respiratory depression in the neonate is very uncommon from in utero magnesium exposure but can occur in low-birth-weight infants with decreased urine output.

β$_2$-Agonists

Ritodrine hydrochloride remains the only tocolytic drug approved by the Food and Drug Administration (FDA), while terbutaline is the most commonly prescribed medication. These are selective β$_2$-receptor agonists which act primarily by inhibiting smooth muscle uterine contractions. β$_2$ receptors may also be found in the bronchioles and blood vessels, and their stimulation results in bronchial relaxation and hypotension. Both drugs are also weak β_1-receptor agonists, and tachycardia is common.

An intravenous solution of ritodrine in 5% dextrose in water (150 mg/500 mL) is the standard concentration of drug in intravenous fluids. A loading dose is unnecessary and maintenance therapy consists of an initial infusion of 100 µg/minute (20 mL/hour) with upward dose adjustments in 50 µg/minute increments to a maximum level of 350 µg/minute (70 mL/hour). Maintenance therapy is titrated according to contraction frequency and may be continued for several days if necessary. It is usually continued for 12 hours after the arrest of labor before the patient is begun on oral therapy.

The most frequent side effects with intravenous ritodrine are cardiovascular. The maternal heart rate may increase up to 40 beats/minute above the baseline, and the pulse pressure may widen up to 20 mm Hg as the intravenous dose is increased. If this results in troublesome symptoms, relief can often be obtained by reducing the dose for a short period of time. It can usually be increased again later without recurrence of symptoms. Pulmonary edema has been reported in patients who are also receiving glucocorticoids or excessive intravenous fluids. Hypotonic solutions or 5% dextrose in water should be used. Transient metabolic problems may include hyperglycemia, hyperinsulinemia, lipemia, ketonemia, hyperlactacidemia, and hypokalemia. Unpleasant side effects may include tremor (10–15%), restlessness (20%), and palpitations (33%).

Although not approved by the FDA for this indication, terbutaline is another beta-agonist which has been used in place of ritodrine in many highly respected institutions. Their mechanisms of action and side effects are similar. While some investigators have claimed greater efficacy and fewer complications in comparison to oral ritodrine, their observations are questioned by other authorities due to lack of information regarding equipotent dosage. The major advantage of terbutaline is its considerably lower cost. A standard subcutaneous dose is 250 µg, while the oral dosage is approximately 5 mg every 4 hours.

Oral therapy is usually started an hour before discontinuing the intravenous regimen and is begun once uterine contractions are barely palpable. Initial oral therapy consists of either ritodrine 10 mg every 2 hours, or terbutaline 5 mg every 2 hours. The dose is then titrated to maintain a maternal pulse of 90–100 bpm and the absence of contractions. It usually ranges from 10–20 mg every 2–6 hours for ritodrine and 5 mg every 2–6 hours for terbutaline.

If labor recurs, the patient should be reexamined carefully. The infusion may be restarted if no contraindications to tocolysis are found. The initial ritodrine infusion will inadequately inhibit labor in approximately 50% of patients. These patients are at high risk for subclinical intrauterine infection, and amniocentesis for Gram stain, culture, and sensitivity may be appropriate. The addition of a simultaneous magnesium sulfate infusion, as outlined above, will result in the successful treatment of half of these patients. However, if labor persists or fetal pulmonary maturity has developed, the medications should be discontinued.

Indomethacin

This prostaglandin inhibitor has been shown to successfully arrest premature labor. There is concern that prolonged use may result in a narrowing or closure of the ductus arteriosus and a persistent fetal circulation. Short-term therapy (less than 72 hours) may occasionally be helpful to allow for steroid treatment to enhance fetal pulmonary maturity in patients refractory to other tocolytics. A 25-mg dose may be given orally or rectally every 4–6 hours.

Neonatal Survival Rates

When premature delivery is anticipated, it is necessary to counsel the patient on the chances that the baby will survive in the intensive care nursery and be discharged home. Listed in Table 3.5 are survival percentages according to gestational age and birth weight for inborn infants admitted to our Intensive Care Nursery between 1986 and 1994. It is appropriate for each institution to develop its own survival statistics in order to render sound therapeutic judgments and to counsel patients adequately.

PREMATURE RUPTURE OF MEMBRANES

Premature rupture of the membranes (PROM) is defined as spontaneous rupture of the amniotic membranes occurring at any gestational age before the onset of labor. A latent period usually lasts at least one hour. The incidence of PROM ranges from 4.5 to 7.6% of all pregnancies. Preterm PROM occurs in approximately 1% of pregnancies and clearly represents a more pressing problem for the obstetrician.

Table 3.5
Neonatal Survival Rates at The University of Oklahoma Medical Center According to Gestational Age and Birth Weight (1981–1994)[a]

Gestational Age (weeks)	% Survivors	Birth Weight (g)	% Survivors
24	20	≤500	0
25	25	501–800	22
26	50	801–1000	75
27	75	1001–1250	82
28	83	1251–1500	94
29	94	1501–1750	97
30	95	1751–2500	98
31	95	>2500	99
32	97		
>33	99		

[a] These rates are for singleton infants without life-threatening anomalies.

Diagnosis requires visualization of amniotic fluid leading from the cervical ostium or in the vaginal vault, testing any fluid for a basic pH (nitrazine positivity), and ferning. This should be accomplished during sterile speculum examination. Cervical cultures for Group B beta-streptococci, chlamydia, and gonorrhea (in certain populations) should be obtained, prolapsed cord ruled out, and cervical effacement and dilatation estimated during this initial examination. The subsequent development of infection has been highly correlated with the interval (in hours) from initial digital examination. Therefore, digital examination should be avoided unless the patient is clearly in labor or a decision has been made to effect delivery. Ultrasound examination is useful to document the gestational age, fetal weight, amniotic fluid volume, fetal presentation, presence of twins, and any fetal malformation. If the diagnosis of PROM remains in doubt, the instillation of 35 mL of sterile fluorescein ophthalmologic solution by amniocentesis, followed by inspection of the vagina under black light illumination for the characteristic fluorescent pattern, will usually resolve the issue.

General Measures

The obstetrician is required to balance the relative risks of prematurity and infection. These risks may vary from population to population and at various gestational ages. When possible, local data should also be considered in formulating an institution's management protocols. Discussion with neonatal staff is essential and maternal transfer to a tertiary care center is urged if a septic premature infant is anticipated. However, it is appropriate to remain cognizant of certain general principles.

Dating is often very difficult after the occurrence of PROM. The resultant oligohydramnios may depress fundal height and impair ultrasonic evaluation. Biparietal diameters and abdominal circumferences may be falsely lowered, but femur length measurements are usually relatively reliable.

A nonreassuring fetal status, particularly from cord compression, is much more common than in idiopathic premature labor. This is especially true if the fetus has a precarious lie (breech, back-up transverse). In those patients whose fetuses have achieved a potentially viable gestational age, initial evaluation should include a prolonged period of electronic fetal monitoring. Subsequently, the gravida should be instructed in daily fetal movement charting, since fetal activity is not impaired with PROM. Prolonged nonstress tests or biophysical profiles should be performed at 24–48-hour intervals.

Many cases of preterm PROM, as well as up to one-third of cases of idiopathic preterm birth, may be due to subclinical intraamniotic infection. Indigenous host products (cytokines) secreted in response to infection can also be identified in the amniotic fluid of these pregnancies. These cytokines, including interleukin-1, interleukin-6, interleukin-8, and tumor necrosis factor (cachectin), are secretory products of macrophage activation.

Surveillance is required to detect potential intraamniotic infection. Maternal temperature should be recorded frequently each day. The presence of an elevated white blood count may provide confirmatory evidence of a clinically suspected infection, but it has been demonstrated repeatedly not to offer any enhanced predictive value over clinical signs. Therefore, the expense of daily blood count monitoring does not appear justified. Although not customarily ordered, a C-reactive protein test may provide further laboratory evidence of infection in the presence of an elevated leukocyte count. Amniocentesis for Gram stain, culture, and sensitivity can be accomplished in approximately 50–60% of women with PROM. The presence of bacteria on a Gram stain of unspun amniotic fluid (or a subsequent positive culture) is associated with clinical evidence of maternal or neonatal infection in 50–60% of patients. Other investigators have reported a persistently decreased amniotic fluid volume, nonreactive nonstress test, or abnormal biophysical profile to have equal or better predictive accuracy for infection in this population.

Patients with PROM frequently demonstrate fetal pulmonary maturity at relatively early gestational ages. If free-flowing fluid can be obtained from the vaginal vault, the lecithin/sphingomyelin (L/S) ratio is usually quite similar to that obtained by amniocentesis, and if phosphatidylglycerol is present, it is always present at amniocentesis. When vaginal fluid cannot be obtained, an amniocentesis should be considered if clinically appropriate.

Most randomized studies have shown little or no benefit from the use of intravenous tocolytics in pregnancies complicated by PROM. Although it is controversial, most obstetric authorities do recommend the use of the corticosteroids in this condition for the enhancement of fetal lung maturity.

At Term

Ninety percent of patients with PROM will enter spontaneous labor within 24 hours and present few management problems. Several studies have demonstrated increased perinatal mortality and group B streptococcal infection when the latent period exceeds 24 hours. We follow a policy of beginning to induce or augment labor within this time interval. On the other hand, aggressive attempts to induce gravidas with long and closed cervices (unfavorable Bishop scores) are associated with higher rates of operative delivery. Therefore, expectant management or use of an intravaginal prostaglandin E_2 product is necessary with careful evaluation for infection and an abnormal fetal heart rate (FHR) pattern.

34–37 Weeks

In this group of patients, the risk of neonatal hyaline membrane disease is very low when 16 hours or more have elapsed since the membranes have ruptured. We utilize oxytocin induction in most instances to attempt to accomplish delivery shortly after 24 hours. If the Bishop score is extremely unfavorable, conservative management is acceptable.

24–33 Weeks

The risk of pulmonary immaturity outweighs the risk of infection in this subpopulation. Conservative measures according to the principles outlined above are practiced. The patient should be advised that even with conservative therapy, approximately 50% of patients will begin labor within 24 hours and 75% within 5 days.

Before 24 Weeks

Any patient with well-documented PROM before the 24th gestational week should be informed that the probability of leaving the hospital with a living normal child is poor, perhaps as low as 25%. Many of these children develop pulmonary hypoplasia and/or orthopaedic deformities, die in utero, or deliver at very early gestational ages. Furthermore, surviving infants weighing 750 grams or less are at high risk for developmental or intellectual impairment. The option of pregnancy termination should be discussed eventually. The patient may elect conservative therapy in the hope that the fetus will grow and mature despite the unfavorable odds.

CORTICOSTEROIDS TO ENHANCE FETAL LUNG MATURITY

The use of corticosteroids offers promise to accelerating fetal pulmonary maturity when preterm delivery is probable. According to a recent National Institutes of Health consensus report, most studies involving the use betamethasone or dexamethasone have revealed significant reductions in incidences of respiratory distress, intraventricular hemorrhage, and neonatal deaths when corticosteroids have been given before anticipated delivery, especially between 26 and 34 weeks. Developmental evaluation of treated fetuses who are now school-age children have not revealed any adverse effects with such short-term therapy.

The anticipated delivery of a premature infant requires a prompt and accurate evaluation of fetal pulmonary maturity by amniotic fluid testing if possible. An L/S ratio of less than 2:1 and the absence of phosphatidylglycerol strongly suggest fetal lung immaturity. A trial of corticosteroid therapy may be useful in enhancing fetal lung maturity, especially between the 24th and 34th weeks of gestation.

When fetal lung maturity testing is not readily available (such as during the night, weekends, or holidays), corticosteroid therapy may be administered empirically if the gestational age is 34 weeks or less and impending delivery is anticipated. Good clinical judgment is necessary, realizing that a time lapse must exist between maternal treatment and a fetal response. The underlying antepartum complication should be expected to remain stabilized; otherwise, delivery should take place regardless of any corticosteroid therapy.

General Considerations

Corticosteroid treatment does appear to be helpful for pregnancies complicated by preterm rupture of the membranes. Most investigators conclude that there is no association between maternal and neonatal infection with the use of short-term corticosteroid therapy. Corticosteroids may increase the white blood count (primarily neutrophils), so clinical criteria and appropriate cultures are especially important to screen for infection.

Hypertension is not exacerbated, and fetal mortality is not increased, with steroid therapy alone. Nevertheless, pregnancy intervention is necessary during such therapy when hypertension worsens.

Corticosteroids may accentuate glucose intolerance because of the increased insulin requirements occurring from the inhibition of glucose utilization, mobilization of amino acids for conversion to glucose and glycogen, and induction of liver enzymes for gluconeogenesis. Steroid therapy is therefore not recommended when preterm delivery of the poorly controlled diabetic is anticipated.

Patients whose pregnancy is complicated by a multifetal gestation are prescribed the same dose as is given for singleton pregnancies. However, the extent of enhancement of fetal lung maturity is less predictable.

Antenatally administered corticosteroids are as helpful in promoting fetal lung maturity in female as in male fetuses. Furthermore, the benefit of corticosteroids is not influenced by race.

Contraindications to Corticosteroid Therapy

Absolute contraindications to corticosteroid therapy are uncommon. Maternal contraindications include febrile illness, tuberculosis, active herpes, or other infections. Corticosteroid therapy is also contraindicated in the presence of intraamniotic infection, imminent delivery, a mature fetal lung test result, or an inability to monitor the fetus.

Steroids may be given with caution in those pregnancies complicated by borderline hypertension, well-controlled diabetes mellitus, hyperthyroidism, placental insufficiency, minimal uterine bleeding, preterm labor adequately treated with tocolytic drugs, or preterm ruptured membranes. Further research is needed to evaluate the risks and benefits of using corticosteroids in women with PROM, and the safety of repeat dosings.

Drug Choice and Dose Regimen

Drugs to enhance fetal lung maturation include betamethasone (12 mg intramuscularly every 12–24 hours for 2 doses) or dexamethasone (4 mg intramuscularly every 8 hours for 6 doses). Each rapidly crosses the placenta, and neither has been clearly shown to offer advantages over the other in promoting fetal lung maturity. Betamethasone is the drug used most commonly because only two dosings are necessary.

The shortest period for the drug to be effective is believed to be 24 hours after the final dose. If 7 or more days have elapsed after completing the drug therapy, a repeat of amniotic fluid testing (with an L/S ratio less than 2 and negative phosphatidylglycerol) may be preferred before prescribing another course of therapy.

MULTIFETAL GESTATION

Although a twin gestation is reportedly found in 1 in 80 pregnancies, the actual incidence is higher, as more multifetal gestations which may abort are diagnosed by ultrasonography in early gestation. Early diagnosis and careful management are recommended for optimal care, since virtually every medical and obstetric complication associated with pregnancy is more common in a multifetal gestation.

Antepartum Management

A high index of suspicion is necessary for early diagnosis. Clues would include the following: older multigravida, maternal family history of dizygotic twins, fertility pills (clomiphene: 6% twinning, Pergonal: 25% twinning), and uterine size greater than menstrual dates (as early as the end of the first trimester). Proper care requires frequent clinic visits (to check cervix, blood pressure, blood count, diabetes screen, etc.), serial ultrasound examinations (approximately every 3–6 weeks), and proper nutrition (folate and iron supplementation; 300 additional calories per day; avoidance of excess salt).

A cervical cerclage for twinning alone is not justified. Guidelines for tocolytic drugs and corticosteroid therapy for the singleton fetus are applicable to the multifetal gestation. Half of twins are born before 34 weeks, so frequent cervical examinations, additional daily rest periods, and perhaps home uterine activity monitoring are justified to reduce the chance of advanced premature labor.

Supportive care and patient education are necessary. Discussions should include pain relief during labor, potential complications before or during labor, and care of the infants after delivery. The infants' doctor should be aware of the pregnancy and informed after hospital admission.

In the event of a preterm fetal demise, immediate delivery is not advisable unless late in gestation. A twin-twin transfusion should be suspected, and delivery should be considered if 28 weeks or beyond. Maternal serum fibrinogen levels should be drawn weekly to search for any coagulopathy.

Fluid from both sacs should be sampled when performing an amniocentesis for genetic testing. Amniotic fluid retrieved from only one gestational sac is usually all that is necessary for fetal lung maturity testing. The sac containing the "healthier" of the two fetuses should be sampled. Criteria for interpreting fetal lung tests is the same as for singleton pregnancies.

The performance and interpretation of many fetal surveillance techniques are more limited with multifetal gestations. As a general rule, if the mother is healthy and fetal growths are appropriate, no further testing is necessary. The same principles of nonstress testing, biophysical profile assessment, and fetal movement charting for the singleton fetus apply for the multifetal gestation. Periodic ultrasound examination is the most useful means for assessing fetal growth and well-being. Ultrasonography is also useful in searching for placenta location, conjoined twins, stuck twin syndrome, monoamniotic twins with cord entanglement, and any space-occupying anomalies.

Intrapartum Management

The anesthesia, neonatal, and obstetric staff should be notified when the patient is admitted to the labor floor. The patient's blood should be typed and cross-matched for possible transfusion. If time permits, a bedside real-time ultrasound examination should be performed to search for two separate sacs, any major anomaly (including conjoined twins), fetal presentations, fetal growth disparity, and placental localization, especially if a cesarean section is planned. Listed below are guidelines for delivery.

Cesarean Section

1. Suggested indications:
   - Twin A: breech
   - Nonreassuring fetal status
   - Prolapsed cord
   - Three or more fetuses
   - Delivery before 33 weeks or estimated fetal weights 1500 g or less
   - Delivery of twin B if abnormal FHR pattern, prolapsed cord, constricted uterine ring (despite halothane), persistent abnormal presentation, or twin B larger with failure to descend adequately
2. Prophylactic antibiotics are indicated
3. Vertical skin and uterine incisions may be necessary for adequate space
4. Epidural anesthesia preferable with uterus displaced off of inferior vena cava

Vaginal Delivery

1. Labor on left side
2. Supplemental oxygen
3. Early amniotomy
4. Electronic monitoring of FHR and uterine contractions
   a. Fetal heart rate:
      internal electrode–twin A
      external transducer–twin B
   b. Uterine contractions: internal uterine catheter connected in series to both monitors
5. If uterine inertia exists, oxytocin may be used cautiously
6. Two obstetricians (including staff) in attendance at delivery
7. Large episiotomy
8. Twin A delivered in the usual manner as a singleton

9. No absolute time for delivery of second twin as long as monitoring fetal heart rate and watching for any excess hemorrhage (possible abruption). Ultrasonic visualization of the second twin may be performed in the delivery room to locate the fetal heart rate, confirm fetal presentation, assist with an external version, and watch the examiner's hand during any extraction procedure.

10. May need halothane to relax uterus to guide the second twin into the pelvis and for partial breech extraction

11. If the second twin is breech, an external version may be accomplished after vaginal delivery of the first twin and before rupturing the second sac

BLEEDING IN SECOND HALF OF PREGNANCY

The most common causes of third trimester bleeding include labor, placental abruption, or placenta previa. Vaginal bleeding at any time during pregnancy may result from cervical erosion, polyps and carcinoma, and trauma. A vasa previa or uterine rupture should also be considered. With the exception of labor or a blood-mucus "show," these conditions are potentially life-threatening to the mother and fetus and frequently result in premature delivery. Successful management requires anticipation of potential complications, intervention to reverse complications, and competent neonatal assistance.

Initial Evaluation

A thorough history is necessary to determine the amount and character of the bleeding, any pain, prior bleeding, trauma, any uterine anomaly, and activity of the fetus. Evaluation of the patient requires careful monitoring of her vital signs. The uterus should be examined for tone, tenderness, and contractions. A digital pelvic examination should be performed only after ultrasonography has ruled out placenta previa. Fetal heart activity should also be sought to rule out the possibility of a demise.

Initial laboratory tests should include a Kleihauer-Betke test, urinalysis, and coagulation studies (PT, PTT, platelet count, fibrinogen, fibrin split products). Any pooled vaginal blood should be obtained to test for fetal blood. The observation of clot formation is often as valuable as more complex coagulation studies. An APT test is performed by many obstetricians by mixing any vaginal blood with an equal part of 0.25% sodium hydroxide. The blood will turn to a light brown color if it is maternal in origin; otherwise, it is of fetal origin.

Depending on the extent of hemorrhage, an infusion of 5% glucose in lactated Ringer's solution is indicated using an 18-gauge or greater catheter. Continuous external FHR monitoring is required to search for any fetal tachycardia, loss of beat-to-beat variability, or bradycardia. Two to four units of blood should be typed and cross-matched.

Ultrasonography should be performed as soon as possible, along with reviewing any prior reports. The diagnosis of a placenta previa may be made using ultrasonography. Elevating the presenting fetal part transabdominally may permit a better view of the placenta in the lower pelvis. A placental abruption may appear as a sonolucent retroplacental mass or an elevation of the membranes which may expand or contract over time depending on the extent of hemorrhage. Often the examination is of no value if hemorrhage has occurred externally, since the sonolucent area is smaller in size and the retroplacental blood is homogeneous with the placenta. During ultrasonic examination, it is also possible to search for fetal malformations, multifetal gestation, and fetal presentation.

Depending on the circumstances, an amniocentesis should be considered for fetal lung maturity testing. Blood within the amniotic fluid suggests the diagnosis of an abruption, and renders the L/S ratio less reliable. However, the L/S ratio of blood is approximately 1.8:1.0, and levels above this value are usually reliable. Testing for phosphatidylglycerol (PG) in addition to the L/S ratio is often necessary.

Tocolytic agents should be used with much caution. The diagnosis should be fairly certain, fetal distress should not be evident, and vaginal bleeding should not be sufficient to cause maternal hypotension.

If the pregnancy is not near term and there is no further bleeding while in the hospital, the patient may be discharged eventually with proper precautions. Ideally, she should usually be within a 30-minute drive with transportation readily available. The patient should be instructed on proper nutrition and discontinue any smoking. Physical activities are to be restricted, and douching and sexual intercourse are contraindicated. She should be seen weekly on an outpatient basis, and a hematocrit test may be performed periodically. The telephone number of the clinic and labor hall should be given to the patient.

Placenta Previa

Factors associated with a placenta previa include multiparity, multifetal gestation, prior cesarean deliveries, uterine contour abnormalities, and induced abortion.

"Silent" placenta previas are diagnosed early in gestation with more frequent ordering of ultrasound examinations. Up to half of all placentas are either low-lying or cover the cervical ostium in the second trimester, but only 2–3% of all placentas remain within the lower uterine segment at term. This occurs most frequently in those patients whose placentas are central or completely cover the internal cervical ostium in the second trimester.

Delivery by cesarean section is generally recommended if a placenta previa is apparent in a patient at 38 weeks or greater (or earlier with evidence of fetal lung maturity). A vaginal delivery with a very marginal placenta is possible, but requires provisions for a cesarean section, cautious pelvic examination, and very close fetal and uterine monitoring.

In the absence of life-threatening hemorrhage, approximately half of patients with a placenta previa remote from term may be treated with conservative therapy. Blood should be replaced and fetal-maternal monitoring initiated as outlined above. The patient usually requires hospitalization for 5 days or more. If bleeding persists, as evidenced by continuous spotting on the perineal pad, she should remain in the hospital with close fetal monitoring. If bleeding subsides, the patient may ambulate gradually. She may be discharged from the hospital once bleeding subsides if there is no evidence of fetal distress, especially if this is her first episode of bleeding.

More specific criteria for outpatient management of a pregnancy with a placenta previa include: (*a*) no active bleeding, (*b*) no severe anemia (hematocrit less than 30%), (*c*) premature fetus, (*d*) patient lives within 30 minutes of hospital, (*e*) patient and relatives understand condition, and (*f*) there is a telephone at home and reliable transportation is available. Precautions concerning proper nutrition and restrictions in physical activity would apply. The patient should be instructed on charting fetal movement and notifying her physician at once if there is any further bleeding, premature labor, fetal inactivity, or fever. While this management protocol has yielded excellent results on our services, other investigators have suggested that gestation is prolonged with continuous hospitalization until near term.

An ultrasound examination is useful for localizing the placenta before a cesarean section. If surgery is necessary, a high transverse or a vertical uterine incision is recommended if the placenta previa sweeps anteriorly. Occasionally, a placenta previa is associated with a placenta invading into the uterus (accreta or percreta), and cesarean hysterectomy may be necessary to control bleeding. It is important to discuss this possibility with the patient when obtaining informed consent for cesarean section.

Placental Abruption

A clinically evident placental abruption occurs in approximately 0.5–1% of pregnancies. It is most commonly associated with conditions leading to chronic uteroplacental insufficiency such as hypertension, smoking, trauma, or cocaine use. It is also found commonly associated with a marginal previa. An abruption severe enough to cause a fetal demise occurs in 1/500 pregnancies. This diagnosis is usually one of exclusion if a placenta previa is not visualized on ultrasound examination. Fetal monitoring is desirable using nonstress tests, biophysical profiles, and fetal movement charting, although the true value of these tests for this acute disorder is limited.

If bleeding is minimal, the preterm pregnancy may be managed expectantly. However, delivery should be considered if the bleeding continues or there is evidence of fetal lung maturity. Liberal use of cesarean section is indicated especially when there is any suggestion of fetal compromise or of hemorrhage severe enough to cause fetal or maternal death. However, approximately half of pregnancies with placental abruption may be managed successfully with vaginal delivery.

An attempt at vaginal delivery is possible, but prolonged labor should be avoided. Prompt and adequate replacement of maternal blood loss is paramount, regardless of the time interval to delivery. An amniotomy is recommended to search for blood in the amniotic fluid, to facilitate labor, and to decrease the risk of thromboplastin release into the maternal circulation. The use of forceps to shorten the second stage of labor is acceptable, unless the risk of trauma is too great a concern. Examination of the pla-

centa is useful, although not always diagnostic, and the pathologist should be notified of the expected diagnosis.

A placental abruption is likely to recur in one-tenth to one-
fourth of subsequent pregnancies. The actual risk is dependent
on associated medical or obstetric complications.

Hemorrhagic Shock

Hemorrhagic shock may follow excessive bleeding from a placenta previa or placental abruption, ischemic necrosis to distant
organs (especially the anterior pituitary and the kidneys), or may
result from the delayed diagnosis and inadequate replacement of
lost blood.

When hemorrhagic shock is suspected, the mother and fetus
should be monitored carefully and delivered promptly. The
mother's vital signs should be monitored and recorded on a flow
sheet. Urine output should be maintained at 25 mL/hour or
greater. A central line may be used with central venous pressure
maintained in the range of 8–15 cm of water. If left ventricular
function is considered abnormal, pulmonary artery pressures may
be determined using a Swan-Ganz catheter (see Chapter 10). Pulmonary artery pressure should be maintained below 18 mm Hg.

Replacement of blood requires the infusion of packed erythrocytes and fresh frozen plasma (all factors except platelets),
in addition to the rapid administration of a 5% glucose and normal saline or lactated Ringer's solution (see Chapter 10). A
plasma expander such as albumin may also be administered to
increase the intravascular volume. Serum electrolytes, calcium,
and arterial blood gases should be determined when fluid, electrolyte, and acid/base imbalances are strongly suspected.

Postpartum Care

Most pregnant patients with third trimester bleeding will do sat-
isfactorily after delivery. Any coagulation difficulties usually correct themselves within a short period. Incisions should be inspected periodically for hematoma formation or infection. Careful
monitoring of the fluid intake and output is necessary to avoid
hypovolemia or hypervolemia. The patient's blood count, electrolyte levels, and urine volume should be monitored, and any
imbalances corrected. Infections of the genital tract are more
common in patients who have had profuse intrapartum vaginal

bleeding. If prophylactic antibiotics have not been started, the patient should be monitored carefully for any endometritis.

POSTDATES

Between 2 and 11% of all pregnancies will remain undelivered for 2 weeks or more beyond the estimated date of confinement. Approximately 40% will have inaccurate dates. This complication of pregnancy represents one of the most frequent abnormalities in routine obstetric care and is a common indication for fetal well-being testing and induction of labor. The placenta is thought to degenerate as gestation advances beyond the 37th week, and the amount of amniotic fluid decreases from 750 mL at 37 weeks to 250 mL at 42 weeks. Between 12 and 43% (approximately 20% overall) of patients with postdate pregnancies deliver infants with classic findings of dysmaturity or postmaturity (long, lean bodies with desquamation of the skin).

With accurate gestational dating and the pregnancy now 2 weeks beyond the estimated date of confinement, a search for other complications and an examination of the cervix are indicated. If there is any other complication (such as hypertension) or if the cervix is "ripe," intervention is recommended by "prophylactic" induction of labor if the fetus is in a cephalic presentation. If accurate dating is not possible, the patient may be managed conservatively with semiweekly clinical visits and fetal biophysical assessments. The clinician should record the dilation of the cervix, fundal height, maternal weight, presence or absence of hypertension, and estimated fetal weight. Half of postdate patients will be expected to go into labor and delivery by 42⅔ weeks, while 90% will deliver by 43 weeks.

Fetal assessment tests at or beyond 41 weeks' gestation should include fetal movement charting daily and a semiweekly modified biophysical profile (FHR testing with a search for oligohydramnios). The contraction stress test is used at many institutions as the initial antepartum FHR test at 42 weeks and is recommended if undelivered by the 43rd week. There is currently no role for umbilical artery Doppler flow studies.

We offer our patients the option of receiving a topical dose of prostaglandin E_2 gel when the cervix is unripe (Bishop score 4 or less), assuming that there is no contraindication to labor. Once easily palpable, the amniotic membranes should be ruptured to permit internal monitoring of the FHR and uterine activity. Internal uterine pressure catheters also permit the amnioinfusion of 1000 mL normal saline in the presence of variable decelerations or early-onset meconium.

There is approximately a 20% chance of a primary cesarean section or need for operative vaginal delivery in postdate patients. This would be explained by the increased incidence of cephalopelvic disproportion and fetal distress. Approximately 25% of postdate pregnancies will have a macrosomic fetus (more than 4000 g). Between 2.5 and 10% of postdate pregnancies will carry a fetus weighing 4500 g or more. Any evidence of an abnormal FHR pattern (usually from umbilical cord compression) requires observation, fetal vibroacoustic stimulation, fetal scalp stimulation or scalp blood sampling, or prompt delivery. A labor protraction disorder would involve less than 1 cm/hour dilation or less than 1 cm/hour descent; an arrest of labor would involve no cervical dilation for 2 or more hours or a failure of descent for more than 1 hour.

Meconium is present in 25–30% of postdate cases (compared to 10–15% at term) and is often thick. Continuous suction should be undertaken to clear the upper airways (at and above the larynx) immediately after delivery of the infant's head. After delivery of the remainder of the body, the upper airway, including the vocal cords, is frequently inspected and suctioned for the presence of any retained meconium. The value of this practice remains a source of debate. Any infant with physical findings of postmaturity requires close observation, since birth asphyxia, hypoglycemia, and hypocalcemia often require admission to the intensive care nursery.

Suggested Readings

American College of Obstetricians and Gynecologists. Diagnosis and management of postterm pregnancy. ACOG Technical Bulletin 130. Washington, DC: ACOG, 1989.

Baltzer J, Regenbrecht ME, Kopcke W, Zander J. Carcinoma of the cervix and pregnancy. Int J Gynaecol Obstet 1990;31:317–323.

Blickstein I. The twin-twin transfusion syndrome. Obstet Gynecol 1990; 76:714–722.

Boyer KM, Gadzala CA, Kelly PD, Gotoff SP. Selective intrapartum chemoprophylaxis of neonatal group B streptococcal early-onset disease, III: interruption of mother-to-infant transmission. J Infect Dis 1983; 148:810–816.

Cox SM, Williams ML, Leveno KJ. The natural history of preterm ruptured membranes: what to expect of expectant management. Obstet Gynecol 1988;71:558–562.

Crowther C, Chalmers I. Bed rest and hospitalization during pregnancy. In: Chalmers I, Enkin M, Keirse MJNC, eds. Effective care in pregnancy and childbirth. Oxford: Oxford University Press, 1989:624–632.

D'Alton ME, Mercer BM. Antepartum management of twin gestation: ultrasound. Clin Obstet Gynecol 1990;33:42–51.

Duff P, Huff RW, Gibbs RS. Management of premature rupture of membranes and unfavorable cervix in term pregnancy. Obstet Gynecol 1984;63:697–702.

Dyson DC, Crites YM, Ray DA, Armstrong MA. Prevention of preterm birth in high-risk patients: the role of education and provider contact versus home uterine monitoring. Am J Obstet Gynecol 1991; 164:756–762.

Evans MI, Littmann L, King M, Fletcher JC. Multiple gestation: the role of multifetal pregnancy reduction and selective termination. Clin Perinatol 1992;19:345–357.

Giuntoli R, Yeh IT, Bhuett N, Chu W, Van Leewen K, Van der Lans P. Conservative management of cervical intraepithelial neoplasia during pregnancy. Gynecol Oncol 1991;42:68–73.

Gonsoulin WJ, Moise KJ Jr, Milam JD, Sala JD, Weber VW, Carpenter RJ Jr. Serial maternal blood donations for intrauterine transfusion. Obstet Gynecol 1990;75:158–162.

Greer BE, Easterling TR, McLennan DA, Benedetti TJ, Cain JM, Figge DC, et al. Fetal and maternal considerations in the management of stage I-B cervical cancer during pregnancy. Gynecol Oncol 1989; 34:61–65.

Hannah ME, Hannah WJ, Hellmann J, Hewson S, Miner R, Willan A. Induction of labor as compared with serial antenatal monitoring in post-term pregnancy: a randomized controlled trial. The Canadian Multicenter Post-term Pregnancy Trial Group. N Engl J Med 1992; 326:1587–1592.

Harman CR, Bowman JM, Manning FA, Menticoglou SM. Intrauterine transfusion—intraperitoneal versus intravascular approach: a case-control comparison. Am J Obstet Gynecol 1990;162:1053–1059.

Kobayashi F, Sagawa N, Nakamura K, Nonugaki M, Ban C. Mechanism and clinical significance of elevated CA 125 levels in the sera of pregnant women. Am J Obstet Gynecol 1989;160:563–566.

Ludomirsky A. Intrauterine fetal blood sampling—a multicenter registry, evaluation of 7462 procedures between 1987–1991. Am J Obstet Gynecol 1993;168 (part 2):318 (abstract 69).

Manning FA, Platt LD, Sipos L. Antepartum fetal evaluation: development of a fetal biophysical profile. Am J Obstet Gynecol 1983; 136:787–795.

Nageotte MP. Prevention and treatment of preterm labor in twin gestation. Clin Obstet Gynecol 1990;33:61–68.

National Institutes of Health Consensus Development Conference on the Effect of Corticosteroids for Fetal Maturation on Perinatal Outcomes; February 28–March 2, 1994; Bethesda, Maryland.

Orr JW Jr, Shingleton HM. Cancer in pregnancy. Curr Probl Cancer 1993;81:1–50.

Phelan JP, Platt LD, Yeh SY, Broussard P, Paul RH. The role of ultrasound assessment of amniotic fluid volume in the management of the postdate pregnancy. Am J Obstet Gynecol 1985;151:304–308.

Rutherford SE, Smith CV, Phelan JP, Kawakami K, Ahn MO. Four-quadrant assessment of amniotic fluid volume: an adjunct to antepartum FHR testing. Obstet Gynecol 1987;70(3 part I):353–356.

Schwartz P. Cancer in pregnancy. In: Gusberg SB, Shingleton HM, Deppe G, eds. Female genital cancer. New York: Churchill Livingstone, 1988:725–754.

Spinnato JA. Hemolytic disease of the fetus: a plea for restraint. Obstet Gynecol 1992;80:873–877.

van der Vange N, van Dongen JA. Breast cancer and pregnancy. Eur J Surg Oncol 1991;17:1–8.

Chapter 4

Perinatal Infections

COMMON VAGINAL INFECTIONS

A vaginal discharge is commonly encountered during pregnancy from hormonal effects and does not necessarily signify ruptured membranes or an inflammatory process. There is no specific therapy for this problem, but most women feel reassured by the knowledge that no infection is present. Most cases of infectious vaginitis result from *Candida albicans, Trichomonas vaginalis,* or bacterial vaginosis. Cervicitis, caused primarily by *Neisseria gonor-rhoeae, Chlamydia trachomatis,* and herpes simplex, is responsible for many patients' complaints of vaginal discharge.

A thorough assessment and an accurate diagnosis are important steps in effecting a cure, since an inaccurate or nonspecific diagnosis is what leads to the majority of treatment failures. Routine tests include determination of vaginal pH, microscopic examination of the vaginal discharge (the wet preparation), and performance of the amine (whiff) test. The vaginal pH can be determined easily by using pH indicator paper that makes distinctions of at least 0.5 between pH 3.5 and 6.0. The wet preparation can be prepared by collecting a sample of vaginal discharge on a cotton-tipped swab and placing it in a test tube containing a small amount of room-temperature normal saline. A drop of 10–20% potassium hydroxide (KOH) can be added to the edge of the original coverslip, or a second slide can be made. The examiner should note whether a "fishy" odor is released (the amine test).

Candida

Candida infections are at least ten times more frequent in pregnant than in nonpregnant women. The increased estrogen production during pregnancy and increased glycogen content of the vagina favor growth. Infection may be asymptomatic, but most often it produces a whitish discharge associated with pruritus and burning of the vulva. Microscopic examination is recommended, and the wet mount has a sensitivity of 40–80%. Sensitivity is improved by adding a drop of 10% potassium hydroxide (KOH) to the wet mount, which dissolves epithelial cells and other debris and allows easier visualization of the diagnostic blastospores. If *Candida* organisms are not demonstrated but the patient is symptomatic, a culture should be considered.

The topically applied imidazole or triazole agents (miconazole, clotrimazole, butoconazole, and terconazole) are superior to nystatin and are the treatment of choice. It appears to make little difference which of these drugs is chosen. A longer course of therapy may be required during pregnancy.

A cream or vaginal suppository taken daily for one week will usually alleviate the symptoms, but recurrence is common. It is worthwhile for a patient to be offered one weekly application of cream for the duration of the gestation to prevent symptomatic recurrence. A five-day course of oral nystatin tablets, 4 times daily, may be helpful in preventing recurrence, because *Candida* reside in the lower intestinal tract and are a source of infection on the perineum and vagina.

There are no known adverse effects from the use of any of these drugs during pregnancy. Rare candidal infections of the placenta are associated with high prematurity and perinatal death rates. Neonatal oral candidiasis and dermatitis are common lesions where there has been contact with the mother at delivery. The oral lesions are recognized as neonatal thrush and usually resolve without incident when treated with antifungal agents.

Trichomonas

Trichomoniasis is one of the most frequently occurring sexually acquired diseases. It has been associated with preterm rupture of membranes, preterm labor, and postsurgical infections. Diagnosis is often not made until there is a profuse, foul-smelling vaginal discharge or an abnormal Pap smear. Up to half of infected women may be asymptomatic. The diagnosis is confirmed by identifying motile, flagellated organisms on a wet preparation using $45\times$ magnification. Because the sensitivity of Pap test diagnosis is only 50%, cytology alone is insufficient for the diagnosis.

The current treatment is metronidazole, 250 mg tablets 3

times daily for 7 days. A single 2-g dose is thought to have a cure rate of 97%, assuming there is no further reinfection. The latter dosing regimen would improve the compliance rate while lowering costs. Concurrent single dose therapy of the male sexual partners is recommended. If a 2-g dose fails, 500 mg twice daily for 7 days should be effective. Gastrointestinal side effects are usually well-tolerated, and resistance to the metronidazole is rare.

Metronidazole has not been shown to be teratogenic in either human or animal studies, but the manufacturer recommends that use of this drug be limited to the second and third trimesters. The understandable concern about the theoretic risk to the fetus can be countered by a strong argument for metronidazole therapy in pregnancy on the basis of the role that trichomoniasis and its associated anaerobic bacterial overgrowth may play in premature rupture of the membranes and postpartum endometritis.

Bacterial Vaginosis

Associations between bacterial vaginosis and several pregnancy-related complications, including premature labor, premature rupture of membranes, chorioamnionitis, and postpartum endometritis, have been described. Bacterial vaginosis is characterized bacteriologically by both *Gardnerella vaginalis* and anaerobic bacterial overgrowth. A symbiotic relationship between these organisms is responsible for the increase in vaginal secretions and "fish" odor. The diagnosis is confirmed microscopically on a saline wet preparation by identifying "clue cells" (vaginal epithelial cells with indistinct cell borders obscured by a large number of attached organisms) and by noting the strong amine odor after alkalinization of the secretions with 10% potassium hydroxide (KOH).

Metronidazole taken in a dosage of 500 mg twice daily for 7 days has proven to be highly effective; however, single dose therapy using 2 g is thought to be less effective. Metronidazole gel may also be administered in a dosage of 400 mg twice daily for 7 days, or 2% clindamycin cream may be used in a 5-g dosage once daily for 7 days. Oral ampicillin therapy has also provided good cure rates. Douches containing an acidifying agent, 1.5% hydrogen peroxide, or povidone-iodine are not recommended during pregnancy. Although controversy remains, most authorities feel that the male sexual partner does not need to be treated.

Group B Streptococci

Group B streptococci (GBS) are common bacteria colonizing the vagina in approximately 15% of pregnant women. The actual attack rate is quite low, however. Group B streptococcal infection is a leading cause of neonatal sepsis with an attack rate ranging between 0.35 and 5.4 per 1000 live births and a mortality rate exceeding 5%. Early diagnosis and treatment are fundamental to improve the outcome of a septic neonate.

The most reliable test for documenting GBS colonization is culture. Ideally, culture samples should be obtained by swab from the lower vagina and rectum and inoculated into Todd-Hewitt broth or onto a selective blood agar. A variety of rapid laboratory tests have been developed to identify GBS. Only the DNA probe has an acceptable sensitivity in detecting lightly colonized women.

Antenatal screening of all pregnant women for GBS colonization is not cost-effective, as there is a very low ratio of neonatal sepsis to colonized mothers (about 0.7%). Screening for GBS colonization (and treatment with penicillin if culture-positive) is indicated for those cases in which a diagnosis has been made of premature labor, preterm ruptured membranes, ruptured membranes for more than 18 hours, intrapartum fever, or prior affected newborn infant. Studies have demonstrated that the intermittently-treated mother often reverts to a carrier state shortly after the antibiotic is discontinued. Administering ampicillin (1–2 mg intravenously every 4–6 hours) during labor to colonized women with these high risk factors has been shown to decrease infection significantly in their infants. It is extremely difficult to determine which neonates are infected because obvious clinical signs, such as pneumonia, are usually not apparent at birth.

Chlamydia

Chlamydia trachomatis is the most common cause of sexually transmitted disease. It is a frequent cause of maternal bartholinitis, endocervicitis, and acute urethritis, as well as neonatal conjunctivitis and pneumonia. Routine monoclonal antibody testing or culturing at the initial prenatal visit does not appear to be cost-effective. Select screening is considered to be worthwhile if there is recurrent abortion, premature labor, preterm ruptured membranes, sexually transmitted infection, abnormal Pap smear, or poor obstetric history. Concurrent infection with *C. trachomatis* should be

suspected when gonorrhea is diagnosed. Penicillin and its derivatives are effective treatments for gonorrhea, whereas chlamydia responds to erythromycin or tetracycline (i.e. doxycycline). The patient's sexual partner should also be treated with erythromycin or
tetracycline. A test of cure is not necessary with the nonpregnant
patient, but is often done with the pregnant patient.

Prenatal transmission of chlamydia is not known to occur,
but an infant delivered vaginally has a 60–70% risk of acquiring
the infection. Approximately 25–50% of exposed infants will develop conjunctivitis in the first 2 weeks, and 10–20% will develop
pneumonia in the first 3–4 months. Although controversial, most
of the literature suggests that there is no increase in adverse pregnancy outcomes when chlamydial infection is not treated during
pregnancy. However, treatment of chlamydial cervicitis with erythromycin during the late weeks of pregnancy is an effective
means of preventing neonatal conjunctivitis and pneumonia.
Erythromycin ointment applied routinely in the infant's eyes at
delivery is effective prophylactic treatment of chlamydial and
gonococcal ophthalmia.

URINARY TRACT INFECTION

Asymptomatic bacteriuria is reported to occur in 2–12% of all
pregnancies. It is most common in black, multiparous patients
with sickle cell trait, but may also be found in women with diabetes, obesity, history of urinary tract infection, urinary tract
anomalies, renal stones, and urethral catheterization. Approximately one-fourth of women with asymptomatic bacteriuria will
subsequently develop a symptomatic urinary tract infection. Bacteriuria may be a manifestation of an underlying chronic renal
disease and is associated with a higher incidence of perinatal loss
and low-birth-weight infants. Any increased risk of premature labor may be related to the release of prostaglandins from the bacterial cell walls.

Diagnosis

Each patient should have a urine culture or urinalysis performed
during the initial prenatal visit. A clean midstream urine specimen
containing more than 100,000 colonies of the same pathogen per
milliliter of urine is diagnostic of bacteriuria. Contamination of
the specimen during collection should be suspected with a smaller

colony count of multiple organisms. Approximately 80% of urinary tract infections are caused by *E. Coli,* 10–15% by *Klebsiella pneumoniae,* 5% or less by group B streptococci or staphylococci. After an initial negative culture, less than 1.5% of those patients will subsequently acquire a urinary tract infection before delivery.

Therapy

Several oral antibiotics are effective for treatment of lower urinary tract infections. When empirical treatment is indicated, ampicillin or amoxicillin is not the optimal selection because of the increasing pattern of resistance among strains of *E. coli* and *K. pneumoniae* to these two antibiotics. A 3-day course of nitrofurantoin (e.g., Macrobid 100 mg twice a day) is usually comparable in efficacy to a 7-day or 10-day course. Patients who have a poor response to this short course of therapy often have a silent upper urinary tract infection and require extended duration of treatment for 2–4 weeks. Trimethoprim-sulfamethoxazole and amoxicillin-clavulanic acid should be reserved for unusually refractory infections by resistant microorganisms. Sulfisoxazole may displace bilirubin from sites of protein-binding in the neonate, but this effect is rarely a problem except in preterm infants.

A urine culture is recommended within 1 week following completion of the drug therapy. If the culture remains positive, the proper drug should be chosen according to the sensitivity pattern of the isolated organism. The risk of recurrence later in pregnancy is 15–25%.

Hospitalization for a urinary tract infection is necessary when there are systemic manifestations of upper urinary tract problems. Along with the intravenous administration of a cephalosporin (e.g., cefazolin), the patient should be watched carefully for any signs of septic shock. A transient decrease in glomerular filtration and a transient form of hemolytic anemia may appear. Acute respiratory distress can develop rarely and is believed to be mediated by bacterial endotoxins. If the patient does not show a response to therapy within 24 hours, an aminoglycoside should be added. Alternatively, if sensitivities are available, they may be utilized to choose a more appropriate antibiotic. Either chronic, low-dose antibiotic suppression (Macrodantin 50 mg twice daily or 100 mg at bedtime) or repeat cultures on a monthly basis are necessary in any pregnant patient with pyelonephritis.

If the culture becomes positive, chronic suppression should

be undertaken. Screening for sickle cell disease is necessary for African-American gravidas who develop pyelonephritis. Any patient with persistent, recurrent, or very severe urinary tract infections during pregnancy should be evaluated. A renal and lower urinary tract ultrasound or intravenous pyelogram, creatinine clearance, and urine culture should be obtained.

HERPES SIMPLEX

The relative infrequency of neonatal herpes (2 in 7500 live births) has made it difficult to study the disease thoroughly. It has been reported that the infection rate of infants born to mothers with symptomatic genital herpes simplex is 50%, with manifestations ranging from subclinical to cutaneous to disseminated (visceral) disease, with or without central nervous system involvement. Of those infected systemically, 60% will die and of those who survive, many are impaired neurologically. The mean onset of symptoms in newborn infants is 6 days, although those who are systemically infected may have delayed onset of clinical signs. The first signs of neonatal herpes infection are variable and range from lethargy to seizures or overwhelming systemic disease.

Antepartum Screening

Virus isolation on tissue culture remains the standard diagnostic procedure. Cultures of the cervix, posterior vaginal fornix, and vulva should be obtained if there is any suspicious vulvar lesion, history of genital herpes, or sexual contact during pregnancy with a person having any visible suspicious genital lesion. Cultures are positive in 92% of colonized cases after 4 days' incubation.

If cultures have not been done previously and the patient is suspected by history or physical examination to have genital herpes, a Pap smear may be helpful and provide information relatively quickly. Cervicovaginal smears have been reported to detect 75% of specimens positive for herpes simplex on culture. Negative cytologic findings do not rule out herpes, however.

Most genital herpes during pregnancy is a recurrence of prior disease. External genital lesions are usually preceded by prodromal symptoms such pruritus, numbness, pain, burning, or paresthesias. The typical course of genital herpes infection involves a prodrome of 1–2 days, vesicle/pustule stage of 2 days, wet ulcer stage of 3 days, and dry crust stage of 7 days. Virus shedding occurs during the 5-day vesicle/pustule/wet ulcer period, and the mean interval between recurrences is 50 days, but may (rarely) be less than 21 days.

Recognition of the low rate of asymptomatic viral shedding (1.4% at term), the short duration of viral shedding during an attack, and the less than 5% incidence of neonatal infection among infants born to mothers with asymptomatic viral shedding has led clinicians to advocate the abandonment of weekly cultures. A cesarean section should be reserved for individuals with symptomatic infection at the time of or during the few days preceding labor.

Treatment goals include the relief of symptoms and promoting reepithelialization. This involves frequent washing with soap and water, thorough drying (blow dryer or heat lamp may be helpful), and dusting with baby powder or corn starch. Any benefit from topical acyclovir on nonmucocutaneous areas during pregnancy is unlikely, although it is considered to be nonteratogenic. Acyclovir should be considered in immunocompetent women who have severe symptoms or in immunosuppressed individuals with unusual debility.

Mode of Delivery

Hematogenous dissemination of herpes simplex virus across the placenta is extremely uncommon. The greatest risk to the fetus occurs during vaginal delivery in the setting of a primary maternal infection. Approximately 40% of infants delivered vaginally under these circumstances become infected. The risk to the fetus when the mother has recurrent infection is much lower, presumably due to the protective effects of passively acquired maternal antibody and the lower viral inoculum associated with recurrent or asymptomatic infection. If overt lesions are present and vaginal delivery occurs, 5% or fewer of infants become infected. If the mother has no overt lesions but is asymptomatically shedding the virus, 1% or fewer of infants are infected.

The following management plan is recommended for treatment of patients with herpes infections during pregnancy: (*a*) persons who have genital herpetic lesions near term, but prior to labor or membrane rupture, should have viral cultures collected at 3–5-day intervals to ensure the absence of virus at the time of birth and thereby increase the likelihood of vaginal delivery; (*b*) asymptomatic patients who have a history of recurrent herpes should be examined carefully at the time of admission to the hospital for labor (if no prodromal symptoms or vesicular lesions are present, vaginal delivery should be anticipated); and (*c*) patients who, at the time they are admitted for labor, have overt vesicular lesions from primary or recurrent infection or have a distinct prodrome, should undergo cesarean delivery regardless of time since rupture of membranes.

Postpartum Infection Control

Mother with Proven or Clinically Suspected Genital Herpes at Term

The Centers for Disease Control and Prevention (CDCP) guidelines do not require isolation of these mothers on the antepartum and postpartum floors. However, from a practical point of view, practitioners are aware that other patients generally become upset when placed in a room with a woman with an active herpes infection. Therefore, isolation is often practiced, using wound and skin precautions. Perineal pads, genital dressings, and bed linen should be double-bagged. The mother may handle and feed her infant if she is out of bed (to reduce the chance of contact with potentially contaminated bed linen), gowned, and follows thorough hand-washing techniques. The infant should be isolated with wound and skin precautions. Contaminated articles should be double-bagged.

The newborn infant may be brought to the mother under supervised conditions as above. Rooming-in is acceptable after the mother has been taught appropriate protective measures. Circumcision should be delayed in proven and suspected cases. A joint committee from the American College of Obstetricians and Gynecologists (ACOG) and the American Academy of Pediatrics recommends that these infants be cultured for the virus (urine, conjunctiva, nasopharynx, other suspicious sites) and have liver function tests and spinal fluid examinations.

Mothers with Nonoral, Nongenital Lesions at Delivery

Cover maternal lesions at all times. Wound and skin precautions with isolation are necessary for the mother. The infant does not require isolation initially but should be isolated and placed on wound and skin precautions after contact with the mother. If there are no lesions in the area of the breasts, the mother may breast-feed; otherwise, she may pump to establish and maintain milk flow. This milk should be discarded until the breast lesions are healed.

Mothers or Medical Personnel with Oral Lesions Only

Exposure to oral herpes (type 1) may be as devastating as genital herpes (type 2) to the neonate. The infected mother and any other infected person exposed to the newborn should cover their lesions with a mask or gauze until they are crusted and should refrain from kissing and nuzzling the infant. The infant does not require isolation, however.

VIRAL HEPATITIS

Hepatitis is one of the most serious infections in pregnancy. Maternal mortality is low in well-nourished populations and is the same as for nonpregnant populations. Other cases of liver dysfunction include noninfectious hepatitis (drug-related), toxemia, cytomegalovirus (CMV) and other viral infections, and gallstones. The onset of liver dysfunction is helpful in formulating the differential diagnosis as follows:

- first trimester: hyperemesis gravidarum, drug reactions
- second trimester: cirrhosis, pyelonephritis, exacerbation of chronic liver disease
- third trimester: cholestasis of pregnancy, eclampsia, preeclampsia, cirrhosis, fatty liver of pregnancy, pyelonephritis.

The laboratory diagnosis of liver disease in the third trimester is outlined in Table 4.1. If helpful, a liver biopsy can be performed during a cesarean section using a True-cut biopsy needle. The risk of hemorrhage is the same as in the nonpregnant patient. We recommend that the liver and gallbladder be palpated at the time of intraabdominal surgery.

Forms of Viral Hepatitis

Characteristics of hepatitis A, hepatitis B, non-A, non-B hepatitis, and hepatitis C are compared in Table 4.2. Acute clinical forms range from being fulminant to severe. Hepatitis B is the most common form during pregnancy.

Mothers who have hepatitis B surface antigen (HB$_s$Ag) with antibody have had a prior infection or immunization and are currently immune, while those who have surface antigen without an-

Table 4.1
Laboratory Diagnosis of Liver Disease in Third Trimester

Condition	SGOT (IU/L)	Bilirubin (mg/dL)	Alkaline Phosphatase
Normal pregnancy	Normal (2–35)	Normal (1.2) to slight increase	2 × increase (normal: 30–96 IU/L)
Infectious hepatitis	500–1000	1.5–5	2–3 × increase
Cholestasis of pregnancy	Normal to slight increase	1.5–5	10 × increase
Toxemia	100–1000	Slight increase	2–3 × increase
Gallstones	Normal to slight increase	Variable	3–10 × increase
Active cirrhosis and chronic active hepatitis	50–150	1.5–5	3 × increase
Fatty liver of pregnancy	300–500	1.5–10	3 × increase

tibody have active infection or are chronic carriers. Mothers who are also carriers of e antigens and who lack the e antibody are infectious and may transmit the virus to the fetus.

The CDCP and ACOG recommend hepatitis B virus screening for all pregnant women. Infants born to mothers who are chronic carriers of HB_sAg may have severe or lethal hepatitis during the first 4 postnatal months and commonly become chronic carriers. While infection rates are higher for infants whose mothers become infected in the third trimester, these infants usually experience milder disease. Hepatitis B immune globulin (HBIG) and hepatitis B vaccine should be administered to decrease the incidence of maternal disease.

Transplacental infection of hepatitis A has not been reported. However, neonatal infection can occur. Therefore, infants born to mothers with active hepatitis A should be treated with immune specific globulin. There is little information about perinatal transmission of non-A, non-B hepatitis.

Hepatitis D is another RNA virus which is dependent on hepatitis B for replication. Diagnosis is made by measurement of the D antigen and identification of an IgM-specific antibody. Acute hepatitis D is usually self-limited and rarely leads to chronic

Table 4.2
Forms of Viral Hepatitis

Characteristics	Hepatitis A	Hepatitis B	Non-A, Non-B	Hepatitis C
Prior terminology	Infectious hepatitis	Serum hepatitis	Unrecognized	Unrecognized
Virus type	RNA	DNA	Unknown	RNA
Incubation time	15–50 days	30–180 days	30–160 days	35–160 days
Transmission route	Fecal-oral	Parenteral or body fluids	Parenteral, close contacts	Transfusion, parenteral, or body fluids
Serologic tests	HA antibody IgM types	HB_sAg, HB_cAg HB_sAb, HB_eAg	None	HC antibody
Maximum infectivity	Prodrome	Prodrome or HB_sAg carriers	Probably prodrome	Prodrome
Incidence of chronicity	None	Chronic persistent hepatitis / Chronic active hepatitis / Asymptomatic carrier	Chronic persistent / Chronic active / Asymptomatic carrier	Chronic persistent hepatitis / Chronic active hepatitis / Asymptomatic carrier
Transmission risk to infant	Rare	1st & 2nd trimester: up to 10% / 3rd trimester: 80–90%	None	44–80%
Infant disease	Rare clinical hepatitis (at 14–30 days of age) / No carriers	Usually mild hepatitis, rarely severe (at 20–120 days of age) / Commonly become carriers	None	Unknown / Also seropositive for HIV
Prophylaxis for infant	ISG—only for infant of mother with acute infection / HBIG—not useful / Vaccine	ISG—not useful / HBIG—useful at birth and at 3 months / Vaccine—useful after HBIG(?)	None needed	None available

disease. Perinatal transmission may occur, and measures to prevent transmission of hepatitis B are effective here.

Proposed Management

1. Establish type of immunologic tests to be performed
2. Institute appropriate isolation and precautions until type of hepatitis is confirmed
3. Determine need for contact prophylaxis with serum globulin preparations
4. Activity—determined by tolerance; rest encouraged
5. Diet—patient preference; parenteral if necessary; high protein
6. Antiemetics—phenothiazines may be used
7. Corticosteroids—not indicated
8. Watch for any mental or sleep disturbance—impending coma
9. Treat any additional medical problems (drug abuse, HIV, etc.)
10. Discharge from hospital after improvement in liver function tests
11. Notify pediatrician before anticipated delivery
12. Attempts should be made at delivery to avoid aspiration by the infant of any maternal blood. Observe blood precautions for predelivery and postdelivery care if HB_sAg is positive
13. If the mother remains infected during delivery, breast-feeding should be avoided. Handle blood or lochia-soaked dressings with gloved hands and disinfect sitz baths

Among health care personnel, obstetricians and gynecologists are considered to be at average risk of acquiring hepatitis B virus infection. Other hospital staff such as nurses, phlebotomists, and i.v. team personnel are at higher risk and should be considered to be candidates for hepatitis vaccine immunization, which is effective and safe. All pregnant women should be tested for HB_sAg and if seronegative, should be vaccinated.

The principal means of preventing hepatitis B virus infection is vaccination. Vaccination appears to confer protection for 5–9 years. Two recombinant DNA vaccines for hepatitis B virus, Recombivax HB (10 μg) and Engerix-B (20 μg), have been developed for intramuscular injection. The combination of passive and active immunization has been particularly effective in reducing the frequency of perinatal transmission of hepatitis B virus.

The CDCP has recommended universal active immunization of all infants born in the United States. The immunization schedule for infants of women who have been screened and are negative should be started preferably before discharge but no later than 2 months of age. Infants of women who are known to be HB-$_s$Ag-positive or whose status is unknown should have treatment started within 12 hours. Infants born to seropositive or untested mothers should also receive HBIG and the recombinant vaccine simultaneously at different intramuscular sites.

HUMAN IMMUNODEFICIENCY VIRUS (HIV) INFECTION

Acquired immunodeficiency syndrome (AIDS) is an infectious disease caused by a retrovirus known as human T-cell lymphotropic virus (HIV). The virus can be transmitted through sexual intercourse, contaminated needles, blood or blood product transfusion, or perinatally from mother to infant. Most mothers are asymptomatic and the latent period lasts for an average of almost 10 years. Once symptomatic, life expectancy is 5 years or less. At least 7000 children are born to HIV-infected mothers each year.

Perinatal Transmission and Screening

The risk of vertical transmission has been associated with advanced stage of disease, low CD4 (T4) lymphocyte count, and increased viral burden. The risk of transmission is 8–30%. Transmission of the virus may occur before, during, or after birth. The virus has been isolated from breast milk of infected women, and breast-feeding may be implicated as a mode of transmission. There is an increase of spontaneous abortion, low birth weight, premature rupture of membranes, and premature delivery. A dysmorphic syndrome with intrauterine HIV infection has been described in infants and children with positive serologic tests. Growth failure, microcephaly, and craniofacial abnormalities have been noted. Follow-up examinations of infants at risk of developing AIDS are limited, but a slow rate of weight gain has been evident. The affected child's age at onset of symptoms does not necessarily correlate with the birth weight, mode of delivery, or status of membranes at the onset of labor.

The CDCP has developed recommendations designed to reduce the risk of perinatal transmission. All women should be counseled with regard to antibody testing if they are pregnant (or may become pregnant). The following groups of women are at high risk of infection: i.v. drug abusers; those born in countries where heterosexual transmission is thought to a play a major role; prostitutes; those who have been sex partners of i.v. drug abusers, bisexual men, men with hemophilia, men born in countries where heterosexual transmission is thought to play a major role, or men who otherwise have evidence of infection with HIV.

Counseling and testing must be conducted in a confidential environment. Serologic screening for antibody by enzyme-linked immunosorbent assay (ELISA) should be performed with the woman's consent after counseling has been provided regarding the risk of infection, the interpretation of the test results, the risk of transmission, and the definite increased likelihood of disease among women infected with HIV. The screening antibody test for HIV is relatively inexpensive. If a repeat test remains positive, confirmation should be obtained by the more expensive Western blot assay to more specifically identify antibodies to antigens.

Counseling Infected Women

Women with positive results for HIV antibodies should be counseled regarding their own risk of developing AIDS and the risk of perinatal and sexual transmission.

1. Advise infected women to delay pregnancy until more is known regarding perinatal transmission
2. Discourage drug use and advise against sharing needles
3. Refer sex partners for counseling and testing
4. Inform couples of protected sexual practices to reduce the risk of HIV transmission to uninfected partners; encourage consistent and proper use of condoms
5. Screen for tuberculosis, sexually transmitted diseases, CMV infection, and toxoplasmosis
6. Immunizations such as an annual influenza vaccine, pneumonococcal vaccine can also be offered, and hepatitis B vaccine can be offered to patients who are hepatitis B-seronegative
7. Interventions, such as elective cesarean delivery, vaginal virucides, reduction in the duration of rupture of mem-

branes, and fetal scalp blood sampling or scalp electrode placement need to be evaluated further
8. Universal precautions to prevent transmission of HIV and other blood-borne agents apply to infected patients and healthcare personnel
9. Advise against breast-feeding
10. Inform couple not to donate blood, organs, or sperm

Drug Therapy

Zidovudine (ZDV) may decrease maternal mortality and delay the onset of opportunistic infections. It is indicated for HIV-infected patients with a CD4 lymphocyte count less than 200 cells/mm^3. The initial oral dosage is 100 mg orally five times daily. Intravenous ZDV administered during labor should consist of a loading dose of 2 mg/kg, followed by a continuous infusion of 1 mg/kg until delivery. Complete blood counts should be performed monthly, and hematologic toxicity may require temporary discontinuation or dose reduction, although the effectiveness of lower doses has not been definitely established. Pancreatitis and a painful sensory neuropathy are major side effects. No malformations have been reported with therapy. Newborns should continue to be treated daily for 6 weeks.

In February 1994, the National Institutes of Health discontinued a clinical trial exploring the effect of ZDV on transmission from HIV-infected women to their infants because of a reduction in vertical transmission of the virus by two-thirds. These were the results of a single, randomized, controlled trial in patients who met well-defined study criteria. Therapy should be discussed and offered to all HIV-infected pregnant women.

Morbidity and mortality are high for HIV-infected women who acquire *Pneumocystis carinii* pneumonia (PCP). Prophylaxis against PCP is indicated when the CD4 count is less than 200 cells/mm^3 or when the percentage of CD4 lymphocytes is less than 20% of the total lymphocyte count. Since fetal and neonatal morbidity are rare with therapy, women at high risk should receive prophylaxis. When considering administration of trimethoprim-sulfamethoxazole during the first trimester or at term, one must discuss with each patient the theoretical risk of teratogenicity or newborn kernicterus and transient hemolysis before initiating therapy. Prenatal exposure to ZDV and trimethoprim-sulfamethoxazole therapy warrants hematologic monitoring of the newborn.

HUMAN PAPILLOMA VIRUS INFECTION

Human papilloma virus (HPV) of the genital tract is the most common sexually transmitted viral infection in the United States. It is known that 1–3% of Pap tests will show cytologically detectable HPV disease (active, productive infection). The biology of HPV infection is not completely understood. The entire lower genital tract may be involved, starting from the perianal area to the perineal body, vulva, vagina, and cervix. Overt condylomata acuminata that are found in 30% of all patients with HPV disease usually appear as a soft, pink or white, vascular, sessile tumor with multiple fine, fingerlike projections.

Management of these infections during pregnancy is difficult. The papillary lesions may proliferate on the vulva and vagina. Transmission to the infant may result from transplacental transmission, direct contact with the infected genital tract at delivery, or postnatal contact with an infected individual. Laryngeal polyps have been described from vertical transmission regardless of route of delivery.

The most important part of clinical management is to help the patient understand that she has acquired an infection that is lifelong and may recur at any time within the lower genital tract. At present, there is no standard approach to treat overt or subclinical HPV infection. A variety of modalities include keratolytic agents (podophyllin, trichloroacetic acid, and 5-fluorouracil cream), physical agents (cryotherapy, laser therapy, and electrocautery), surgical resection, and immunotherapy (autologous vaccine, dinitrochlorobenzene, and interferon).

Topical therapy is best used during pregnancy. Only visible lesions are amenable to treatment. Trichloroacetic acid acts by precipitation of surface proteins. Application on external lesions should be done with a cotton-tipped swab. Therapy is usually repeated in 2–3 weeks. Cryotherapy and electrocautery have reported cure rates of 63% and 90% respectively when performed in an outpatient setting with or without local anesthesia. Carbon dioxide laser therapy may be more effective, although controlled clinical trials are necessary. The time, cost, and morbidity rates from laser vaporization exceed those of other treatments, and advanced training in colposcopy and laser therapy is necessary.

Large and friable lesions may cause extensive vaginal damage and bleeding at delivery and may necessitate scheduling a cesarean section. There is no consensus regarding the protective benefit to the neonate of cesarean versus vaginal delivery. Because years of latency may precede the appearance of lesions, the risk of perinatal exposure has been difficult to assess.

GONORRHEA

The incidence of gonococcal infections in pregnant patients has been reported to range from 3 to 6%. Most studies have involved indigent patient populations, and the incidence in the general population is probably lower. Acute salpingitis is a rare event after the third gestational month, because the cervical mucus plug blocks the access of the ascending Gram-negative diplococcus to the upper genital tract. However, the incidence of disseminated gonorrhea is higher during pregnancy.

Every pregnant woman should be cultured for gonorrhea at her initial prenatal visit, and again if recurrent infections remain a possibility. Prompt treatment is necessary to prevent maternal complications, infection of the patient's sexual partner, gonococcal ophthalmia neonatorum, and infection of the upper genital tract at the time of delivery. If the incidence of gonococcal infection in the third trimester is greater than 1% in the given population, the CDCP recommends routine repeat culturing at 34–36 weeks' gestation.

Treatment for undisseminated, uncomplicated gonorrhea is the same as for the nonpregnant patient and may be undertaken on an outpatient basis, in accordance with the following guidelines:

1. Treat with an adequate dose of an appropriate antibiotic as outlined in Table 4.3
2. Reculture cervix and rectum as a test of cure in 3–7 days and retreat if necessary. Culture again at 34–36 weeks' gestation
3. Examine and treat sexual contact(s)
4. Examine patient for other sexually transmitted diseases (chlamydia, syphilis, herpes) and treat accordingly
5. Before delivery, notify pediatrician of maternal culture results. Consider gonorrhea cultures, serologic tests for syphilis, etc., on infant when appropriate

SYPHILIS

Approximately 100,000 cases of adult syphilis and 300–400 cases of congenital syphilis are reported in the United States each year. The rise of infection in female patients has led to an increased in-

Table 4.3
Single Dose Therapy for Women with Uncomplicated Gonorrhea

Drugs of choice:
  Ceftriaxone[a,b] 125 mg i.m. (deltoid)
  OR
  Amoxicillin[c] 3 g orally **plus** probenecid 1 g orally
Alternatives:
  Penicillin G procaine 4.8 million U i.m. (divided into 2 injections at one
    visit) **plus** probenecid 1 g orally
  Spectinomycin[a,d] 2 g i.m.
  Cefoxitin 2 g i.m. **plus** probenecid 1 g orally

[a] Effective against penicillin-resistant strains; recommended in treatment failure.
[b] Drug of choice for pharyngeal isolates.
[c] Less effective against anal or pharyngeal gonorrhea.
[d] Recommended for penicillin-allergic patients.

cidence of congenital syphilis. It is now understood that the risk to the unborn child is present throughout gestation, although the fetus is unable to mount an immune response to the spirochete until mid-gestation. Untreated patients with primary or secondary disease have a vertical transmission risk of approximately 50%. Half of these patients will deliver preterm or have a stillbirth. Early latent syphilis transmission rates are approximately 40%, but only 20% of these pregnancies result in preterm delivery or perinatal mortality. This risk to the fetus is reduced when mothers have latent disease and decreases further with late syphilis.

Primary, usually painless, lesions (chancres) will develop 21 days after exposure (range, 10–90 days). Within a few weeks to several months after the primary lesion, secondary syphilis resulting from widespread dissemination is characterized by low-grade fever, malaise, sore throat, headache, adenopathy, and the cutaneous or mucosal rash on the soles of the feet or palms of the hands. The most common manifestation of tertiary syphilis is benign syphilis (gumma) affecting mostly skin, bone, and mucosa. Serious cardiovascular and neurologic manifestations of tertiary syphilis occur in approximately 5–20% of patients.

Diagnosis

Nonspecific antibody tests such as the VDRL or RPR are used for initial screening. When a positive serologic test is obtained, further evaluation as shown in Figure 4.1 is indicated. A primary le-

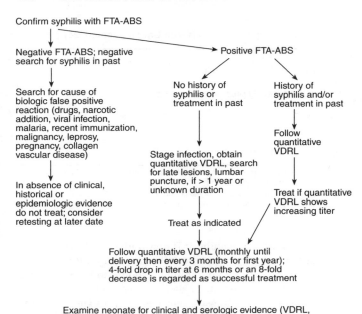

Confirm syphilis with FTA-ABS

Negative FTA-ABS; negative search for syphilis in past → Positive FTA-ABS

Search for cause of biologic false positive reaction (drugs, narcotic addition, viral infection, malaria, recent immunization, malignancy, leprosy, pregnancy, collagen vascular disease)

No history of syphilis or treatment in past

History of syphilis and/or treatment in past

In absence of clinical, historical or epidemiologic evidence do not treat; consider retesting at later date

Stage infection, obtain quantitative VDRL, search for late lesions, lumbar puncture, if > 1 year or unknown duration

Follow quantitative VDRL

Treat if quantitative VDRL shows increasing titer

Treat as indicated

Follow quantitative VDRL (monthly until delivery then every 3 months for first year); 4-fold drop in titer at 6 months or an 8-fold decrease is regarded as successful treatment

Examine neonate for clinical and serologic evidence (VDRL, FTA-ABS) of congenital syphilis at birth and first weeks of life (maculopapular eruption, IUGR, saddle nose, hepatosplenomegaly, jaundice)

Figure 4.1. Evaluation of a positive serologic test for syphilis during pregnancy.

sion consists of a chancre. Late or latent infection is difficult to suspect on physical examination alone.

Treatment

Treatment for syphilis is indicated in the pregnant patient in the following conditions:

1. The previously uninfected patient who now has active disease
2. Treatment judged to be inadequate by history, e.g., noncompliant patient with early syphilis
3. Current treatment regimen judged to be inadequate because of unsatisfactory pattern of serologic response
4. Presumed reinfection because of a rising titer
5. Previous delivery of a congenitally syphilitic infant despite presumed adequate treatment

Therapy is the same as for the nonpregnant patient. Benzathine penicillin remains the drug of choice, and serial quantitative VDRL determinations are necessary to test for therapeutic efficacy. As tetracyclines are contraindicated during pregnancy and erythromycin provides inadequate treatment for the fetus, a patient who is allergic to penicillin should be hospitalized and sensitization should be attempted. Table 4.4 outlines the means for differentiating and treating the various stages of syphilis.

CYTOMEGALOVIRUS

Cytomegalovirus (CMV) infection is the most common congenital infection in the United States, affecting approximately 1% of neonates. Congenital infection may occur with either primary or recurrent maternal infection, but is much more common and serious with the former. Approximately 40% of infants delivered to mothers with primary CMV infection will become infected. On average, 10% of these neonates will have obvious clinical findings including hepatosplenomegaly, jaundice, thrombocytopenia, microcephaly, deafness, chorioretinitis, optic atrophy, cerebral calcifications, and hydrocephalus.

Approximately 60–70% of adults have serologic evidence of previous CMV infection. Most CMV infections in children and adults are subclinical, and routine screening during pregnancy is not indicated. The diagnosis of maternal CMV infection can be made by culturing the virus from urine or genital tract secretions. The detection of IgM-specific antibody is usually indicative of acute or recent CMV infection. Documentation of a positive IgG-specific antibody titer in a patient who previously was seronegative also is confirmation of infection. Detection of CMV in amniotic fluid and demonstration of fetal anomalies by ultrasonography correlate more precisely with severity of fetal infection than IgM detected by cordocentesis.

There is no antiviral agent that is effective in treating subclinical or mildly symptomatic CMV infection or in preventing congenital infection.

TOXOPLASMOSIS

Serologic tests of *Toxoplasma gondii* are not performed routinely during pregnancy, since intrauterine infections are quite uncommon and often difficult to determine. Between 25 and 33% of all women have been infected previously and are therefore immune

Table 4.4
Treatment and Follow-up of Syphilis in Pregnancy

Syphilis State	Drug(s) of Choice	Alternative	Follow-up
Healthy Contact[a] or **Early** (primary, secondary, or latent 1 year)	Benzathine penicillin G 2.4 million U, i.m. once (half dose in each hip)	Erythromycin[b] 500 mg orally 4 times per day for 15 days	Serial VDRL titer monthly (every 3 months after delivery for 1 year)
Late (more than one year's duration, benign gummatous, cardiovascular)	Benzathine penicillin G as above, weekly for 3 doses	Erythromycin as above for 30 days	CSF normal[c] no signs or symptoms of neurosyphilis: serial VDRL titer as above then every 6 months for 1–2 years. Repeat annually
Late (neurosyphilis)	Penicillin G 12–24 million U every 4 hours for 10–14 days **Or** Procaine penicillin G 2–4 million U, i.m. (half dose in each hip) **plus** probenecid 500 mg orally 4 times per day, **both** for 10–14 days	None	CSF abnormalities or signs and symptoms of neurosyphilis[d]: follow-up as for normal CSF; also repeat LP every 3–6 months until count and protein normal
Congenital As above, depending on stage	Procaine penicillin G 50,000 U/kg i.m. daily for 10 days, **OR** (only if CSF is normal) benzathine penicillin G 50,000 U/kg, i.m. once	None	

[a] Contact with active skin or mucous membrane lesion.
[b] Poor transplacental diffusion; postpartum penicillin treatment of infant recommended.
[c] CSF VDRL negative; normal protein, no pleocytosis.
[d] May be asymptomatic.

during any reactivation of the infection. Infected newborn infants may be asymptomatic or demonstrate hydrocephaly, chorioretinitis, microphthalmia, and mental retardation. Initially asymptomatic infants may develop sequelae of infection months to years later.

The oocysts may be acquired from the maternal ingestion or handling of raw meat or exposure to feces of infected predator cats. Toxoplasmosis should be suspected with persistent flu-like illness. Lymphadenopathy may be found occasionally. Susceptible pregnant women should be advised to avoid undercooked meat. They should wash their hands after handling raw meat and thoroughly clean countertops and dishes. Patients who own cats should be instructed to keep their cats indoors and to avoid contact with the litter box.

A positive serologic test (Sabin-Feldman) indicates prior infection, and any rise in titer usually represents only a reactivation of infection. A minimum fourfold increase in titers over a 4-week period or the presence of IgM toxoplasma antibodies is necessary to diagnose a recent infection. The placenta should be examined microscopically for any oocysts.

Several methods have been used to diagnose fetal infection. Amniotic fluid may be obtained by amniocentesis and then injected into mice or incubated in tissue culture. Fetal blood can be aspirated and assayed for total IgM concentration and IgM-specific antibody after 21 weeks of gestation. Ultrasonographic findings consistent with several fetal infections include microcephaly, ventriculomegaly, growth retardation, visceromegaly, and hydrops.

If acute fetal infection is documented, patients may be offered pregnancy termination or antibiotic treatment. Investigations in France have confirmed the value of sulfadiazine, pyrimethamine, and spiramycin in treatment of fetal toxoplasmosis. The pediatric staff should be notified at the time of diagnosis before delivery. Physical contact with an infected patient is unlikely to result in transmission of infection, so special handling precautions of an infected infant are unnecessary.

TUBERCULOSIS

Exposure to tuberculosis is common in urban populations and less-developed countries. Up to 12.5% of gravidas may be tuberculin sensitive. A tuberculin skin test becomes positive (10 mm or more) 4–12 weeks after exposure (cell-mediated delayed sensitivity) and will remain positive for life.

We routinely screen for tuberculosis to prevent both spread of any active or reactivated disease and fetal infection. Evaluation of a positive skin test is shown in Figure 4.2. This precaution is appropriate in populations at risk even though pregnancy, birth, puerperium, and lactation do not predispose to a relapse, and congenital tuberculosis is rare. Administration of a BCG vaccine will cause the tuberculin skin test to remain strongly positive. Guidelines for BCG administration in the nonpregnant state also apply during pregnancy.

The risk of untreated tuberculosis to the pregnant woman and fetus outweighs the risk of treatment. Standard agents for treating tuberculosis include isoniazid (INH), rifampin, ethambutol, and pyrazinamide. The first three have been widely used in pregnancy without adverse maternal or fetal consequences. Active disease should be treated promptly, but the possibility of an in-

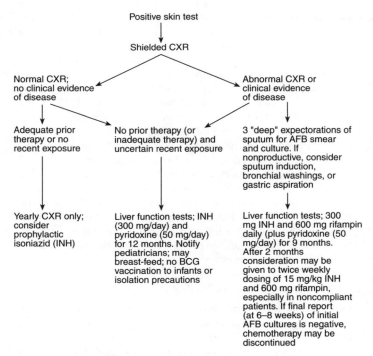

Figure 4.2. Evaluation after a positive tuberculin skin test.

creased risk of INH hepatotoxicity in pregnancy leads some physicians to defer prophylaxis with this agent until after delivery.

For patients not suspected of having drug-resistant tuberculosis, therapy with the two drugs isoniazid and rifampin is recommended as initial treatment. Isoniazid, rifampin, and ethambutol have been used successfully during pregnancy with a relatively low risk of teratogenesis or maternal toxicity. Nearly all pregnancies treated with one or more of these agents deliver healthy term infants. The greatest range of experience is available for isoniazid and ethambutol. While some fetuses born to women treated with rifampin may demonstrate blood dyscrasias and limb malformations, malformation rates associated with rifampin are no greater than background rates in otherwise normal women.

IMMUNIZATIONS

The diagnosis of viral infections during pregnancy is often inexact and usually by exclusion. Furthermore, pregnant patients infected by theses viruses are often asymptomatic. Except for influenza, the organisms listed in Table 4.5 are associated with an increased risk of abortion or congenital and neonatal disease. Viruses at conception may linger and affect the embryo and fetus, and the risk to the fetus is greatest during organogenesis in the first trimester. Signs suggesting that the newborn was infected with a virus in utero include head size abnormalities, hepatosplenomegaly, prematurity, growth retardation, hemolytic anemia, and thrombocytopenia.

TORCH titers in the mother are useful only in determining whether she has had a prior exposure. When acute and convalescent sera are compared, a fourfold increase in virus-specific IgG antibody titer is diagnostic. Virus-specific IgM titers suggest recent infection.

Accurate gestational dating is necessary, since pregnancy termination should be offered only if the diagnosis is certain, risks are understood, and gestational age is less than 24 weeks. These criteria are met uncommonly, however. The pediatrician should be notified at delivery about any suspected prenatal viral infection, and the placenta should be sent for histologic examination as live vaccines theoretically have the ability to cross the placenta and infect the fetus. Vaccinations using inactivated or dilute viruses (influenza, hepatitis) may be used if there is a serious underlying condition. There are currently no vaccinations for Cox-

Table 4.5
Recommendations for Exposure to Specific Infections during Pregnancy

	Influenza	Rubella	Tetanus-Diphtheria
Maternal risk if infected	Possible increase in morbidity and mortality during epidemic of new antigenic strain	Low morbidity and mortality, not altered by pregnancy; symptomatic in only 1/3 cases	Severe morbidity; tetanus mortality 60%; diphtheria mortality 10% in respiratory cases
Fetal/neonatal risk if infected	Unclear; reports contradictory; rare transplacental transmission	Congenital rubella syndrome, severe fetal anomalies if mother infected during first trimester	Neonatal tetanus mortality 60%
Vaccine	Inactivated virus vaccine formulated according to antigenic types expected each year	Live, attenuated virus vaccine	Combined tetanus diphtheria toxoids preferred
Fetal risk from vaccine	Unconfirmed; has been isolated in placenta	None confirmed, theoretical risk	None confirmed
Indications for vaccination during pregnancy	Recommended only for patients with serious underlying chronic diseases	Contraindicated	Lack of primary series or no booster within past 10 years
Dose/schedule	Adults: 0.5 mL i.m. (may depend on previous immunization)	—	Primary: 3 doses of 0.5 mL i.m. at 3–8-week intervals; booster after 5 years
Comments	Vaccination of pregnant women left to physician's discretion	IG is not recommended for post-exposure prophylaxis, except for women who would not consider therapeutic abortion	Updating of immune status should be part of antepartum care

Table 4.5 (Cont.)

	Varicella Zoster (Chickenpox)	Mumps	Measles
Maternal risk if infected	Low morbidity and mortality; not altered by pregnancy; pneumonia is greatest danger	Low morbidity and mortality; not altered by pregnancy	Significant morbidity (heart failure, pulmonary edema); low mortality; not altered by pregnancy
Fetal/neonatal risk if infected	Rarely affected; strictures of extremities in second trimester; increased if maternal infection 5 days before delivery and direct viral contact with neonate	Abortion; fetal damage; questionable fibroelastosis in neonate	Risk of moderate to severe disease; association with increase in abortion rate; low birth weight; one study reports malformations
Vaccine	Varicella zoster immune globulin 625 U i.m. or convalescent zoster plasma within 72 hours of exposure	Live, attenuated virus vaccine	Live, attenuated virus vaccine
Fetal risk from vaccine	None reported	None confirmed	None confirmed
Indications for vaccination during pregnancy	VZIG may prevent or modify maternal disease; for newborns with maternal infection 5 days before and 2 days after delivery	Contraindicated	Contraindicated
Dose/schedule	—	—	—
Comments	CDCP is maintaining surveillance of varicella during pregnancy; varicella zoster immune globulin (VZIG) 625 U i.m. for infant if maternal illness 5 days before or 2 days after delivery	—	Use immune globulin (IG), 0.25 mL/kg; maximum dose 15 mL

sackie, Epstein-Barr (mononucleosis), echovirus, herpes, HIV, or cytomegalovirus infections.

Suggested Readings

Adler SP. Cytomegalovirus and pregnancy. Curr Opin Obstet Gynecol 1992;4:670–675.

Alford CA, Stagno S, Pass RF, Britt WJ. Congenital and perinatal cytomegalovirus infections. Rev Infect Dis 1990;12(7 Suppl): 5745–5753.

American Academy of Pediatrics Committee on Infectious Diseases and Committee on Fetus and Newborn. Guidelines for prevention of group B streptococcal (GBS) infection by chemoprophylaxis. Pediatrics 1992;90:775–778.

American College of Obstetricians and Gynecologists. Antimicrobial therapy for obstetric patients. ACOG Technical Bulletin 117. Washington, DC: ACOG, 1988.

Centers for Disease Control. Rubella vaccination during pregnancy—United States, 1971–1988. MMWR 1989;38:289–293.

Corey L, Whitley RJ, Store EF, Mohan K. Difference between herpes simplex virus type 1 and type 2 neonatal encephalitis in neurological outcome. Lancet 1988;1:1–4.

Daffos F, Forestier F, Capella-Pavlovsky M, Thulliez P, Aufrant C, et al. Prenatal management of 746 pregnancies at risk for congenital toxoplasmosis. N Engl J Med 1988;318:271–275.

Dobbins JG, Stewart JA, Demmler GJ. Surveillance of congenital cytomegalovirus disease, 1990–1991. Collaborating Registry Group. MMWR CDC Surveill Summ 1992;41:35–39.

Dunlow S, Duff P. Prevalence of antibiotic-resistant uropathogens in obstetric patients with acute pyelonephritis. Obstet Gynecol 1990;76: 241–244.

Dunn DT, Newell ML, Ades AE, Peckham CS. Risk of human immunodeficiency virus type 1 transmission through breastfeeding. Lancet 1992;340:585–588.

European Collaborative Study: Mother-to-child transmission of HIV infection. Lancet 1988;2:1039–1043.

Foulon W, Naessen A, Mahler T, de Waele M, de Catte L, de Meuter F. Prenatal diagnosis of congenital toxoplasmosis. Obstet Gynecol 1990;76:769–772.

Fowler KB, Stagno S, Pass RF, Britt WJ, Boll TJ, Alford CA. The outcome of congenital infection in relation to maternal antibody status. N Engl J Med 1992;326:663–667.

Gibbs RS, Mead PB. Preventing neonatal herpes—current strategies. N Engl J Med 1992;326:946–947.

Hohlfeld P, Vial Y, Maillard-Brignon C, Vaudaux B, Fawer CL. Cytomegalovirus fetal infection: prenatal diagnosis. Obstet Gynecol 1991;78:615–618.

Miles SA, Balden E, Magpantay L, Wei L, Leiblein A, Hofheinz D, et al. Rapid serologic testing with immune-complex-dissociated HIV p[24] antigen for early detection of HIV infection in neonates. Southern California Pediatric AIDS Consortium. N Engl J Med 1993;328: 297–302.

Minkoff HL, DeHovitz JA. Care of women infected with the human immunodeficiency virus. JAMA 1991;266:2253–2258.

Muno ND, Sheppard S, Smithels RW, Holzel H, Jones G. Temporal relations between maternal rubella and congenital defects. Lancet 1987;2:201–204.

Prober CG, Hensleigh PA, Boucher FD, Yasukawa LL, Au DS, Arvin AM. Use of routine viral cultures at delivery to identify neonates exposed to herpes simplex virus. N Engl J Med 1988;318:887–891.

Prober CG, Sullender WM, Uasukawa LL, Au DS, Yeager AS, Arvin AM. Low risk of herpes simplex virus infections in neonates exposed to the virus at the time of vaginal delivery to mothers with recurrent genital herpes simplex virus infections. N Engl J Med 1987;316: 240–244.

Roos T, Martius J, Gross U, Schrod L. Systematic serologic screening for toxoplasmosis in pregnancy. Obstet Gynecol 1993;81:243–250.

Sperling RS, Stratton P. Treatment options for human immunodeficiency virus-infected pregnant women. Obstetric Gynecologic Working Group of the AIDS Clinical Trials Group of the National Institute of Allergy and Infectious Diseases. Obstet Gynecol 1992;79: 443–448.

Stagno S, Pass RF, Cloud G, Britt WJ, Henderson RE, Walton PD, et al. Primary cytomegalovirus infection in pregnancy: incidence, transmission to fetus and clinical outcome. JAMA 1986;256:1904–1908.

Yancey MK, Armer T, Clark P, Duff P. Assessment of rapid identification tests for genital carriage of group B streptococci. Obstet Gynecol 1992;80:1038–1047.

Fetal Surveillance Techniques

ULTRASONOGRAPHY

There is considerable controversy surrounding the issue of routine ultrasound screening in pregnancy. Arguments supporting the routine use of ultrasonography include the early detection of multiple gestation, improved dating, and the detection of unsuspected fetal anomalies in low-risk patients. If performed in the first trimester, ultrasonography may be useful in finding ectopic pregnancy or missed abortion before it is apparent clinically. However, screening ultrasonography in low-risk pregnancies does not improve perinatal outcome. There is no increased incidence of abnormalities among offspring with in utero exposure to ultrasonography, and long-term follow-up studies have also supported the safety of ultrasonography.

Gestational Age Determination

Many fetal body measurements can be determined which help to assess gestational age. Measurements to be taken at certain times of gestation are shown in Table 5.1. These measurements are limited by the obstetrician's or radiologist's experience and the quality of the ultrasonographic equipment. The earlier in gestation (26 weeks or less), the more accurate the dating parameter measurement. A biparietal diameter (BPD) or femur length (FL) measurement during the third trimester is often inaccurate. Accuracy is improved with more than one measurement with at least a 3-week interval between measurements. Confidence in dating is also improved when multiple dating parameters are measured and averaged to yield a composite ultrasonographically-predicted gestational age.

Table 5.1
Gestational Age Determination Using Fetal Anatomic Measurements[a]

Time of Gestation	Growth Pattern
Gestation sac 5–10 weeks	Increases 7 mm/week 2 cm at 6 weeks 5 cm at 10 weeks
Crown-rump length (CRL) 8–14 weeks	Increases 1 cm/week 1 cm at 7 weeks 7.5 cm at 14 weeks
Biparietal diameter (BPD) 15–40 weeks	Increases 3 mm/week between 16–29 weeks Increases <2 mm/week between 30–40 weeks
Cerebellum diameter 15–40 weeks	Increases 1 mm/week between 15–25 weeks Increases 2.5 mm/week between 26–35 weeks Increases 2 mm/week between 36–39 weeks
Head circumference (HC) 15–40 weeks	Increases 13 cm/week between 23–31 weeks Increases 1 cm/week between 32–40 weeks
Abdominal circumference (AC) 15–40 weeks	Increases 1.1 cm/week between 14–28 weeks Increases 1 cm/week between 29–40 weeks
Femur length (FL) 15–40 weeks	Increases 3 mm/week between 14–25 weeks Increases 2.3 mm/week between 26–40 weeks

[a] The accuracy (95% confidence interval) with one measurement is within 7 days at 16 weeks, 10 days at 17–26 weeks, 14 days at 27–28 weeks, and 21 days beyond 28 weeks.

The BPD is measured from the outer to the inner edges of the cranium. The cranium should appear oval, with no orbits in view, and with the falx cerebri at midline. The thalamus and the genu of the corpus callosum should also be visualized. In contrast, the abdominal circumference (AC) and occipitofrontal (OF) measurements are taken from outer edges.

Threatened Abortion

Visible milestones include seeing the gestational sac as early as 5 weeks, the embryo at 7 weeks, and fetal heart motion at 8 weeks.

A blighted ovum or missed abortion is to be suspected if there is no growth or a regression of the sac over a 2-week period and no fetal limb or heart motion is seen after the 8th week. However, if fetal cardiac activity is observed, the probability of continued pregnancy without abortion is greater than 94%.

The main advantage of transvaginal scanning in this circumstance is the proximity of the transducer to the organ of interest, which allows the use of higher frequency. Transvaginal ultrasonography has rendered obsolete the need for a full bladder because, by transducer location, transvaginal ultrasonography reduces or eliminates the problems posed by obesity or the presence of bowel.

Fetal Malformation

As more ultrasound examinations are performed on pregnant women, a higher proportion of major fetal malformations will be detected before delivery. A fetal malformation may be seen for the first time during a genetic amniocentesis or may be suggested by polyhydramnios or oligohydramnios. Visualization of internal structures (cerebral ventricles, cerebellum, cisterna magna, four-chambered heart, heart valves, stomach, bowel, kidneys, bladder) along with surface anatomy (head, neck, limbs, bone texture and contour, spine, male genitalia) is possible. Under most circumstances, it is best to have the ultrasound examination repeated by a highly experienced ultrasonographer for purposes of documentation, education, and additional useful information.

When fetal malformations are suspected, it is suggested that the ultrasound examination be performed in the presence of a staff neonatologist or pediatrician who can then provide further counseling to the parents, plan for the care of an infant deemed salvageable, and discuss the case with the appropriate pediatric surgical service.

Uterine Size Less than Dates

Conditions to consider include inaccurate dates, intrauterine growth retardation (IUGR), oligohydramnios (secondary to IUGR, infection, ruptured membranes, renal anomaly), and fetal descent into the pelvis. Delayed fetal growth should initially be suspected when a bimanual examination shows the uterine size to be less than estimated gestational age.

Suspected IUGR

The following findings on ultrasound examination may strengthen the suspicion of IUGR or permit a more accurate dating of the pregnancy.

Biparietal Diameter (BPD)

1. The BPD measurement is frequently not helpful and can even be misleading in the evaluation of IUGR, because fetal head growth is usually relatively spared in this condition
2. Consider microcephaly if the body size and cerebellum are appropriate but BPD and HC measurements are small
3. Look for a low profile or late flattening pattern of the skull
4. IUGR is rare when BPD is more than 50th percentile for gestational age

Oligohydramnios

1. A normal amount of amniotic fluid is unusual in pregnancies complicated by IUGR
2. Failure to observe a pocket of fluid measuring at least 2 cm (in perpendicular dimensions), or an amniotic fluid index (AFI) of less than 5, suggests oligohydramnios, which is present in approximately half of all cases with IUGR

Femur Length (FL)

1. Useful if dating is uncertain or if dwarfism or IUGR are suspected
2. Need to compare with BPD measurements
3. After 22 weeks the ratio of femur length to abdominal circumference (FL:AC) is equal to $0.22 \pm .02$ in normally growing fetuses. A FL:AC of more than 0.24 is suggestive of IUGR

Head Circumference/Abdominal Circumference (HC/AC)

1. Ratio decreases with gestational age
2. Equivalent measurements at 36 weeks
3. Asymmetric IUGR in 60% of cases if HC/AC value is in 95th percentile for age
4. Failure of the AC to increase by at least 10 mm over a 14-day period is highly suggestive of IUGR

Estimated Fetal Weight

1. Accurate gestational age determination is necessary
2. Measurements of the BPD or FL and AC are necessary for weight prediction using published tables
3. Less accurate if there is oligohydramnios, multifetal gestation, fetal malpresentation, maternal obesity, or fetal weight more than 2500 g

Uterine Size Greater than Dates

Conditions to consider if uterine size is greater than predicted include inaccurate dates, large-for-gestational-age (LGA) fetus, multifetal gestation, polyhydramnios, pelvic mass (uterine fibroid, ovarian tumor), and hydatidiform mole. These abnormalities may be suspected during the bimanual examination and confirmed by ultrasound examination.

Multifetal Gestation

1. Usually can see two sacs in the first trimester, but 20% of twins seen on early ultrasound scan "vanish" or regress spontaneously
2. Three percent of twins may be monoamniotic (1 sac only), which is associated with a 50% perinatal mortality from umbilical cord entanglement, twin-twin transfusion, birth trauma, congenital anomalies, and conjoined twins
3. After 24 weeks, repeat scans every 3–6 weeks to search for:
   a. BPD growth—in normally growing twins is essentially the same as for singletons
   b. Intertwin growth discordance (25% weight difference)—search for differences in BPDs (more than 5 mm), HCs (more than 5%), ACs (more than 5%), or weights (more than 15%). Prognosis is poorer if discordance is present before 28 weeks
   c. Twin-twin transfusion—differences in amniotic fluid volume, fetal size, fetal heart rate
   d. Anomalies
   e. Biophysical profile—breathing patterns, limb motion, muscle tone, amniotic fluid volume

Third Trimester Bleeding

Placenta Previa

1. Placental location and margin may be seen in almost all pregnancies

2. Posterior placenta may be shadowed by fetus
3. Exact localization of cervix is necessary but may be difficult
4. Need postvoid film if full maternal bladder (may "push" anterior placenta toward cervix)
5. Placenta "migrates" during pregnancy due to development of lower uterine segment; consequently, most second trimester previas disappear by term
6. If central previa is found during the first half of pregnancy, repeat scan in third trimester

Placental Abruption

1. Very difficult to diagnose with ultrasound
2. May appear as an echo-free area behind a convex placenta, a thickened placenta because of a heterogeneous clot, or a rounded elevation of membranes by the clot
3. Sonolucent area behind the placenta is usually a normal second trimester artifact
4. A thickened placenta (more than 5 cm) may also result from diabetes, Rh isoimmunization, syphilis, nonimmune fetal hydrops, chorioangioma, or trophoblastic disease

Additional Uses

1. Before, during, or after special procedures: amniocentesis, cervical cerclage, fetal transfusion, external version of breech fetus, locating the fetal heart during heart rate monitoring, locating placenta before cesarean section
2. Fetal presentation determination
3. Intrauterine fetal demise (IUFD) diagnosis: no fetal heart or limb motion, collapsed cranium
4. Localizing fetal heart and other body parts during the delivery of a second twin
5. Visualizing intrauterine cavity when delayed postpartum or postabortal hemorrhage
6. Determining fetal sex by visualizing penis as early as 16 weeks
7. Assessing fetal maturity (biometry, placental grade) as described in Chapter 1

DOPPLER FLOW STUDIES

The combination of real-time sonography and Doppler equipment permits a noninvasive measurement of fetal blood flow, especially in the umbilical vessels and the descending aorta. Sonographic localization of the umbilical arteries in the fetal abdomen is followed by Doppler measurement of blood velocity. This investigational technique may improve the accuracy of prediction of physiologic reserve, especially for high-risk pregnancies such as those with hypertension or fetal growth retardation in which chronic uteroplacental insufficiency is likely.

Diminished umbilical artery blood flow may be an early sign of fetal compromise and placental vascular resistance. An elevated umbilical artery systolic/diastolic (S/D) ratio may offer insight into fetal compromise. The absence of blood flow diastole or reverse flow in diastole reflects extreme placental vascular residue and is considered ominous. Doppler flow studies may provide a reflection of the amount of oxygenation, since the fetus, placenta, and umbilical cord have a great capacity to shunt blood to vital organ centers (brain, heart, adrenal glands) during periods of relative hypoxia. Whether reduced umbilical blood flow is the cause or result of chronic fetal hypoxia is unclear at this time.

M-Mode Echocardiography

Imaging the fetal heart and directly measuring parameters that reflect myocardial contractility and ventricular size are possible as early as 18 weeks' gestation with real-time directed M-mode echocardiography. The ability to noninvasively assess fetal cardiac disorders can provide information which is useful in appropriate management of the pregnancy and delivery and in planning specialized neonatal care. This technique also has potential use in the prenatal investigation of fetal cardiac spatial anatomy and cardiac rhythm disturbances.

The standard echocardiogram involves viewing the long axis, great vessels, short axis, four chambers, and aortic arch. Fetal cardiac failure can be detected, its etiology can be better clarified, and serious cardiac malformations may be excluded. Dysrhythmias may also be better characterized in the atria and ventricles. Adjacent structural abnormalities that may impinge on cardiac function include, but are not limited to, intrathoracic cysts or tumors, diaphragmatic hernias, and abdominal wall defects.

ANTEPARTUM FETAL HEART RATE TESTING (AFHRT)

Antepartum fetal heart rate testing (AFHRT) has gained popularity in the biophysical assessment of fetal well-being. Data are readily interpretable and provide timely results. The nonstress test (NST) measures indirectly the intactness of the fetal autonomic and central nervous systems during fetal movement, while the contraction stress test (CST) reflects the respiratory and nutritive reserve (baroreceptors and chemoreceptors) of the fetoplacental unit during the stress of spontaneous or oxytocin-induced uterine contractions.

These tests are quite useful in predicting fetal well-being. Favorable results are associated with a low probability of antepartum stillbirth. Any suspicious result requires a thorough clinical reassessment, good clinical judgment, and additional testing as necessary. In general, the nonstress test has replaced the contraction stress test as the initial FHR test. It is a test of convenience, however, and any suspicious finding requires a CST (or repeat NST) later that day.

Nonstress tests are performed during outpatient visits in most cases. The tests may be performed at any time during the third trimester (28 weeks or more) with the realization that an abnormal result requires follow-up. Most tests are usually not performed until 32 weeks or later.

These tests are indicated when there is any suggestion of uteroplacental insufficiency. Pregnancies complicated by postdates, discordant twins, diabetes, suspected IUGR, preeclampsia, chronic hypertension, collagen vascular disease, or documented fetal inactivity are associated with chronic uteroplacental insufficiency and would benefit from FHR testing.

Techniques

NST

1. Place patient in a semi-Fowler's or lateral tilt position
2. Determine FHR variability and reactivity in association with fetal and uterine activity
3. Instruct mother on fetal movement recording

CST

1. Same as steps 1–3 above
2. If there is no spontaneous uterine or fetal activity, ask the mother to gently palpate a nipple to promote uterine contractions

3. In the unlikely event that nipple stimulation does not result in an adequate contraction pattern, begin oxytocin infusion (0.5–1.0 mU/minute). The dose should be doubled every 15 minutes until there are at least three contractions every 10 minutes, repetitive late decelerations, or hypertonic uterine contractions

4. After discontinuing the oxytocin, observe for any persisting uterine contractions

Interpretation

Standard definitions of a nonreactive or reactive NST and a negative, suspicious, or positive CST are shown in Table 5.2. Considerations during test interpretation should include physician experience, prolonged maternal supine positioning, maternal obesity, polyhydramnios, excess fetal activity or inactivity, physiologic fetal rest period (20 minutes to 1 hour), abnormal fetal lie, and instability of any underlying complication(s).

Nonstress test results are not influenced by maternal weight, caffeinated beverages, ambulation, or a recent meal. Instead, FHR reactivity is more dependent on the fetal activity pattern and the primary underlying complication. Preterm rupture of the membranes does not affect the reliability of NST results.

A nonreactive NST requires more prolonged testing, vibroacoustic stimulation (VAS) using an artificial larynx device for 3

Table 5.2
Interpretation of Antepartum Fetal Heart Rate Tests

NST	
Reactive:	2 or more adequate FHR accelerations (15 beats/minute above baseline, lasting 15 seconds or more) during a 20–40-minute period
Nonreactive:	0–1 adequate accelerations during the 20–40-minute test period
CST	
Negative:	No late deceleration with uterine contractions (3 in 10 minutes)
Suspicious:	Any decelerations which are not persistent (coincident with 50% or less of adequate contractions)
Positive:	Repetitive late decelerations (coincident with more than 50% of contractions)

seconds above the fetus, or a CST. If the NST result is reactive, it is generally safe to wait up to 1 week before repeating the test. However, any acute change in the underlying antepartum complication (such as worsening diabetes), an umbilical cord accident, or a placental abruption may lead to acute fetal compromise. Decelerations of the FHR may be related to maternal positioning or hypotension. If decelerations are repetitive despite a reactive result, a CST is indicated because there may be cord compression or fetal hypoxia.

A CST is contraindicated in the presence of a vertical uterine scar, prior premature labor, multifetal gestation, third trimester bleeding, or preterm rupture of the membranes. If a NST is nonreactive and a CST is contraindicated, a fetal biophysical profile (fetal breathing movement, fetal muscle tone and motion of limbs, amniotic fluid volume, and placental morphology) using ultrasonography should be performed.

A positive CST is more likely to be truly worrisome if a nonreactive pattern was present, a deceleration was seen on a prior NST, the fetus remains inactive, or the obstetric or medical condition is deteriorating. A cesarean section is not absolutely necessary after a positive CST, however. Depending on the clinical condition, a trial of labor with an early amniotomy and internal monitoring may be preferred.

BIOPHYSICAL PROFILE

The earliest attempts to evaluate fetal well-being by ultrasound were based on anatomic considerations. The vitality of the fetal central nervous system may be inferred indirectly from heart rate testing or movement charting. Because antepartum FHR testing methods are time-consuming and may yield falsely positive results, obstetricians have included ultrasound visualizations in certain circumstances to more thoroughly assess fetal status. Evaluation of fetal activity, muscle tone, and breathing movements also provides useful information in predicting fetal well-being. However, each parameter considered alone may be falsely abnormal, and results may be unreliable in predicting fetal outcome.

A "biophysical profile" (BPP) includes results of the nonstress test and observation of fetal activity, fetal muscle tone, fetal breathing, and amniotic fluid volume. Determination of a composite score is shown in Table 5.3. Each biophysical variable is given a score of 2 if normal or 0 if abnormal. Therefore, the max-

Table 5.3
Technique and Interpretation of Biophysical Profile Scoring

Biophysical Variable	Normal (score = 2)	Abnormal (score = 0)
Fetal breathing movements	One or more episodes of ≥30 seconds in 30 minutes	Absent or no episode of ≥30 seconds in 30 minutes
Gross body movements	Three or more discrete body/limb movements in 30 minutes (episodes of active continuous movement considered as single movement)	Two or fewer episodes of body/limb movements in 30 minutes
Fetal tone	One or more episodes of active extension with return to flexion of fetal limb(s) or trunk; opening and closing of hand considered normal tone	Either slow extension with return to partial flexion, or movement of limb in full extension or absent fetal movement
Nonstress test	Reactive pattern	Nonreactive pattern
Amniotic fluid volume	One or more vertical pockets of fluid measuring ≥2 cm	Less than one 2-cm pocket

imum possible score is 10 and the lowest possible score is 0. Studies have shown that this profile provides a better prediction of a nonreassuring fetal status, low 5-minute Apgar score, and perinatal mortality than any other method used alone.

If the composite score is 8–10, the test may be repeated in 1 week unless the underlying complication worsens. There is no indication for promptly delivering the fetus if the score is 8 or greater. If the composite score is 4–6, there is cause for concern, and delivery should be considered if fetal pulmonary maturity is demonstrated. A score of 0–2 would require the pregnancy to be delivered without delay.

AMNIOTIC FLUID VOLUME

Amniotic fluid volume can be estimated during an ultrasound examination as normal, abnormally increased (polyhydramnios), or abnormally decreased (oligohydramnios). A semi-quantitative way to describe amniotic fluid volume is the amniotic fluid index. The amniotic fluid index is calculated by dividing the uterus into four quadrants as defined by the linea nigra and the umbilicus.

In each of the four quadrants the largest vertical pocket of amniotic fluid free of umbilical cord and fetal parts is measured, and
these four numbers are added together. Although the normal
values vary by gestational age, values of 24 or greater and 5 or less
are always abnormal.

Many centers perform a modified BPP rather than complete
testing. Most authorities agree that these are the two most significant predictors of fetal well-being. Furthermore, most would
agree that in many clinical situations, such as postdate pregnancy, a decreased amniotic fluid volume is an indication for delivery even if there is a reactive NST or an otherwise normal BPP.

FETAL MOVEMENT CHARTING

The monitoring of fetal activity is a convenient surveillance technique in high-risk pregnancies. Although not a direct test of placental function, it serves as a signal of impending fetal jeopardy
and possibly death. The maternal awareness of a recent decrease
or loss of propulsive fetal motion has been traditionally regarded
as a warning sign, especially in pregnancies complicated by hypertension, diabetes, or Rh isoimmunization, where chronic
uteroplacental insufficiency is suspected. No costs are incurred
when this technique is used outside of the clinic setting.

Technique

Many testing schemes have been developed, and the superiority
of any one method has not been clearly established. Described
below is a daily fetal movement charting (DFMC) technique
which we have found to be practical.

1. Fetal movement charting may begin at any time during the
   second half of pregnancy; however, it is particularly useful
   during the third trimester.
2. The patient is asked to rest, preferably in a lateral recumbent
   position, in a quiet room. The recording may be discontinued after 10 movements are counted (the "count-to-10 technique").
3. Strong or propulsive fetal movements ("rollovers," "balling
   up," "kicks," but not "flutters" or "hiccups") are recorded on
   a standard fetal movement chart. Clusters of movements
   should be counted as one.
4. The patient should also be asked to report any concern about

a significant decrease in the total number or in the strength of fetal movements.

5. A new chart should be given to the patient with each return visit, and the previous chart should be placed in the prenatal record.

Interpretation

Most fetuses are perceived to move 10 times within 30 minutes. This rate does not decrease significantly near term. As long as the fetus is healthy, this average does not decrease markedly despite the presence of an antepartum complication. It should be remembered that each fetus has its own activity pattern, and no two pregnancies are alike.

A fetus is considered to be active if 10 movements are perceived per hour. Fetal inactivity is defined on our service as fewer than 10 movements perceived per hour for 2 consecutive hours. An excessively active fetus (40 movements or more per hour over a prolonged period) is not a worrisome sign.

Evaluation of Fetal Inactivity

The decision to intervene in the presence of fetal inactivity should not be based on fetal movement studies alone. Any patient complaining of a decrease in fetal activity on routine questioning should be instructed to chart fetal movement. A reported cessation or documented fetal inactivity should be a warning which requires further investigation, although a seemingly slow but continuously moving fetus may be doing quite well. An NST or modified BPP may be used to evaluate fetal inactivity. In addition, described in Table 5.4 is an ultrasonographic means of evaluating the fetus perceived to be inactive.

FETAL LUNG MATURITY TESTS

Respiratory distress syndrome (RDS), or more specifically, hyaline membrane disease, is found in approximately 15% of infants with birth weights of 2500 g or less. Prevention of RDS may be unavoidable if the patient is delivered prematurely for obstetric or medical complications. Respiratory insufficiency results from a deficiency of surfactant, a material that provides a stable surface tension within the alveolar spaces. Alveolar surface tension is diminished with insufficient surfactant, and the lungs collapse during expiration.

Table 5.4
Ultrasonographic Evaluation of Fetus Perceived to be Inactive

Real-time ultrasonography	*Vigorous movement seen*
Determine viability	Reassure
Observe for fetal cardiac motion, lower limb and trunk motion, breathing activity	Assess patient's ability to perceive fetal motion using ultrasound
Search for a malformation	Resume fetal movement counting and other fetal assessment methods
Characterize placental morphology and amniotic fluid volume	*Lack of vigorous movement seen*
	Further testing by FHR or BPP
	No movement
	Consider delivery

Surfactant is composed of phospholipid compounds that include phosphatidylcholine (lecithin), phosphatidylglycerol (PG), phosphatidylinositol (PI), and disaturated phosphatidylcholine (DSPC). Although other amniotic fluid tests have been used in predicting fetal maturity, the most reliable means of quantitating pulmonary surfactant involves a measurement of these abundant phospholipids.

Types of Tests

Lecithin/Sphingomyelin Ratio (L/S)

This ratio is the most standardized and widely used determination of fetal pulmonary maturity. The assay technique is critical, since variations in centrifugation, activation of thin layer plates for separation of phospholipids, moisture, and densitometer precision affect test results.

As a general rule, a mature L/S ratio (2:1 or greater) is predictive of fetal lung maturity (and lack of subsequent neonatal RDS) in 97% of cases. A ratio of 1.5–1.9 is associated with respiratory distress in half of infants, while a value below 1.5 is associated with a 73% risk of respiratory distress. These percentages vary depending on the laboratory and clinical criteria used in the interpretation of respiratory distress.

Phosphatidylglycerol (PG)

This phospholipid may be measured despite the presence of meconium or blood in the amniotic fluid or after preterm rupture of the membranes. This determination is useful and reliable in conjunction with L/S measurements in pregnancies with Rh isoimmunization or diabetes in which a "mature" L/S ratio may be erroneous and misleading. Phosphatidylglycerol does not generally appear until 35 weeks' gestation but increases in quantity until the 40th week.

Other Tests

Although less often reported, other reliable tests to assess fetal lung maturity include:

1. Optical density measurements at 650 nm (a value of 0.15 or greater correlates with a mature L/S ratio)
2. Microviscosity from the high relative lipid concentration of amniotic fluid
3. "Shake" test or foam stability index (FSI) to determine whether pulmonary surfactant is present in adequate amounts to generate a stable foam in the present of ethanol
4. Measurement of disaturated phosphatidylcholine (DSPC)
5. Monoclonal antibody testing against phosphatidylglycerol

In all tests, a positive test result is reassuring, but falsely decreased or "immature" results are frequently reported. An advantage of some of these tests is that they may be performed without sophisticated laboratory facilities.

General Recommendations

The L/S ratio has been widely recognized as the "gold standard" for assessing fetal lung maturity. If there is a condition that would suggest a falsely mature L/S value or if the test result is borderline, the L/S ratio alone may be inadequate. Two conditions commonly associated with a falsely mature L/S ratio are diabetes mellitus and Rh isoimmunization, in which there is a relative fetal hyperinsulinemia. The use of another test would be recommended in such cases.

These test results should be used only as additional information when preterm pregnancy intervention or repeat cesarean section is anticipated. A laboratory result should not replace good clinical judgment when the management of a high-risk pregnancy is considered.

Examination of the infant is essential to assess the predictability of the amniotic fluid test. Evidence of respiratory distress includes definite clinical findings (tachypnea, nasal flaring, chest retractions) and chest x-ray findings (reticulogranular pattern), and the need for supplemental oxygen therapy.

Suggested Readings

American College of Obstetricians and Gynecologists. Ultrasonography in pregnancy. ACOG Technical Bulletin 187. Washington, DC: ACOG, 1993.

Druzin ML, Fox A, Kogut E, Carlson C. The relationship of the nonstress test to gestational age. Am J Obstet Gynecol 1985;153:386–389.

Druzin ML. Antepartum fetal heart rate monitoring: state of the art. Clin Perinatol 1989;16:627–642.

Ewigman BG, Crane JP, Frigoletto FD, LeFevre ML, Bain RP, McNellis D. Effect of prenatal ultrasound screening on perinatal outcome: RADIUS study group. N Engl J Med 1993;329:821–827.

Moore TR, Cayle JE. The Amniotic fluid index in normal human pregnancy. Am J Obstet Gynecol 1990;162:1168–1173.

Smith CV, Phelan JP, Platt LD, Broussard P, Paul RH. Fetal acoustic stimulation testing, II: a randomized clinical comparison with the nonstress test. Am J Obstet Gynecol 1986;155:131–134.

U.S. Department of Health and Human Services, Public Health Service, National Institutes of Health. Diagnostic ultrasound imaging in pregnancy. NIH publication no. 84–667. Washington, DC: U.S. Government Printing Office, 1984.

Chapter 6

Fetal Disorders

INTRAUTERINE GROWTH RETARDATION

An infant whose birth weight is less than the 10th percentile for that gestational age is classified as having undergone intrauterine growth retardation (IUGR). Depending on the population, 5–7% of infants will be growth retarded. These infants are at increased risk for perinatal mortality, neonatal acidosis, hypoglycemia, hypocalcemia, and polycythemia. The lower the birth weight percentile, the greater the likelihood of fetal jeopardy.

Growth retardation may be characterized further as being symmetric (early onset, usually from a genetic or teratogenic insult) or asymmetric (late onset, usually due to inadequate fetal nutrition either from inadequate maternal nutrition or diseases limiting placental transfer of nutrients). Infants with asymmetric growth retardation usually have a good long-term prognosis if neonatal complications are adequately controlled, while the prognosis for a symmetrically growth retarded infant is more guarded. Etiologies of intrauterine growth retardation are listed in Table 6.1.

Diagnosis

Clinical Evaluation

Most truly growth retarded infants have an obstetric, medical, nutritional, or social history suggesting a risk for IUGR. A knowledge of gestational age and a high index of suspicion are necessary. Abnormally low fundal height measurements have an 86% sensitivity and a 90% specificity for IUGR.

Ultrasound Evaluation

Ultrasound has enhanced our ability to evaluate potentially growth retarded infants. While many tests have been proposed,

Table 6.1
Examples of Causative Factors of Intrauterine Growth Retardation

Chromosomal	*Maternal vascular disease*
Turner's syndrome	Toxemia
Trisomy 21, 18, 13	Chronic hypertension
	Renal disease
Drugs, chemicals	Cyanotic heart disease
Heroin	Severe diabetes (Class D, F, R)
Methadone	Collagen vascular disease
Cocaine	
Alcohol	*Maternal anemia*
Phenytoin	Iron deficiency
Tobacco	Folate deficiency
	Hemoglobinopathy
Infection	
TORCH agents	*Other*
	Maternal malnutrition
Antepartum hemorrhage	Multifetal gestation
Abruptio placentae	
Placenta previa	

the optimal diagnostic accuracy is obtained by employing multiple ultrasound parameters.

The biparietal diameter (BPD) tends to remain in the same growth quartile (less than the 25th percentile, the 25th to the 75th, or more than the 75th). A drop from the upper groups to the low group is highly suggestive of growth retardation. The diagnosis is unlikely if the BPD is greater than the 50th percentile. Failure of the BPD to increase over 3 weeks is a poor prognostic sign. Additionally, a delay in biparietal diameter, head circumference, or abdominal circumference in relation to the cerebellar diameter is indicative of IUGR.

A head/abdominal circumference ratio greater than the 95th percentile suggests asymmetric IUGR. An increase in the abdominal circumference of less than 10 mm over a 14-day period may be the most sensitive ultrasound marker for IUGR. Frequently, this is associated with a femur length/abdominal circumference ratio greater than the 95th percentile (i.e., greater than 0.24).

Many pregnancies complicated by IUGR have decreased quantities of amniotic fluid. Although most demonstrate an amniotic fluid index (AFI) of 5 or more, those pregnancies with intact membranes and with lower measurements are commonly found to have an IUGR fetus.

Amniotic Fluid Maturity Evaluation

Many IUGR infants demonstrate accelerated pulmonary maturity. This fact is useful in differentiating the truly IUGR from the misdated pregnancy. The diagnosis of IUGR is more strongly suspected when phosphatidylglycerol is detected and the BPD measures less than 8.7 cm.

Management

Medical Treatment

1. Frequent reclining on left side
2. Stop smoking
3. High caloric diet (2500 calories/day)
4. Fetal movement charting in combination with either NSTs, CSTs, or biophysical profiles
5. Ultrasound scan every 3–4 weeks until third trimester, then as often as weekly for a modified biophysical assessment
6. Weekly or semi-weekly exams after 32 weeks

Appropriately Timed Interruption of Pregnancy

Several investigators advocate delivery when the fetus is mature (lecithin/sphingomyelin (L/S) ratio greater than 2, or phosphatidylglycerol (PG) present). This form of management removes the fetus from the hostile environment but increases the risk of cesarean section. Others feel that the benefit of this routine approach has not been documented. As cesarean section rates are high, the patient should instead be followed until there is either a more favorable Bishop cervix score, abnormal fetal biophysical assessment result, or worsening of any maternal disease.

Delivery of the immature fetus, despite an absence of risk factors or a stable underlying condition, is indicated only if antepartum tests are clearly abnormal. If a test result is suspicious, the test should be repeated within 24 hours as long as the condition is stable. Corticosteroid therapy is recommended if delivery is anticipated before 34 weeks or if the L/S ratio is known to be less than 2:1.

Careful Management of Labor

1. Lateral position of the recumbent mother
2. Oxygen to mother by face mask or nasal prongs as necessary
3. Electronic fetal monitoring; selective scalp pH sampling if appropriate
4. Be prepared to perform a cesarean section if a nonreassuring fetal status worsens
5. Early clamping of umbilical cord, since these fetuses tend to be hemoconcentrated
6. Obtain umbilical artery blood gases determination

Meticulous Neonatal Care

1. Pediatrician in attendance
2. Orderly resuscitation
3. Diagnosis and management of hypoglycemia, hypocalcemia, hyperviscosity, meconium aspiration, renal problems (if asphyxia), altered thermoregulation
4. Proper nutrition to improve growth
5. Suspect genetic or infectious etiology if no other known risk factors
6. Placenta for careful histologic examination if growth delay is severe, unexplained, or accompanied by preterm delivery.

FETAL MACROSOMIA

A macrosomic fetus is defined as having a weight in the upper 10th percentile at term (greater than 4000 g). Clinical suspicion is necessary, since the disorder is associated with diabetes mellitus, Rh isoimmunization, and postdate gestation. Mechanical difficulties and trauma during labor and delivery should be anticipated.

Diagnosis

Estimation of fetal weight is dependent on clinical and ultrasound examinations. A weekly bimanual pelvic examination is useful within 2 weeks of the estimated due date to determine the presenting part, condition of the cervix, adequacy of the pelvis, and estimation of fetal weight. Ultrasound examinations are limited in diagnosing fetal macrosomia but may permit measuring the femur length, biparietal diameter, abdominal circumference, and amniotic fluid volume. A BPD greater than 10.5 cm at term is strongly suggestive of fetal macrosomia or hydrocephaly, and a chest-biparietal diameter difference of 1.4 cm or greater is suggestive of fetal macrosomia in a diabetic pregnancy.

Management

When a large-for-gestational-age fetus is suspected, glucose tolerance testing is indicated, and the maternal blood type and antibody screen should be determined. In the presence of gestational onset diabetes, insulin therapy and closer glucose monitoring are recommended as early in gestation as possible as an attempt to lower the birth weight. Other conditions associated with fetal macrosomia include large parents, a space-occupying anomaly, α-thalassemia, nonimmune fetal hydrops, postdates, and Beckwith-Wiedemann syndrome. Many infants are healthy and have no obvious reason for their large size.

Macrosomia is associated with an increased risk of a traumatic vaginal delivery such as shoulder dystocia, brachial plexus injury, clavicular fracture, and maternal soft tissue injury. Any pregnancy in which macrosomia is suspected should be monitored closely during labor using internal uterine catheters and fetal heart rate monitoring devices. A cesarean section is recommended if there is early evidence of failure to descend adequately during labor, fetal compromise, or breech presentation. Conflict remains about the value of routine cesarean section without a trial of labor for suspected fetal macrosomia alone if an especially large fetus (greater than 4500 g) is anticipated or if the fetus is 4000 g or more in a diabetic pregnancy.

If a macrosomic infant is delivered, it should be followed carefully for hypoglycemia. Determination of maternal serum hemoglobin A_{Ic} is recommended to screen for any previous glucose intolerance.

NONIMMUNE FETAL HYDROPS

Fetal hydrops not related to maternal isoimmunization was first described in 1943. The widespread application of diagnostic ultrasound scanning has resulted in a dramatic upsurge in the antenatal diagnosis. Causes of nonimmune fetal hydrops are listed in Table 6.2. While the prognosis is usually poor (90% perinatal mortality) because of pulmonary hypoplasia or coexisting major anomalies,

Table 6.2
Etiology of Nonimmune Fetal Hydrops

Fetal
  Hematologic
    Fetomaternal or twin-twin
      transfusion, α-thalassemia,
      G6PD deficiency
  Multiple gestation with parasitic fetus
  Cardiovascular
    Congenital heart disease
      (ASD, VSD, hypoplastic
      left heart, pulmonary insufficiency,
      intracardiac tumor, Ebstein's
      anomaly, subaortic stenosis,
      tricuspid valvular dysplasia,
      tetralogy of Fallot, premature
      closure of foreman ovale)
    Tachyarrhythmias (SVT, arterial
      flutter, heart block)
    Fibroelastosis
    Myocarditis
  Pulmonary
    Cystic adenomatoid malformation
    Pulmonary lymphangiectasia
    Pulmonary hypoplasia

Idiopathic
  Renal
    Congenital nephrosis
    Renal dysplasia
    Renal vein thrombosis
  Intrauterine infection
    TORCH
    Parvovirus
    Leptospirosis
    Congenital hepatitis
    Chagas' disease
  Miscellaneous
    Meconium peritonitis
    Fetal neuroblastoma
    Small bowel volvulus
    Disseminated intravascular
      coagulation
    Chromosomal—trisomy 18,
      trisomy 21, Turner's
      syndrome, XX/XY
      mosaicism
    Achondroplasia
    Tuberous sclerosis
    Storage disease
    Polycystic ovaries
    Sacral teratoma

Placental
  Umbilical vein thrombosis
  Chorionic vein thrombosis
  Chorioangioma

Maternal
  Diabetes mellitus

some infants may be salvaged with careful antepartum surveillance involving the fetus, placenta, or mother. Shown in Table 6.3 are tests to be performed in the antepartum and neonatal periods.

Therapy

Before 24 weeks

Treat any fetal cardiac arrhythmia and offer termination if any chromosome abnormality or potential life-threatening anomaly is present.

Between 24 and 32 Weeks

Treat any fetal cardiac arrhythmia. Corticosteroid therapy may enhance fetal lung maturity. Deliver if hydrops (pleural or pericardial effusion) worsens.

After 32 Weeks

Deliver in the event of fetal lung maturity, further fetal compromise, or progressive hydrops.

Table 6.3
Tests to Perform in the Antepartum and Neonatal Periods

Antepartum	*Neonatal*
Accurate gestational dating	Complete blood count with differential
Blood type and antibody screen	
Serologic test for syphilis (VDRL)	Blood type and Coombs' test
TORCH screen	VDRL
Kleihauer-Betke test	Serum IgM level
Diabetes screen	Liver function tests
Ultrasonography, serial (chest, abdomen, neck, surface anatomy, placenta, umbilical cord, amniotic fluid volume)	Renal function tests
	ECG, echocardiography
	Chromosomal analysis
	Cultures (bacterial and viral), TORCH screen
Fetal echocardiography	X-rays (chest, abdomen, long bones, skull)
Nonstress tests	
Fetal movement charting	Diagnostic paracentesis and/or lung thoracentesis
Amniotic fluid for viral cultures and karyotype (if delivery not anticipated soon), maturation (if beyond 32 weeks)	Placental anatomy and histologic evaluation
	Retrieve blood samples before any transfusions

Before Delivery

Notify pediatrician well in advance of delivery. Expect birth asphyxia, anemia, and hypovolemia, and plan on resuscitation.

POLYHYDRAMNIOS

Polyhydramnios is defined as 2 liters or more of amniotic fluid. The incidence is reported to be 0.4% of all pregnancies. The etiology is variable, but conditions are similar to those contributing to nonimmune fetal hydrops (Table 6.2). Diabetes, isoimmunization, multifetal gestation, and congenital abnormalities are frequently present. In more than half of cases no definite cause is identifiable, but many malformations associated with polyhydramnios may be visualized prenatally.

An acute rather than chronic onset has a less favorable prognosis. The more severe the polyhydramnios, the higher the probability of a fetal anomaly. Clinical suspicion is best confirmed by ultrasound examination. Methods to evaluate the mother and fetus are listed in Table 6.4.

Antepartum Management

1. If etiology is unknown, wait until L/S is 2 or greater. Concentrations of amniotic fluid PG, creatinine, etc., may be falsely low.

Table 6.4
Evaluation of Polyhydramnios

Maternal
    Accurate pregnancy dating
    1-hour post 50-g glucola diabetes screen (3-hour GTT if abnormal)
    Irregular antibody screen
    Observe weight gain and fundal height
Fetal
    Ultrasound scan to rule out multifetal gestation and to examine:
        Head size: BPD, ventricle-to-hemisphere ratio
        Fetal swallowing and neck width
        Chest cavity (heart rate, valve action, pericardial effusion, pleural effusion, breathing motion, thoracic mass)
    Abdomen (masses, bowel atresia, wall masses, kidney outline, bladder filling)
    Skeletal system (especially vertebral volume and limb length)
    Echocardiography

---

2. Perform amniocentesis if the fetus is immature and there is maternal respiratory compromise, premature labor, or marked uterine distension. Using an 18-gauge spinal needle or angiocath and an intravenous infusion set connected to a sterile container (such as a thoracentesis bottle) on the floor, 500–2000 mL of fluid should be removed slowly at approximately 500 mL/hour. A higher gauge needle should not be used, because drainage may be too slow or the system may become clotted. Fetal heart rate monitoring should be performed after the amniocentesis (immediately if blood is retrieved). The amniocentesis may be repeated, usually in 1–3 weeks, depending on the patient's symptoms.

3. An alternative to repeated transabdominal amniocenteses with withdrawal of fluid is the therapeutic use of prostaglandin synthetase inhibitor. This approach is based on the known decreased rate of urinary flow in the premature fetus exposed to indomethacin. Mothers have been treated with indomethacin 2.2–3.0 mg/kg body weight per day, either orally or rectally. The treatment is started between 22 and 31 gestational weeks and continued for 2–11 weeks (usually 3 weeks or less) until the 35th week. Fetal urine output, observed by serial bladder ultrasonography, has been found to decline significantly, especially during the first week of therapy.

4. Bed rest in lateral recumbent position.

5. Frequent examinations are necessary for measurement of maternal abdominal circumference, fundal height, weight, and for signs of congestive heart failure.

6. Frequent maternal serum electrolyte and protein determinations should be made.

7. Weekly ultrasound examinations are recommended to assess fetal growth and activity, placental morphology and integrity, and amniotic fluid volume.

8. Biophysical profiles, fetal movement charting, and fetal heart rate testing should be conducted, even though each is often of limited value (poorly discernible tracing, cord compression patterns).

9. If labor is premature, a tocolytic agent may be used if etiology remains unknown, or if L/S ratio is immature and there are no other complications.

10. Deliver if the fetus is mature or there is biophysical evidence of fetal compromise.

11. Notify pediatricians after diagnosis is confirmed and before anticipated delivery.

Intrapartum Management

1. Baseline complete blood count
2. Type and screen mother's blood
3. Slowly remove 500–2000 mL of fluid before any induction; carefully control release during labor
4. Watch for placental abruption, umbilical cord prolapse, and postpartum uterine atony
5. Placenta to be sent to pathology
6. Cesarean section if unable to monitor FHR or any nonreassuring pattern, fetal malpresentation, suspected space-occupying anomaly, or placental abruption

FETAL HYDROCEPHALY

The diagnosis of fetal hydrocephaly should be considered during ultrasound examination when the lateral ventricles are found to extend more than halfway from the midline falx cerebri to the lateral skull table. Since asynclitism can frequently distort the relationship between various intracranial structures, the diagnosis of hydrocephalus should always be confirmed by an experienced obstetric ultrasonographer. The diagnosis is made occasionally before the late second trimester when the option of therapeutic abortion is still an alternative. However, hydrocephalus may be an unanticipated finding during an ultrasound examination in the latter half of the pregnancy.

Infants with other congenital abnormalities (approximately 85% with intracranial or extracranial anomalies such as open spinal defects), a shift of the midline intracranial structures, a cerebral mantle thickness less than 10 mm, an expansion of the hydrocephaly, or a head circumference greater than 50 cm have a poorer prognosis for normal neurological function. An absolute correlation between ultrasound findings and subsequent neurological function is unclear. If any cerebral mantle remains and no other abnormalities are present, the fetus should probably not be subjected to a destructive procedure to facilitate vaginal delivery. Attempts at intrauterine ventricular amniotic shunts have been unsuccessful.

A neonatologist and a neurosurgeon should be notified before delivery. The route of delivery and initial evaluation of the newborn infant are important for subsequent therapy and genetic counseling. The treatment and prognosis of hydrocephalus are based on whether it is a communicating or noncommunicating lesion (Table 6.5). After the initial evaluation, the pregnancy is followed with bi-weekly ultrasonic examinations to determine whether the hydrocephalus is progressive or stable.

Progressive change is evidenced by further ventricular enlargement and cerebral cortex compression. A cesarean delivery is probably the preferred route unless there is no remaining mantle, asymmetric ventriculomegaly, or satisfactory progress during labor with a reassuring FHR pattern. Decompression of the fetal head with an 18-gauge spinal needle (transvaginally if possible) is undertaken rarely when progressive changes are severe and vaginal delivery is planned. If the hydrocephaly remains stable, delivery is customarily delayed until there is amniotic fluid evidence of pulmonary maturity.

FETAL ARRHYTHMIAS

Up to 15% of fetuses have some form of cardiac arrhythmia. Diligent evaluation of the maternal history and physical examination, as well as of the fetus, is required to identify a fetus whose cardiovascular function is severely compromised. Most infants with arrhythmias (especially irregular or "skipped" heart beats) do well during the antepartum and intrapartum periods. These arrhythmias often convert to a normal sinus rhythm at or shortly after birth. Fetal heart rate abnormalities may be classified into three major groups: tachycardia, bradycardia, and irregular.

Table 6.5
Etiology of Fetal Hydrocephaly

Noncommunicating	Communicating
Aqueductal stenosis (may be X-linked recessive)	Arnold-Chiari malformation
Dandy-Walker cyst	Encephalocele
Intracranial mass	Inflammation of the leptomeninges
	Lissencephaly
	Congenital absence of arachnoid granulations
	Choroid plexus papilloma

Tachycardia

(Atrial tachycardia, atrial flutter, complete AV block, supraventricular tachycardia)

Evaluation

1. Fetal echocardiography to characterize the arrhythmia, outline any structural defect, or search for any pericardial effusion or thoracic anomaly
2. Serial ultrasound examinations to search for polyhydramnios, hydrops, and body size dimensions
3. Fetal well-being tests, such as movement charting, ultrasound visualization, and NST (if FHR is less than 200 bpm)
4. Careful neonatal observation and evaluation

Management

1. Notify pediatrician or pediatric cardiologist
2. Maternal digoxin therapy—usually 0.25 mg daily if there is evidence for fetal heart failure (verapamil or propranolol if there is no response to digoxin)
3. Early delivery if fetal lung maturity or signs of fetal compromise and no response to maternal medication
4. If conversion is successful, await spontaneous labor with close monitoring during stress of uterine contractions
5. A vaginal delivery may initiate a vagal response and convert the rapid heart rate to a more normal rate

Bradycardia

(Complete heart block)

Evaluation

1. Fetal echocardiography
2. Serial ultrasonography to search for polyhydramnios, hydrops, delayed fetal growth, pericardial effusion
3. Fetal well-being tests such as movement charting and ultrasound visualization
4. Amniocentesis for fetal karyotype if delivery is not imminent
5. Serum antinuclear antibodies (ANA), since many mothers will have or develop systemic lupus erythematosus

Management

1. Notify pediatricians
2. Maternal isoproterenol or digoxin therapy if fetal immaturity and signs of distress or heart failure
3. Early delivery if fetal lung maturity or evidence of distress, and no intrauterine response to medication
4. Careful neonatal observation and evaluation (may require a pacemaker)

Irregular

(Premature atrial contractions, premature ventricular flutters)
Evaluation and management same as for bradycardia

RECURRENCE RISKS OF MALFORMATIONS

Between 2 and 4% of all infants will have one or more major malformations at birth. Most are not life-threatening but may be disfiguring. The diagnosis is usually made at delivery after an unremarkable prenatal course. Often malformations are isolated and multifactorial in nature, but a karyotype is recommended if there is any question of diagnosis, if an associated chromosomal abnormality is suspected, or if more than one major anomaly is found.

Along with a discussion of treatment alternatives by the infant's physician, new parents should be reassured that the risk of recurrence is low. Recurrence risks of certain malformations are listed in Table 6.6. Ultrasound examinations and maternal serum alpha-fetoprotein (MSAFP) testing are recommended in subsequent pregnancies, although many of these malformations cannot be visualized. A genetic amniocentesis is unnecessary, however, unless the previous infant had a known chromosomal abnormality, an open neural tube defect, or a detectable inborn error of metabolism.

THE STILLBORN INFANT AND REPEATED ABORTION

The stillbirth rate in the United States is 9–10 per 1000 live births. When possible, it is important to determine the etiology of the fetal death. Of equal importance is protection of the maternal and family psychosocial health.

Historical and physical data may provide important clues. Helpful information includes accurate gestational dating, medical or obstetric complications, maternal blood type and antibody

Table 6.6
Recurrence Risk of Specific Malformations with One Affected Child

	Recurrence risk (%)
Cleft lip with or without palate	4
Cleft palate only	2
Open neural tube defects	2–4
Hydrocephaly	1
Congenital heart disease (VSD, ASD, PDA, PS, AS, T of F, transposition, coarctation)	2–4
Clubfoot	3
Congenital hip dislocation	4–5
Pyloric stenosis	3
Hypospadias	3
Abdominal muscle deficiency (prune belly)	1
Arthrogryposis (congenital contractures)	5–15
Craniosynostosis	1–2
Renal agenesis, bilateral (Potter's syndrome)	1–3

screen, exposures to noxious agents (drugs, x-rays, infections), outcome of prior pregnancies, ethnic background and genetic histories, and occupations. A total body x-ray or photograph of the fetus is recommended for the permanent records, the patient, and the referring physician. An instamatic camera may be found in most labor and delivery room areas.

The placenta, cord, and membranes should be examined carefully. A description of the gross appearance of the placenta should be recorded in the medical record. The placenta should be prepared in formalin and appropriate clinical information gathered (including the patient's registration number and delivery date) before being sent to pathology.

An autopsy of the products of conception is recommended for detailed analysis of morphology and visceral and somatic growth. Along with an assessment of craniofacial proportions and specific organs, body measurements should include the crown-rump, crown, heel, arm, leg, and foot lengths. Specimens of preferably amniotic fluid or fresh tissues (skin, amnion, or liver) should be placed in a sterile container with saline and sent promptly to a genetics laboratory for karyotyping. Chromosomal aberrations are associated with 50–60% of all first trimester abortions and 5–10% of stillbirths. Autosomal trisomy comprises approximately 50% of chromosomally abnormal abortuses and monosomy X occurs in 25% of abortuses. Parental karyotyping is suggested for cases of repeated pregnancy loss for determination of any balanced translocation or inversion.

Testing of the mother should include a Kleihauer-Betke test (at the time of stillbirth), thyroid function test, glucose tolerance screening, renal function tests, serum immunologic testing (ANA, anticardiolipin antibody, lupus anticoagulant, partial thromboplastin), and toxoplasmosis titer. The cervix should be cultured for *Listeria, Chlamydia,* and *Mycoplasma.* A hysterosalpingogram, after menses have resumed, may provide helpful information.

With repeated first trimester pregnancy losses, the patient should be instructed on basal body temperature charting, and a serum progesterone determination is recommended after conception is suspected. If test results do not provide a possible explanation for repeated abortion, an immunologic etiology should be considered. The likelihood of another spontaneous abortion is at least 25% and may be greater if the abortus had a normal chromosomal complement or if there have been no other live-born offspring.

Grief Response

An immediate and a delayed grief response by the expectant parents is natural and to be anticipated. Half of all women who experience a perinatal death will require prolonged psychiatric treatment or hospitalization within the next 12 months. The psychological effects on the father are less well documented. Facilitation of the grieving process at the time of death and during the first 6 postpartum weeks may decrease the incidence of psychiatric complications.

The mother should be warned that she may have difficulty with normal daily functions such as eating and sleeping. She may also dream about the infant and imagine that she hears or sees the infant. These are not signs of significant psychiatric illness; rather, they are a part of normal grieving process.

The couple may be counseled that in American society, most adults do not perceive the death of a fetus or child less than 1 year of age in the same light as they would perceive the death of an older person. Therefore, acquaintances may make what appear to be somewhat callous comments such as, "Don't worry about it. You can have another one."

It may be beneficial also to explain to parents that other children frequently experience sibling rivalry toward the unborn fetus and may consider the death to be a result of these feelings. Therefore, the death should be discussed specifically with the children, and they should be told that they had nothing to do with its cause.

If the family decides to name the infant or have a funeral, these actions may provide reality and closure to the event. However, the family should not be forced to take these actions if they do not feel they are appropriate. Bodies sent to pathology or for autopsy are usually cremated. It is frequently helpful to see the family for a prolonged interview approximately one month postpartum, and preferably again later, to assess their adaptation to the loss, discuss any autopsy or placental findings, and describe implications for future pregnancies. Pregnancy should not be encouraged until the couple is ready both psychologically and emotionally.

Suggested Readings

American College of Obstetricians and Gynecologists. Fetal macrosomia. ACOG Technical Bulletin 159. Washington, DC: ACOG, 1991.

American College of Obstetricians and Gynecologists. Diagnosis and management of fetal death. ACOG Technical Bulletin 176. Washington, DC: ACOG, 1993.

American College of Obstetricians and Gynecologists. Early pregnancy loss. ACOG Technical Bulletin 212. Washington, DC: ACOG, 1995.

Brook CO. Consequences of intrauterine growth retardation. Br Med J 983;286:164–167.

Cowchock FS, Reece EA, Balaban D, Branch DW, Plouffe L. Repeated fetal losses associated with antiphospholipid antibodies: a collaborative randomized trial comparing prednisone with low-dose heparin treatment. Am J Obstet Gynecol 1992;166:1318–1323.

Holzgreve W, Curry C, Golbus M, Callen P, Filly R, Smith J. Investigation of nonimmune hydrops fetalis. Am J Obstet Gynecol 1984;150:805–811.

Larsen T, Larsen J, Petersen S, Griesen S. Detection of small-for-gestational-age fetuses by ultrasound screening in a high-risk population: a randomized controlled study. Br J Obstet Gynecol 1992;99:469–475.

Lockshin MD. Antiphospholipid antibody syndrome. JAMA 1992;168:1451–1453.

Moise K. Indomethacin therapy in the treatment of symptomatic polyhy-
    dramnios. Clin Obstet Gynecol 1991;34:310–325.

Smith C, Plumbeck R, Rayburn W, Albaugh K. Relation of mild idio-
    pathic polyhydromnios to perinatal outcome. Obstet Gynecol
    1992;79:
    387–393.

Chervenak F, Berkowitz R, Romero R, Tortora M, Mayden K, Duncan C,
    Mahoney M. The diagnosis of fetal hydrocephalus. Am J Obstet Gy-
    necol 1983;147:703–710.

Kleinman C, Copel V, Weinstein E, Santulli T, Hobbins J. In utero diag-
    nosis and treatment of fetal supraventricular tachycardia. Semin
    Perinatal 1985;9:113–127.

Chapter 7

Special Procedures

GENETIC AMNIOCENTESIS AND GENETIC COUNSELING

Certain genetic disorders may be diagnosed by prenatal genetic counseling and diagnostic testing. The availability of amniotic fluid sampling in early pregnancy is widespread, and normal results are reassuring. Primary indications for genetic amniocenteses include: maternal age 35 years or older, prior infant with inborn error of metabolism, prior infant with or strong family history of open neural tube defects, mother known to be a carrier of an X-linked disorder, prior infant with a chromosomal disorder, history of habitual abortion, elevated maternal serum alpha-fetoprotein (MSAFP), or positive screen for Down syndrome. Maternal serum screening between 15 and 18 weeks for neural tube defects and chromosomal problems are discussed in Chapter 1.

Any patient 35 years or older is at increased risk for delivering an infant with a chromosomal abnormality (Table 7.1). The likelihood of there being a cytogenetic abnormality at age 35 is 1/180, which exceeds the generally accepted risk of fetal demise or abortion following amniocentesis (less than 1/200). A patient who has previously delivered a child with an autosomal or sex chromosomal trisomy has a 1–2% risk of delivering another affected child. A parent may be found to be a balanced translocation carrier after karyotype evaluation for infertility or repeated pregnancy wastage. These individuals usually appear normal but may produce offspring with chromosomal translocations. The risk of delivering an infant with an unbalanced translocation depends on the chromosomal site involved. The risk for D/G is 4% if the father is a carrier, and 9–11% if the mother is a carrier.

X-linked recessive disorders such as Duchenne muscular dystrophy and hemophilia are transmitted by women carrying the

171

Table 7.1
Chromosomal Abnormalities per 1000 Live Births

Maternal Age	Down Syndrome Alone	Any Chromosomal Abnormality
30	0.9–1.2	2.6
31	0.9–1.3	2.6
32	1.1–1.5	3.1
33	1.4–1.9	3.5
34	1.9–2.4	4.1
35	2.5–3.9	5.6
36	3.2–5.0	6.7
37	4.1–6.4	8.1
38	5.2–8.1	9.5
39	6.6–10.5	12.4
40	8.5–13.7	15.8
41	10.8–17.9	20.5
42	13.8–23.4	25.5
43	17.6–30.6	32.3
44	22.5–40.0	41.8
45	28.7–52.3	53.7
46	36.6–68.3	68.9
47	46.6–89.3	89.1
48	59.5–116.8	115.0
49	75.8–152.7	149.3

From Hook EB Rates of chromosome abnormalities at different maternal ages. Obstet Gynecol 1981;58:282.

trait to 50% of male fetuses but is not transmitted to female fetuses. Therefore, an amniocentesis for karyotype determination is useful to determine the sex of the fetus. An absolute diagnosis can be made only by sampling fetal blood.

An amniocentesis may be useful in diagnosing a fetus affected by sickle cell anemia or thalassemia. Genetic mapping by DNA fragment analysis of retrieved amniotic fluid cells has been helpful in determining mutations of the β-globulin chain. Using restriction endonuclease enzymes, the DNA may be more discernible at specific base sequences to determine any abnormal fragments.

Most biochemical genetic disorders are autosomal recessive in inheritance. The recurrence risk for a couple to deliver another affected infant is 25%. However, a few biochemical disorders (e.g., osteogenesis imperfecta) are autosomal dominant with a recurrence risk of 50%. More than 100 of these biochemical disorders may be diagnosed prenatally by analysis of cellular enzymes responsible for mucopolysaccharide, carbohydrate, lipid, or amino acid metabolic derangements. Table 7.2 lists biochemical disorders that may be diagnosed prenatally.

A pregnant patient with a prior history of an infant with an open neural tube defect (NTD) carries a 2% recurrence risk and

Table 7.2
Biochemical Disorders That May Be Detected Prenatally

Disorder	Biochemical Defect
Adrenogenital syndromes	Metabolites of 11-, 17-, or 21-steroid hydroxylase
Chronic granulomatous disease	Granulocyte NBT reduction
Cystic fibrosis	MUGB-reactive proteases
Ehlers-Danlos syndrome, type IV	Unknown (lack of type III collagen)
Fabry's disease[a]	Ceramide trihexoside galactosidase
Galactosemia	Galactose-1-phosphate uridyl transferase
Glycogen storage disease, type II (Pompe's disease)	α-1,4-glucosidase
Hemoglobinopathies	Synthesis of abnormal hemoglobin
Hemophilia A[b]	Factor VIII deficiency
Hemophilia B	Factor IX deficiency
Hunter's syndrome	Iduronate-2-sulfatase
Hurler's syndrome	L-iduronidase
Hyperammonemia, type II	Ornithine carbamoyltransferase
Hyperthyroidism	Unknown (reverse tri-iodothyronine level)
Hyperthyroidism	Multiple (reverse tri-iodothyronine level)
Krabbe's disease	Galactocerebroside β-galactosidase
Maple syrup urine disease	Branched-chain ketoacid decarboxylase
Niemann-Pick disease	Sphingomyelinase
Phenylketonuria	Phenylalanine hydroxylase
Placental sulfatase deficiency[a]	Placental sulfatase
Porphyria (acute intermittent)[a]	Uroporphyrinogen I synthetase
Sandhoff's disease	Hexosaminidase A and B
Tay-Sachs disease	Hexosaminidase A
α-Thalassemia	Decreased synthesis of α-chain hemoglobin
β-Thalassemia	Decreased synthesis of β-chain hemoglobin

[a] Autosomal dominant
[b] X-linked

would be a candidate for an amniocentesis. A patient with a first-degree family relative having an offspring with an NTD has a 1–2% chance of delivering a similarly affected infant. Pregnant patients in whom there is an NTD in an indirect family member (nieces, nephews, or cousins) are also candidates for an MSAFP determination (Chapter 1). Occult spina bifida may produce a falsely normal amniotic fluid AFP determination.

Before an amniocentesis is performed, usually between 14 and 18 weeks, a discussion of the indications and risks of the procedure is necessary. It is useful for this discussion to be conducted by an experienced genetic counselor, and preliminary information such as blood type, gestational age, and genetic history should be obtained. The risk of fetal loss (1–4%), vaginal spotting or fluid leakage (1–2%), chorioamnionitis (0.1%), prematurity, complications of pregnancy or delivery, congenital anomalies or physical injury, or developmental problems of the infant is not increased because of this procedure. Fetal injuries are usually of a minor cutaneous variety. Immediately before the procedure, the patient is again encouraged to ask questions and to be aware that results are not usually available until 1–2 weeks later (depending on the test and laboratory).

Technique

1. An ultrasound examination is routinely performed before, during, and after the amniocentesis to increase the likelihood of a successful initial tap and perhaps lower the risk of bleeding, fetal loss, or premature delivery. By localizing the placenta, the chance of a bloody tap is decreased, thereby minimizing the risk of fetomaternal hemorrhage and of a falsely elevated amniotic fluid AFP result. The target site for needle insertion is identified on the gravid abdomen after the fetal head and thoracic wall have been isolated.

2. Local anesthesia may be used but is not usually necessary during the insertion of the 22-gauge spinal needle. Approximately 20 mL of amniotic fluid is withdrawn from the intrauterine sac, which is 14–16 weeks' size. The initial 1–2 mL of fluid should be discarded to decrease the chance of maternal cell contamination. The total volume of amniotic fluid ranges from 100 mL at 14 weeks, 200 mL at 16 weeks, to 300 mL at 18 weeks. Brown fluid (old blood) is associated

with an abnormal pregnancy outcome in approximately half of cases.

3. When an inadequate specimen is retrieved or the fluid is very bloody, a second needle insertion may be necessary. Ultrasonography with the transducer adjacent to the sterile field is used during the procedure to better localize the needle during insertion. More than two needle insertions should be avoided, and the needle should not be wider than 19-gauge. Although the placenta should be avoided during needle insertion whenever possible, passage of the needle through an anterior placenta is necessary in approximately one-third of cases and has not been associated with an increased risk of complications.

4. A multifetal gestation is discovered in 2% of cases, and each sac may be tapped by inserting the needle under ultrasound guidance in 95% of cases. A careful search for two sacs is necessary. Indigo carmine (2–3 mL) may be diluted with sterile saline (1:10) and instilled in the first sac.

5. After the needle is withdrawn, an ultrasound examination is performed again, primarily for patient reassurance. Any bleeding usually subsides in a few minutes. The patients may continue their daily routines and expect only mild, transient uterine cramping. Any symptoms of vaginal bleeding, severe cramping, fluid loss, or fever should be reported. Rh-negative, unsensitized patients should receive one vial (300 mg) of anti-D immune globulin.

Results

Amniotic fluid is obtained in 94% of cases with the first needle insertion. Cell culturing is successful in 99% of cases. Alpha-fetoprotein results are usually available in a few days and karyotype results by two weeks. Abnormal karyotypes are found in 1–2% of all cases and communicated directly to the patient's physician instead of to the patient initially. Fetal-to-maternal bleeding is present in 5–10% of taps.

Chorionic Villus Sampling: An Alternative

Prenatal diagnosis by chorionic villus sampling (CVS) is performed at many perinatal centers between 8 and 13 weeks' gestation. CVS has been advantageous in that it may be performed earlier in gestation. The time from direct preparation of the chorionic villi until cytogenetic results is similar to that of amniotic fluid testing. Along with chromosomal studies, other fetal disorders that may be diagnosed include sickle cell disease, β-thalassemia, and enzymatic diseases (e.g., 21-hydroxylase deficiency). Despite these diagnostic possibilities, the applicability of CVS has not been determined for widespread clinical use. Retrieval of chorionic villi and minimizing pregnancy loss are dependent on physician experience. Procedure-related fetal loss rate appears to be 1%. Patients considering CVS are counseled that there is probably a slightly higher risk of pregnancy loss from CVS than from amniocentesis, especially from the transcervical approach. The frequency of otomandibular-limb hypogenesis appears to be more common after CVS, especially for CVS performed before 9 menstrual weeks.

The procedure is safely performed at 8–13 weeks with the highest success rate at 9–11 weeks. Mild postprocedure bleeding is common, but there are minimal maternal sequelae. The sampling is performed transcervically using polyethylene tubing with a wire obturator or transabdominally with a 21-gauge spinal needle. Later in pregnancy, when a fetal malformation or intrauterine growth retardation (IUGR) is associated with severe oligohydramnios, transabdominal CVS is an alternative method of invasive sampling.

The catheter is guided under ultrasound visualization, and villi are aspirated into 5 mL of tissue culture medium in a 20–30 mL syringe. Between two and four aspirations are performed for each patient. Retrieval of tissue has been reliable, and karyotype data have been reported in more than 95% of cases at certain centers. The false negative diagnosis rate is 0.1%; however, there is a 1% frequency of falsely abnormal karyotypes when direct preparations are examined. This may be the result of fetal karyotypic mosaicism, confined placental mosaicism, or pseudomosaicism. Therefore, abnormal karyotypes should usually be confirmed by amniotic fluid or umbilical blood sampling.

CERVICAL CERCLAGE

An incompetent cervix is defined historically as painless dilation and effacement of the cervix during pregnancy. Its reported incidence varies from 1 in 54 to 1 in 1850 pregnancies. It is identified most commonly during the second trimester (usually 18–26 gestational weeks) and less reliably in the early third trimester.

Cervical incompetence should be suspected if premature rupture of membranes or premature labor occurs repeatedly in the second trimester or early third trimester. Women with known maternal diethylstilbestrol (DES) exposure, prior trauma from an overly vigorous dilation and curettage (D & C), conization, or laceration, or in whom an abnormal cervix or uterine cavity has been identified, are at increased risk for cervical incompetence.

The diagnosis of an incompetent cervix is suspected when an 8-mm Hegar's dilator can be easily passed through the internal cervical ostium in the nonpregnant state. Hysterosalpingography before a subsequent pregnancy may be helpful to search for uterine anomalies. Ultrasound scanning of the lower uterine segment during pregnancy may provide useful information such as whether there is a downward protrusion of the amniotic membranes, funneling of the cervix in relation to the upper vagina, thinning of the lower uterine segment, dilation of the cervical ostium, or shortening of the cervix. Any such changes on serial ultrasound examinations are suggestive of an incompetent cervix.

A cervical cerclage is intended to reinforce the incompetent cervix. Successful pregnancy rates after cervical cerclage range from 50 to 85%. Controversy continues about the value of a prophylactic cervical cerclage in patients with a history of in utero DES exposure or those with recurrent hemorrhage from a placenta previa.

Procedure

1. Before a suture is placed, ultrasound examination is helpful to accurately date the pregnancy, rule out multifetal gestation, localize the placenta, and establish fetal viability.
2. Most cerclages are performed between the 14th and 16th gestational weeks, after any chance for early spontaneous abortion has been excluded and when the risk of infection is lowest. The procedure is usually performed on an outpatient basis.
3. The type of cerclage, McDonald or Shirodkar, is dependent on the individual surgeon's preference, as both are equally effective. The McDonald cerclage is used primarily, since there is less trauma, blood loss, operative time, and scarring.
4. Fetal heart tones should be sought before and after the procedure to rule out the possibility of intrauterine demise.
5. A No.2 nylon or No.5 Mersilene silk suture is used for McDonald cerclages. Whether one or two sutures are placed is

dependent on the individual surgeon's preference and the extent of cervical effacement. The suture should be cut several centimeters long to allow easy visibility when the cerclage is removed at or beyond the 38th week. Mersilene tape is used for the Shirodkar procedure.

6. A subdural (saddle) or epidural anesthetic block is as acceptable as general anesthesia.

7. If an emergency cerclage is performed with bulging membranes, general anesthesia is administered with the patient in a steep Trendelenburg position. A transabdominal amniocentesis may be necessary to decompress the bulging membranes. The vagina is not cleansed. Several stay sutures using No. 2-0 silk are attached to the edge of the effaced cervix. The herniated membranes should fall back into the uterine cavity or may be pushed in using a moist sponge or finger. Two purse-string sutures should then be placed.

8. Antibiotics, tocolytics, or sedatives are not absolutely required but are often prescribed.

Special Considerations

1. Despite the increased risk of premature labor, the finding of a bicornuate or septate uterus or a multifetal gestation alone does not necessitate a cervical cerclage.

2. If there is a history of third trimester premature delivery preceded by premature labor, a cervical cerclage is not necessary. Instead, more frequent cervical exams are recommended. A cerclage should be promptly placed if there is any dilation of the internal cervical ostium, if the index finger can be passed into the cervical ostium, or if ultrasound scanning reveals shortening of the cervix, funneling of the membranes, or thinning of the myometrium.

3. Coital activity may resume approximately one week after a prophylactic McDonald procedure. The vaginal incisions of the Shirodkar procedure require 4–6 weeks to heal. The suture may cause penile discomfort.

4. If chorioamnionitis is suspected later, an amniocentesis is helpful to search for any polymicrobial infection.

5. An IUD string retriever is sometimes helpful in retrieving the suture during removal.

6. Placement of a transabdominal cervicoisthmic cerclage is to

be considered if the cervix is too short or if a prior trans-vaginal cerclage has been unsuccessful.

MIDTRIMESTER ABORTION

Patients desiring a pregnancy termination for medical or obstet-ric indications between 13 and 24 weeks often go through a process of grief which involves denial, sadness, guilt, anger, and finally acceptance. This is especially true in patients who request abortion for a genetically abnormal or malformed fetus. These patients are more likely to be older, often married, and desirous of a favorable pregnancy outcome. Furthermore, these patients have usually visualized a living fetus on ultrasound examination before an amniocentesis, and fetal quickening has left an in-creased feeling of attachment.

Once the decision for pregnancy termination has been made, it should be accomplished with minimal delay, since com-plications increase with advancing gestational age. Methods avail-able to terminate the pregnancy should be discussed with the pa-tient in an open and honest manner, with advantages and disadvantages being presented in detail. The two most common methods for pregnancy termination involve prostaglandin E_2 vaginal suppositories or surgical dilation and evacuation.

Prostaglandins

Prostaglandin E_2 vaginal suppositories are useful for the removal of an intact fetus for morphologic examination and other diag-nostic testing to confirm any suspected genetic abnormality or body malformation. Disadvantages to the use of prostaglandin vaginal suppositories include the discomfort of labor, side effects from drug use (nausea, diarrhea, fever), labor, prolonged initia-tion to delivery interval (mean 14 hours, range 10–22 hours), de-livery of a liveborn fetus (5%), failure to effect delivery in 24 hours (10%), incomplete passage of tissue (10–15%), and re-tained placenta for 2 or more hours requiring operative inter-vention. Conditions in which prostaglandins should be used with caution or are contraindicated are listed in Table 7.3.

To shorten the initiation-to-abortion time, two to four lami-naria tents may be wedged within the cervical ostium 4 hours or more before they are removed and a suppository is inserted to ini-tiate cervical dilation. Because of side effects from the medications,

Table 7.3
Conditions in which Prostaglandin Therapy Should be Used with Caution or is Contraindicated

Used with Caution	Contraindications
Asthma	Hypersensitivity
Hypertension	Active pelvic inflammatory disease
Hypotension	Unfavorable fetal position (transverse lie)
Cardiovascular disease	Placenta previa, complete
Renal disease	
Peptic ulcer disease	
Anemia	
Jaundice	
Diabetes mellitus	
Seizure disorder	
Prior uterine surgery	
Fever	

premedication involves an antidiarrheal agent (Lomotil 5 mg orally) and an antiemetic (prochlorperazine 10 mg i.m.). Meperidine (50 mg i.m.) and acetaminophen (350-mg rectal suppositories) are often necessary to relieve uterine contraction discomfort and to control fevers of 38°C or greater. Administration of further suppositories should be delayed until the maternal temperature is less than 38°C. Otherwise, profound hyperthermia may occur.

A Prostin 20-mg suppository should be inserted up to the vaginal apex every 3–5 hours. Monitoring of uterine contractions is necessary, and an intrauterine pressure catheter may be helpful. If intense and sustained contractions are noted, a cervical tear or uterine rupture may occur. Persistent sustained contractions may be reversed by removing the suppository and, if necessary, infusing a β-adrenergic tocolytic drug (e.g., terbutaline 250 μg intravenously or subcutaneously). If uterine contractions remain inadequate, low doses of oxytocin may be administered simultaneously.

Dilation and Evacuation (D & E)

Before 16 weeks' gestation, surgical termination is the preferred method, although it may be considered up to 20 weeks in some circumstances. The procedure is rapid and relatively painless, and it can be performed on an outpatient basis, thereby decreasing medical costs. Disadvantages to dilation and evacuation procedures include the inability to adequately examine the fetus, risks requiring surgical expertise, and potential injury to the cervix or uterine perforation.

Appropriate surgical technique requires sufficient cervical dilation. Three or more medium-sized laminaria are usually inserted at least 4 hours before the procedure. The diameter of dilation should be equal to the number of weeks of gestation plus 2 mm (for example, 18 mm dilation at 16 menstrual weeks). Instruments necessary for sufficient evacuation include Hegar's dilators, a nonflexible 16-mm vacuum system, and heavy crushing forceps (e.g., Sopher forceps).

Most patients prefer to be asleep during the procedure, so low concentrations of inhalation agents or intravenous sedation and analgesia are usually administered. Uterine evacuation may also be adequately performed with regional or paracervical anesthesia and sedation. Oxytocin (20 U per liter i.v. fluid) or Methergine (0.2 mg i.v. slowly) is used routinely during the operation and shortly thereafter to reduce blood loss and risk of infection.

General Precautions

1. Unless uterine evacuation is completed over a short period of time, most patients are prescribed oral tetracycline (such as doxycycline) or ampicillin to reduce postabortion infection rate.

2. The risk of spontaneous abortion or premature labor in subsequent pregnancies is thought to be very low despite the mechanical cervical dilation during these procedures.

3. Rh isoimmunization may result from a pregnancy termination, since the incidence of sensitization is only slightly less at mid-gestation than at term. All Rh-negative unsensitized patients should receive a full dose (300 mg) of Rh immune globulin, unless fetal blood obtained during a surgical procedure is found to be Rh-negative.

4. Major abdominal operations such as a hysterectomy or hysterotomy are rarely necessary unless other methods of pregnancy termination are either unavailable or unsuccessful or if a gynecologic complication is present.

5. Intraamniotic prostaglandin F_2, hyperosmolar urea, or hypertonic saline are no longer used alone because of undesired side effects.

SICKLE CELL ANEMIA TRANSFUSION

Sickle cell anemia has been associated in the past with extremely high neonatal and maternal mortality and morbidity rates. To improve the outcome of pregnancies, simple or partial exchange transfusions in gravidas with SS, SC, or S-thal disease are available. Such transfusions may be undertaken routinely beginning at mid-gestation or the end of the second trimester or may be reserved for complications such as crisis, infection, or symptomatic anemia. The reported risk of maternal morbidity is 1% following exchange transfusion. A cell separator machine allows the patient's plasma, platelets, and leukocytes to be returned with washed compatible donor red cells with Hb AA.

With careful management, a greater than 95% perinatal salvage rate is to be expected with Hb SS, SC, and S-thal. Advantages and disadvantages to partial exchange transfusion are shown in Table 7.4. Close antepartum monitoring is necessary, of the mother (crisis, thrombosis, pyelonephritis, worsening anemia, hypertension), and of the fetus (abortion, stillbirth, premature birth, IUGR). Maximum benefit occurs in the first 6–8 weeks following transfusion and declines thereafter because of the shortened life-span of the stored erythrocytes.

Procedure

1. Notify blood bank personnel well in advance of an anticipated transfusion in the morning (outpatient transfusion may be considered).

Table 7.4
Value of Partial Prophylactic Exchange Transfusions

Advantages	Disadvantages
Decreased hemoglobin-S concentration	Blood group incompatibility
Increased hemoglobin-A concentration	Allergic reaction
Increased oxygenation	Anaphylaxis
Reduced chance of sickling	Hepatitis, HIV
Decreased erythropoiesis	Isoimmunization
Improved sense of well-being	Febrile reaction
Improved reproductive outcome	Premature labor (?)
Useful in anemia? congestive heart failure?	Cost, limited benefits
Decreased maternal infection	Psychologic dependence
Less prolonged hospitalization	
Decreased maternal mortality	

2. Determine hematocrit, hemoglobin A (Hb A), and type and cross-match before anticipated transfusion.
3. Initiate i.v. with lactated Ringer's solution, to be infused until 200–400 mL are given.
4. Phlebotomize 500 mL blood into vacutainer (30 minutes).
5. Give 2 units (150–300 mL/unit) of buffy coat–poor, washed red cells (warmed, under pressure over 1–2 hours).
6. Repeat procedure in afternoon and allow overnight equilibration (total of 4 units of washed erythrocytes).
7. Obtain hematocrit and Hb A determinations next morning if inpatient; otherwise, repeat at next clinic visit
8. Discharge patient if hematocrit is over 35% and Hb A over 40%; if not, repeat procedure until desired levels are obtained or clinical course is improved
9. Schedule clinic visits every 1–2 weeks, with determination of reticulocyte count, hematocrit, and hemoglobin electrophoresis
10. Repeat entire procedure: (*a*) at 36–38 weeks; (*b*) when hematocrit is less than 26% and Hb A is less than 20%; (*c*) if crisis occurs; or (*d*) during labor if necessary.

EXTERNAL BREECH VERSION

Approximately one-fourth of fetuses will be in a breech presentation in the early third trimester, but only 3–4% will remain breech at term. Of those pregnancies with a breech fetus at 37 weeks, only 18% will convert to cephalic presentation before delivery. Management of the breech fetus at term involves consideration of the following alternatives: routine cesarean section, selective vaginal delivery, or external cephalic version. External version usually lasts no more than 5 minutes, and the fetus usually remains in a cephalic position if the version is successful.

Patient Selection

Contraindications for external cephalic version include the following: complications predisposing to uteroplacental insufficiency, twin gestation, fetus with an obvious malformation or suspicious heart rate tracing, fetus that is suspected to be small or large for gestational age, prior uterine surgery, placenta previa, or suspected placental abruption.

Although not a contraindication, more difficulties are likely with an obese or primigravid patient. An inadequate amount of amniotic fluid on ultrasonic examination is also a less favorable prognostic sign. The patient should understand the unlikely but potential risks of the procedure (labor, uterine rupture, cord compression, fetal heart rate abnormality, preterm delivery if performed before 37 weeks) and should be made aware that 35–45% of all attempts will be unsuccessful.

The procedure should be performed at or near labor and delivery units. A reassuring real-time ultrasound examination and a reactive nonstress test should be demonstrated beforehand. A β-adrenergic drug should be given (e.g. terbutaline 250 μg intravenously or subcutaneously) to relax the uterus. The maternal heart rate, maternal blood pressure, and fetal heart rate should be monitored frequently.

A backward flip of the fetus is usually attempted before a forward roll is undertaken. A second examiner should be available to assist in the manipulation. A second attempt after an initial failure may be undertaken only if the mother and fetus remain stable.

The procedure should be discontinued after two or three failed attempts, fetal bradycardia or decelerations, or patient discomfort. If a cesarean section is planned under conduction anesthesia, another attempt at external version may be successful. Fetal heart rate decelerations are uncommon with a successful version. After the fetus is turned, it should be maintained in the new attitude for several minutes. A post-procedure ultrasound examination and a nonstress test are recommended to identify fetal position and any potentially compromised fetus.

NONGENETIC AMNIOCENTESIS

The most common indication for an amniocentesis during the second half of pregnancy is fetal lung maturity testing. It may also be performed to better evaluate pregnancies complicated by Rh isoimmunization or pelvic infection (usually during persistent premature labor or after preterm ruptured membranes). Ultrasound visualization of the fetal vital parts and the placenta permits the selection of a relatively safe pocket of amniotic fluid. After determining that amniocentesis is indicated in select patients, the following risks of the procedure should be explained: infection, fetal trauma, subplacental hemorrhage, umbilical cord insertion, and fetal death. An operative permit should then be completed. A non-emergent procedure should be scheduled on weekday mornings to ensure that results will be available later that same day.

Technique

The procedure is similar to that described in Chapter 1 for an early gestation genetic amniocentesis. Ultrasonography is used before the procedure to determine fetal presentation, fetal biparietal diameter (BPD), fetal heart rate (FHR), placental and umbilical cord localization, and site for needle insertion. Ultrasonography is often used during the procedure to visualize the needle tip. The transducer may be placed near the needle insertion site with a surgical soap or sterile gel applied to the patient's abdomen. A site away from the placenta, umbilical cord, fetal heart, and fetal thorax is ideal. The end of a straw may be used to press gently on the maternal skin to mark a target site.

Aseptic technique is used, but a mask, cap, or gown is unnecessary. Local skin anesthesia is recommended for insertion of a 20-gauge spinal needle but not for a 22-gauge needle. In pregnancies complicated by a multifetal gestation, amniotic fluid should be retrieved from the sac containing an appropriately-sized and apparently healthy fetus.

Documentation of the FHR by auscultation or ultrasound visualization is necessary before and after the procedure. Nonstress testing is recommended if bloody or meconium-stained amniotic fluid is retrieved. If a nonstress test is already planned, it should be scheduled after the amniocentesis. Patient instruction about fetal movement charting may be helpful after the procedure. The full (300 μg) dose of Rh immune globulin is to be administered for all Rh-negative unsensitized women (exception: known Rh-negative father), particularly if any blood is retrieved or if the needle is inserted through the placenta.

Suggested Readings

American College of Obstetricians and Gynecologists. Chorionic villus sampling. ACOG Committee Opinion 160. Washington, DC: ACOG, 1995.

American College of Obstetricians and Gynecologists. Genetic Technologies. ACOG Technical Bulletin 208. Washington, DC: ACOG, 1995.

American College of Obstetricians and Gynecologists. Down syndrome screening. ACOG Committee Opinion 141. Washington, DC: ACOG, 1994.

American Medical Association, Council on Scientific Affairs. Induced termination of pregnancy before and after Roe v. Wade. Trends in the mortality and morbidity of women. JAMA 1992;268:3231–3239.

Atrash HK, Mackay HT, Binkin NJ, Hogue CJ. Legal abortion mortality in the United States: 1972 to 1982. Am J Obstet Gynecol 1987;156: 605–612.

Baerthlein WC, Moodley S, Stinson SK. Comparison of maternal and neonatal morbidity in midforceps delivery and midpelvis vacuum extraction. Obstet Gynecol 1986;67:594–597.

Christian SS, Brady K, Read JA, Kopelman JN. Vaginal breech delivery: a five-year prospective evaluation of a protocol using computed tomographic pelvimetry. Am J Obstet Gynecol 1990;163:848–855.

Davison L, Easterling TR, Jackson JC, Benedetti TJ. Breech extraction of low-birth-weight second twins: can cesarean section be justified? Am J Obstet Gynecol 1992;166:497–502.

Hakim-Elahi E, Tovell HM, Burnhill MS. Complications of first-trimester abortion: a report of 170,000 cases. Obstet Gynecol 1990;76:120–135.

Kirz DS, Haag MK. Management of the third stage of labor in pregnancies terminated by prostaglandin E2. Am J Obstet Gynecol 1989;160: 412–414.

Koonin LM, Smith JC, Ramick M, Lawson HW. Abortion surveillance— United States, 1989. MMWR CDC Surveill Summ 1992;41(5):1–33.

Mahomed K, Seeras R, Coulson R. External cephalic version at term: a randomized controlled trial using tocolysis. Br J Obstet Gynaecol 1991;98:8–13.

Mazze RJ, Kallen B. Reproductive outcome after anesthesia and operation during pregnancy: a registry study of 5,405 cases. Am J Obstet Gynecol 1989;161:1178–1185.

Report of National Institute of Child Health and Human Development Workshop on Chorionic Villus Sampling and Limb and Other Defects, October 20, 1992. Am J Obstet Gynecol 1993;169:1–6.

Robertson AW, Kopelman NJ, Read JA, Duff P, Magelssen DJ, Dashow EE. External cephalic version at term: is a tocolytic necessary? Obstet Gynecol 1987;70:896–899.

Rosen DJ, Illeck JS, Greenspoon JS. Repeated external cephalic version at term. Am J Obstet Gynecol 1992;167:508–509.

Smidt-Jensen S, Permin M, Philip J, Lundsteen C, Zachary JM, Fowler SE, et al. Randomized comparison of amniocentesis and transabdominal and transcervical chorionic villus sampling. Lancet 1992;340: 1237–1244.

Ward BE, Gersen SL, Carelli MP, McGuire NM, Dackowski WR, Weinstein M, et al. Rapid prenatal diagnosis of chromosomal aneuploidies by fluorescence in situ hybridization: clinical experience with 4,500 specimens. Am J Hum Genet 1993;52:854–865.

Winkler CL, Gray SE, Hauth JC, Owen J, Tucker MMJ. Mid-second-trimester labor induction: concentrated oxytocin compared with prostaglandin E2 vaginal suppositories. Obstet Gynecol 1991;77: 297–300.

Chapter 8

Intrapartum Monitoring

INDUCTION OF LABOR

Labor is induced rather than spontaneous in 15–25% of all pregnancies. Indications include postdates, abnormal FHR pattern, intrauterine growth retardation, premature rupture of membranes by more than 12–24 hours, suspected intraamniotic infection, and removal of a mature fetus from a potentially hostile environment (preeclampsia, poorly controlled diabetes, significant cardiac or pulmonary disorders, neoplasia, postdates). Elective induction for simple convenience is not acceptable.

Successful induction requires both sufficient cervical compliance and adequate uterine contractions. The fact that cervical compliance may be the major factor limiting successful induction has led to the development of several protocols for ripening the unfavorable cervix. Adequate uterine contractions can usually be accomplished through administration of oxytocin.

Initial Assessment

To justify induction, there should be a reasonable assurance of fetal pulmonary maturity, obvious evidence of fetal compromise, or significant threat to the mother's life or long-term health. It is generally believed that the fetus should be in a vertex presentation. While some obstetricians feel that induction with a fetus in a breech presentation may be acceptable, most authorities favor cesarean section.

Caution should be employed in the presence of twin gestation, fetal macrosomia, polyhydramnios, a prior low transverse cesarean section, or grand multiparity, because of the risk of uterine rupture. Documented fetal/pelvic disproportion, a previous vertical or classical uterine incision, a previous full-thickness my-

Table 8.1
Bishop Score for Assessing the Cervix before Induction

	0	1	2	3
Dilation (cm)	0	1–2	3–4	5–6
Effacement (%)	0–30	40–50	60–70	80–100
Station	−3	−2	−1, 0	+1, +2
Consistency	Firm	Medium	Soft	
Position	Posterior	Mid	Anterior	

omectomy, untreated gonorrhea, or active herpes infection are considered absolute contraindications to an induction.

The probability of successful induction can be predicted by the Bishop method of cervical scoring (Table 8.1). A Bishop score of 9 or more is almost always associated with successful induction. A score of 4 or less is consistent with an unfavorable cervix and carries a poor prognosis.

Cervical Priming

The Bishop score (especially cervical dilation) and the probability of a successful induction have been shown to improve with the use of any of the following methods: (a) intracervical application of 0.5 mg of a prostaglandin E_2 gel; (b) stripping of membranes; (c) nipple stimulation or warm soaks to nipples for a half-hour three times daily for several days prior to the procedure; or (d) mechanical dilation (laminaria or Foley catheter), usually 12 hours prior to the procedure.

Prostaglandins are 20-carbon compounds formed by the action of the enzyme prostaglandin synthetase, which is found in most cells. Prostaglandins E_2, E_1, and $F_{2\alpha}$ are released from decidual and myometrial cells. They act on specific receptors to alter or inhibit the action of adenyl cyclase, subsequently inhibiting formation of cAMP (adenosine 3',5'-cyclic monophosphate) to eventually bring about changes in smooth muscle tone and modulation of hormonal activity. The intracervical (0.5 mg, Prepidil) or intravaginal (10 mg, Cervidil) application of prostaglandin E_2 has been the subject of much interest. Cervices ripened in this way have led to spontaneous labor, shortened labor, less oxytocin, and lower cesarean section rates for failed induction.

The patient should not be febrile or have vaginal bleeding. A Bishop score of 4 or less is considered to be unfavorable. Other prerequisites to prostaglandin E_2 therapy include a reassuring fetal heart rate tracing (preferably a reactive nonstress test), absence of regular uterine contractions (every 5 minutes or less), and a complete explanation to the patient.

The drug is inserted either at or near the labor and delivery suite, where continuous uterine activity monitoring and FHR monitoring can be performed. Outpatient dosing offers more convenience and less cost, but further study about its safety is necessary. Using the specially designed catheter, intracervical insertion requires direct inspection using a speculum. The patient is expected to remain recumbent for at least 30 minutes and may then be transferred elsewhere in the absence of uterine activity.

The onset of contractions, which are usually irregular and infrequent, is similar to that seen in spontaneous labor. This wide variation in contractions may be explained by differences in individual responsiveness, parity, dosage rate, absorption, initial cervical size, and state of the membranes. Contractions usually become apparent in the first hour, show peak activity in the first 4 hours, and initiate labor in approximately half of all cases (range, 25 to 76%). If any regular uterine contractions persist, electronic monitoring is to be continued, and maternal vital signs should be recorded at least hourly for the first 4 hours.

A minimum time interval between dosing and beginning oxytocin has not been established. The effects of prostaglandin E_2 may be exaggerated with oxytocin, so a postdosing observation period should be at least 4–6 hours. Oxytocin should be deferred or used with great caution in low doses if the patient continues to have uterine activity from the prostaglandin E_2 gel.

If insufficient cervical change (Bishop score change 3 or less) or uterine activity has occurred, another alternative may be a second prostaglandin E_2 dose. Less is known about the value of sequential prostaglandin E_2 dosing versus a single application followed by an equal period of observation. Prerequisites for first dosing also apply. The manufacturer of the commercially available gel recommends a maximum cumulative dose of 1.5 mg of dinoprostone in a 24-hour period.

Oxytocin Administration

Oxytocin is an octapeptide with a half-life of 3–4 minutes and a duration of action of approximately 20 minutes. The mechanism by which this agent facilitates smooth muscle contractions is not fully understood, but it is thought to bind to receptors on myometrial cell membranes where cAMP is eventually formed for a dose-dependent increase in the amplitude and frequency of uterine contractions. The goal of augmentation or induction of labor is uterine contractions occurring every 2–3 minutes and lasting approximately 45–60 seconds. An intrauterine pressure catheter is often helpful in interpreting uterine activity, and a 50 mm H_2O recording is considered to be evidence of an adequate contraction.

An intravenous crystalloid solution should be administered through an 18-gauge intravenous catheter. The oxytocin solution is piggybacked into this main intravenous line and administered by an accurately calibrated infusion pump. The initial infusion rate of 1–2 mU/minute is usually doubled at 30–60-minute intervals. The maximum rate of infusion for augmentation is usually no more than 8 mU/minute while inductions do not generally exceed 20 mU/minute. The uterine response will likely not improve if the rate is 30 mU/minute or more.

Once sufficient uterine activity has led to adequate progress in labor, the dose of oxytocin should not be increased; rather, it may need to be decreased or stopped to allow labor to continue spontaneously. A hyperstimulatory pattern with contractions overlapping each other may be reversed by discontinuing or decreasing the infusion rate of oxytocin while closely observing the fetal heart rate (FHR). If more than 20 mU/minute is required, the dose should be increased by 2 mU every 20 minutes.

Electronic FHR monitoring is recommended shortly before and throughout an induction or augmentation of labor. Internal monitoring techniques are preferred when possible. As a general rule, three contractions should occur every 10 minutes and should not last longer than 60–90 seconds. If internal monitoring is used, uterine pressures should not exceed 75 mm Hg during a contraction and 30 mm Hg between contractions. Another means of describing uterine activity is to use Montevideo units (the number of uterine contractions in 10 minutes multiplied by the mean intensity in mm Hg). A Montevideo score of 200 units or more is desirable.

Serial Inductions

Less is known about the value of serial inductions when delivery has not occurred within 48 hours. Many patients do not have pressing indications for induction of labor. Pregnancies must be reevaluated for any worsening of the underlying complication, cephalopelvic disproportion, and infection to make certain that further delay is safe for mother and fetus. In doing so, the need for cesarean delivery with accompanying surgical risks may be reduced.

Failure of a committed induction attempt is especially common for preterm deliveries. Studies to evaluate oxytocin requirements in this situation are few and difficult to interpret, since the reason for induction may involve several variables, which alone can alter uterine sensitivity. In general, the preterm uterus is less sensitive to oxytocin and may require larger doses or serial inductions. The response to uterine stimulants seems to increase slowly during pregnancy until it becomes relatively stable after 33 weeks' gestation.

INTRAPARTUM FETAL HEART RATE MONITORING

Intermittent auscultation and electronic monitoring are the two methods available to monitor the FHR during labor. Most authorities recommend electronic fetal monitoring in high-risk situations that require close intrapartum surveillance. Conditions that require close intrapartum surveillance and routine electronic fetal monitoring are listed in Table 8.2. Any additional benefit from electronic fetal monitoring over intermittent auscultation in low-risk patients remains controversial, although

Table 8.2
Intrapartum Conditions Requiring Electronic Fetal Monitoring

Meconium staining

Use of oxytocin or prostaglandin

Delivery of an anticipated premature, postmature, Rh sensitized, growth retarded, or macrosomic infant

Medical complications associated with uteroplacental insufficiency (hypertension, diabetes, severe anemia, heart disease, renal disease)

Presence of abnormal auscultatory findings

Prior cesarean section

Other intrapatrum obstetric complications (failure to progress, excessive vaginal bleeding)

---

nurses and especially physicians often desire electronic monitoring during active labor.

Recommendations

1. Both methods of FHR monitoring during labor should be discussed with the patient during the antepartum period and on admission to the labor floor. Her wishes, concerns, and questions about risks, benefits, and limitations should be addressed in an open manner.

2. We recommend and routinely perform a 20-minute tracing on all of our patients admitted in early labor. A reassuring FHR pattern coincident with contractions is a favorable prognostic sign of fetal tolerance to labor.

3. Auscultation of the FHR for 30 seconds every 15 minutes in the active phase of the first stage of labor and every 5 minutes during the second stage of labor is acceptable for monitoring women at low risk. Fetal heart rate changes, particularly bradycardia (less than 120 beats/minute), should be sought when the heart rate is auscultated during and immediately after a uterine contraction.

4. Family-centered care and electronic FHR monitoring are not mutually exclusive.

5. Electronic monitoring should not be a substitute for good clinical judgment. The patient's underlying obstetric condition, blood pressure, laboring position, blood loss, and extent of cervical dilation and fetal descent must also be assessed carefully.

6. In general, direct monitoring by scalp electrode placement provides a more accurate tracing. This technique should be considered when the external tracing is inadequate or suggests fetal compromise. Aseptic technique with the least trauma should be practiced during the placement of the electrode or intrauterine pressure catheter.

7. The relation between any FHR abnormalities and uterine contractions should always be sought. When this relation is questioned, an intrauterine pressure catheter should be inserted.

8. Prolonged supine positioning and immobility of the mother should be avoided. The best laboring positions are ambulating or a semi-recumbent, left lateral position.

9. The relation between early, late, and variable FHR decelerations and uterine contractions is shown in Figure 8.1.

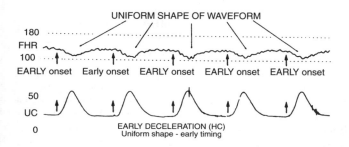

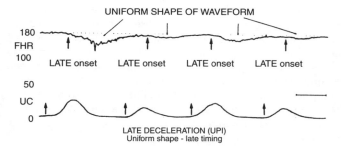

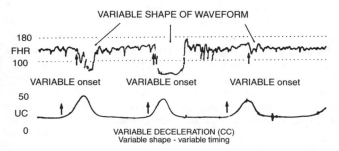

Figure 8.1. Fetal heart rate decelerations in relation to uterine contractions. (Reprinted with permission from Hon, EH. An atlas of fetal heart rate patterns. New Haven, Harty Press, 1968.)

10. Fetal scalp pH determinations are uncommonly used but may be helpful as an adjunct to electronic monitoring when a worrisome FHR pattern is found well before an imminent delivery.

Interpretation

Interpretation of any worrisome FHR pattern requires a prior knowledge of the cervical dilation, station, and uterine contractility. The patient's blood pressure and position and any medications must be known. The FHR pattern should be described and interpreted in terms of baseline and periodic changes. Terms such as fetal jeopardy should be avoided, since they are nondescriptive and difficult, if not impossible, to define. Examples of nonreassuring FHR patterns may include those with absent short-term variability, moderate or severe bradycardia, or severe repetitive variable decelerations. Absent short-term variability (beat-to-beat variability) may indicate compromise of the fetal autonomic system. Moderate bradycardia (80–100 beats/minute) or severe bradycardia (less than 80 beats/minute for more than 3 minutes) may indicate impending fetal demise. Variable decelerations with slow return to FHR baseline (deceleration less than 60 beats/minute) and severe repetitive variable decelerations (more than 60 beats/minute for more than 60 seconds) also represent nonreassuring FHR patterns.

In the presence of nonreassuring FHR patterns, several modes of evaluation should be considered. If fetal membranes are intact, amniotomy and placement of internal electronic fetal monitors may be considered. Initial conservative measures may include change in maternal position to the left lateral position, administration of oxygen, correction of maternal hypotension, and discontinuation of oxytocin if appropriate. Amnioinfusion, fetal scalp stimulation, or fetal scalp blood sampling for acid-base status may also be considered. If these tests remain nonreassuring, delivery should be expedited. All the maneuvers described above are directed toward improving oxygen delivery to the fetus. In the presence of FHR variability, irreversible fetal hypoxia has not taken place.

VAGINAL BIRTH AFTER CESAREAN

The notion that "once a cesarean section, always a cesarean section" is no longer a dominant practice of American obstetrics.

Concern over rising cesarean section rates and recognition that a trial of labor with a transverse uterine scar carries a prognosis significantly different from that with a classical scar has led most obstetricians to offer an attempt of a vaginal birth in many circumstances. The National Institutes of Health Consensus Committee on Cesarean Section and the American College of Obstetricians and Gynecologists have recommended that a trial of labor is permissible among select patients with a prior cesarean section.

Antepartum Considerations

1. Uterine rupture occurs in 1% of patients attempting vaginal delivery after cesarean section and leads to a perinatal mortality rate of 1/1000 births. Uterine scar interruption may be asymptomatic and has been found incidentally in up to 2% of patients. A classical cesarean section is associated with a significantly greater risk of uterine rupture.
2. Approximately 70% (range, 50–90%) of all patients allowed a trial of labor will deliver vaginally. Those patients who have undergone a prior vaginal delivery or whose prior cesarean section was performed for a nonrecurrent indication have the greatest likelihood (between 80 and 90%) of delivering vaginally.
3. There is no increased risk of uterine rupture with two prior cesareans. There is very little information regarding outcome in patients with more than two cesareans.
4. Refresher childbirth courses are to be encouraged.
5. Intravenous analgesia should be used cautiously, particularly during the latent phase of the first stage of labor. Epidural analgesia during the active phase of labor has gained more widespread acceptance.
6. Patients should understand that a hysterectomy may be necessary if the uterus ruptures, but this is a complication in only approximately 1/1000 trials of labor.
7. Clinical pelvimetry is essential during the last few weeks before delivery, but x-ray pelvimetry alone is of little or no value in predicting the likelihood of successful vaginal delivery.
8. The desire for a tubal ligation should be sought as routine prenatal care but this alone should not affect the final decision to attempt a vaginal delivery.

Intrapartum Considerations

1. An intravenous line should be inserted once labor is established.
2. Oxytocin may be used to induce or augment labor, and close monitoring of uterine contractions (especially using intrauterine catheters) is recommended.
3. Electronic FHR monitoring is recommended. The most common sign of uterine rupture is abrupt changes in FHR pattern, including bradycardia or prolonged decelerations.
4. The anesthesiologists should be notified.
5. There is no evidence to support the prophylactic use of forceps.
6. The same expectations of normal progression of labor should be applied to patients with a prior cesarean section.
7. Exploration of the uterus after delivery of the placenta is not essential, and the prognostic significance of assessing scar integrity is uncertain.

DELIVERY AT LESS THAN 25 WEEKS

Perinatal mortality rates among very low birth weight infants have dropped dramatically in the last 10 years. Among the infants who survive, many suffer significant short-term and long-term morbidity. Currently, 25 weeks' gestation appears to be the critical point at or beyond which a reasonable number of infants can be expected to survive with intensive nursery care. Aggressive intrapartum management or cesarean section is not routinely justified below this gestational age.

Dating of the pregnancy is extremely important. A falsely low gestational age determination or estimated fetal weight is frequently related to a poorer neonatal outcome. It is important to recall that ultrasonographic parameters of fetal age and growth tend to be smaller among fetuses in premature labor or with preterm ruptured membranes than among fetuses of similar gestational age who ultimately deliver at term. This may lead to an underestimation of the true gestational age. The neonatal staff should be notified in advance of impending delivery. They should also be given the opportunity to talk to the patient along with the staff obstetrician while management plans are formulated. The patient should be aware that gestational age assessment and the chances of infant survival are more accurately determinable after delivery.

The preferred route of delivery is vaginal unless obstetrically contraindicated. If dating is uncertain and labor is already established, perinatal survival is not enhanced by cesarean delivery. Uterine activity monitoring is necessary during labor. Continuous FHR monitoring is not performed routinely but may be beneficial in changing the mother's position or in the decision to give her oxygen in order to correct any heart rate abnormality.

The initial response of any infant weighing 600 g or more to resuscitative maneuvers is the most important determinant of the infant's chance of survival. A liveborn infant deemed too immature for resuscitation may remain with the parents if they so desire, with staff approval. In most cases, such an infant will be brought to the neonatal treatment room for observation in a dignified manner.

In cases of intentional pregnancy termination at a relatively advanced gestational age (e.g., progressive hydrocephalus, bilateral renal agenesis, anencephaly), the attending physician should carefully plan the procedure to ensure fetal demise before delivery, or if clinically appropriate, discuss with the patient and her family the possible outcome of a liveborn infant. Physicians should be aware of the statutory definitions and legal requirements governing the reporting of abortions, stillbirths, and immature live births of the state in which they practice. Any liveborn infant will require a birth certificate regardless of length of life.

After the delivery of a stillborn fetus or an infant who dies shortly after birth, the obstetric staff should write a note including detailed description of the fetus as an aid to future counseling and care of the patient. A photograph and body x-ray of the infant are quite often helpful. After delivery, careful inspection of the placenta and the lower genital tract is useful to search for any uterine or placental abnormality. Finally, a grief response by both parents should be anticipated and supportive care provided.

MAGNESIUM SULFATE

Magnesium sulfate is important for seizure prophylaxis in patients with severe preeclampsia or eclampsia. In pharmacologic doses, it acts on the central nervous system. Its curariform action at the neuromuscular junction apparently interferes with the release of acetylcholine at motor nerve terminals. Magnesium may also replace calcium at the neuromuscular junction, thereby altering membrane potential and neuromuscular transmission and excitation.

Dosing Regimens

Magnesium sulfate should be given intravenously using a 4–6-g loading dose over 10–20 minutes. The usual 2 g/hour maintenance dose is dependent on the clinical condition of the patient. The patient given magnesium sulfate should be monitored closely for any neuromuscular, respiratory, or cardiac impairment. The following parameters should be monitored carefully: (*a*) deep tendon reflexes every hour (if absent, the dosage should be lowered); (*b*) respiratory rate every hour (should be above 12/min); and (*c*) urine output (should exceed 100 mL every 4 hours, since magnesium is excreted only in the urine).

Serum magnesium levels need not necessarily be obtained routinely. However, a serum magnesium concentration should be drawn when the therapy is continued for more than 24 hours, deep tendon reflexes are hypoactive, or oliguria is present. A concentration between 4 and 7 mEq/L is desired. A level between 8 and 10 mEq/L is associated with a loss of deep tendon reflexes, while respiratory paralysis develops when concentrations exceed 13 mEq/L. Cardiac conduction is affected when serum magnesium concentrations exceed 15 mEq/L.

An antidote to hypermagnesemia is calcium gluconate or calcium chloride in a 10% solution. A 10 mL (1 g) dose injected intravenously will usually correct the hypermagnesemia rapidly. Since eclamptic seizures may occur postpartum, intravenous magnesium is customarily continued for 24 hours along with careful observation of the mother.

Additional Considerations

1. Although magnesium decreases the intrinsic resistance in the uterine vessels, a hypotensive effect does not usually occur or is present only transiently.
2. If a grand mal seizure occurs, magnesium sulfate 4–6 g intravenously over 20–30 minutes or diazepam 10 mg intravenously over 2 minutes should be infused. If the seizure begins despite a maintenance dose of 1–3 g/hour, a serum magnesium level may be subtherapeutic and 3 g/hour would be necessary. Concerns about diazepam therapy include its

potential respiratory depression and the delayed elimination of the principal metabolite.

3. Using seizure prophylaxis doses, magnesium sulfate is thought to have no remarkable effect on impending uterine contractility. Doses used for tocolysis are usually twice those for seizure prophylaxis.

4. The effect of magnesium on the fetus is thought to be minimal, even though serum levels in the fetus rapidly approach those of the mother. Serum magnesium levels in the newborn remain elevated for up to 2 days after delivery. Signs of hypermagnesemia (hypotonicity, lethargy, respiratory depression) occur most frequently when there has been continuous infusion of magnesium sulfate for more than 24 hours and when urinary output is inadequate in the infant. The neurologic and respiratory performances of the neonate do not necessarily correlate with cord magnesium levels. Neonatal calcium levels are unaffected by intrapartum magnesium therapy.

5. Magnesium therapy should be continued during a cesarean section. A lower dose of a muscle relaxant is usually necessary.

6. A number of investigators have provided preliminary data about intravenous phenytoin to prevent or treat seizures of eclampsia. Although the drug may control convulsions, low 5-minute Apgar scores and recurrences requiring magnesium sulfate are concerns.

PROPHYLACTIC ANTIBIOTICS FOR CESAREAN SECTIONS

There has been a fourfold increase in the incidence of cesarean sections within the past 25 years. It is common to expect an increased incidence of postpartum febrile morbidity from infections and prolonged hospitalizations in this group of patients. The newer, more expensive antibiotics do not appear to be more beneficial, and certain products can cause hypoprothrombinemia and bleeding, presumably from impairment of vitamin K synthesis. Factors predisposing to endometritis and wound infection include antecedent labor, ruptured amniotic membranes for 6 hours or more, multiple vaginal examinations, and lower socioeconomic status.

Advantages to prophylactic antibiotic therapy include a lowered incidence of febrile morbidity related to endometritis, wound infection, and urinary tract infection when compared with no therapy. Furthermore, patient discomfort, prolonged hospitalization, and patient inactivity are less frequent with antibiotic therapy. A short course of a penicillin or cephalosporin antibiotic induces changes within the bacterial flora, but serious infections caused by anaerobic bacteria are probably not eliminated.

Limitations to prophylactic antibiotic therapy include cost, inability to avoid serious postoperative infections, and questionable value for low-risk surgical patients. Adverse effects from ampicillin or a cephalosporin product are uncommon but may involve hypersensitivity, which is reversed with drug discontinuation.

Recommendations

1. Prophylactic therapy must be individualized whenever possible. Infectious control precautions and proper surgical technique with sufficient dilation of the lower uterine segment are essential.
2. An ideal protocol for prophylactic antibiotic therapy has not been established. A single antibiotic with broad spectrum coverage such as 1 g of a first-generation cephalosporin (e.g., cefazolin, cefoxitin, cephalothin) appears to be as effective as two or more antibiotics combined.
3. The administration of a drug shortly after cord clamping or surgery is considered to be as effective as administering the drug preoperatively. This protects the unborn infant from antibiotic exposure and avoids masking of neonatal infection.
4. The antibiotic should be administered for less than 24 hours postoperatively, since cost and potential drug complications are reduced. Febrile morbidity is not significantly greater than if the drug were given for 24 hours or more.

Suggested Readings

American College of Obstetricians and Gynecologists. Fetal heart rate patterns: monitoring, interpretation, and management. ACOG Technical Bulletin 207. Washington, DC: ACOG, 1995.

American College of Obstetricians and Gynecologists. Induction of labor. ACOG Technical Bulletin Washington, DC: ACOG, 1995.

Chelmow D, Laros RK Jr. Maternal and neonatal outcomes after oxytocin augmentation in patients undergoing a trial of labor after prior cesarean delivery. Obstet Gynecol 1992;80:966–971.

Flamm BL, Goings JR. Vaginal birth after cesarean section: is suspected fetal macrosomia a contraindication? Obstet Gynecol 1989;74: 694–697.

Flamm BL, Newman LA, Thomas SJ, Fallon D, Yoshida MM. Vaginal birth after cesarean delivery: results of a 5-year multicenter collaborative study. Obstet Gynecol 1990;76:750–754.

Jones RO, Nagashima AW, Hartnett-Goodman MM, Goodlin RC. Rupture of low transverse cesarean scars during trial of labor. Obstet Gynecol 1991;77:815–817.

O'Driscoll K, Foley MM. Correlation of decrease in perinatal mortality and increase in cesarean section rates. Obstet Gynecol 1983;61:1–5.

Pruett KM, Kirshon B, Cotton DB, Poindexter AN 3d. Is vaginal birth after two or more cesarean sections safe? Obstet Gynecol 1988;72:163–165.

Rosen MG, Dickinson JC, Westhoff CL. Vaginal birth after cesarean: a meta-analysis of morbidity and mortality. Obstet Gynecol 1991;77: 465–470.

Scott JR. Mandatory trial of labor after cesarean delivery: an alternative viewpoint. Obstet Gynecol 1991;77:811–814.

Chapter 9

Intrapartum Complications

ABNORMAL LABOR

An evaluation for progress during labor should be based on a comparison with carefully established normal ranges. The strength of uterine contractions depends on their frequency and duration and on the indentability of the uterus. Adequate contractions leading to progressive cervical dilation usually occur every 2–3 minutes and last 45–60 seconds, and the firm uterus is not indentable.

The first stage of labor occurs from the onset of true labor to complete cervical dilation and typically lasts 6–18 hours in nulliparous and 2–10 hours in multiparous women. The second stage from complete dilation of the cervix until birth usually lasts 30 minutes to 3 hours in nulliparous and 5–30 minutes in multiparous women.

Protracted or arrested cervical dilation may develop during the early (latent) and late (active) phases of the first stage and during the second stage. Diagnostic criteria and proposed treatment for abnormal labor patterns are described in Table 9.1. Caput formation of the fetal scalp, a failure of fetal descent into the pelvis, fetal macrosomia, and a poor fetal heart rate (FHR) response to stressful uterine contractions are often present. Intervention before prolonged abnormal labor should minimize fetal compromise and reduce the incidence of neonatal morbidity.

MECONIUM

The passage of meconium-stained amniotic fluid during labor occurs in 20–25% of all vaginal deliveries and may indicate a nonreassuring fetal status. Although there may be no apparent FHR

Table 9.1
Abnormal Labor Patterns, Diagnostic Criteria, and Treatment

Labor Pattern	Nullipara	Multipara	Treatment
Prolonged latent phase	> 20 hours	> 14 hour	Rest or oxytocin
Protraction disorders			Oxytocin, if contractions are inadequate
Dilation	< 1.2 cm/hour	< 1.5 cm/hour	
Descent	< 1.0 cm/hour	< 2.0 cm/hour	
Arrest disorders			Oxytocin, if contractions are inadequate
Dilation	> 2 hour	> 2 hour	Forceps, vacuum, or cesarean delivery
Descent	> 1 hour	> 1 hour	

sign, it may be a consequence of hypoxia or anoxia leading to a relaxation of the fetal anal sphincter and rectum with increased bowel peristalsis and intrauterine gasping. Unlike term and post-date fetuses, the premature fetus infrequently or rarely passes meconium and has an extraordinary capacity to withstand signs of severe distress for many hours until intrapartum death.

Other conditions in which meconium is observed include breech presentation, cord entanglements, prolonged labor, toxemia of pregnancy, and postdate pregnancies. These neonates require resuscitation, respiratory support, and antibiotics more frequently than the general newborn population.

Recommendations

1. Expedient or operative delivery is not indicated because of meconium staining alone. A search for any antepartum or intrapartum complication(s) is necessary.

2. The passage of meconium in breech presentations is caused by pressure of uterine contractions on the fetal intestines and is not necessarily a sign of fetal distress.

3. When meconium is passed at any time during labor, electronic FHR monitoring is necessary. Thick or early heavy meconium is especially associated with asphyxia and acidosis.

4. Should there be a significant alteration in the fetal heart rate, immediate delivery may be needed to save the infant.

5. Aspiration of meconium is thought to be an antepartum event. Despite this, a DeLee suction trap is routinely used to suction the infant's oropharynx, nasopharynx, and gastric aspirate before delivery of the infant's shoulder. A DeLee suction trap should be located in each laboring room in case labor is too rapid for maternal transport to the delivery room.

6. If meconium is thick and the infant is depressed, intubation and suctioning are necessary before the initiation of positive-pressure ventilation. If meconium is thick and the infant is active, management is less precise; both endotracheal intubation and suctioning or observation are accepted therapeutic options.

7. Not all green amniotic fluid is meconium. This may instead consist of vomited bile secondary to a gastrointestinal obstruction.

BREECH DELIVERY

The overall incidence of breech presentation at term is approximately 3%. The incidence is substantially higher at earlier gestational ages, being 40% at less than 28 weeks and 17% between 28 and 31 weeks. Breech-presenting fetuses are at increased risk of perinatal morbidity and mortality not only from birth trauma but also because the presentation is associated with conditions or complications such as prematurity, low birth weight for gestational age, prolapsed cord, congenital malformations, placenta previa, and abruptio placentae.

Many vaginal deliveries occur when the mother presents in late labor and the cervix is nearly completely dilated. In cases in which there is sufficient time for a decision, most authorities believe that carefully selected breech fetuses can safely deliver vaginally, and house officers are provided the opportunity to acquire skills in vaginal breech delivery. The hazards of breech delivery must be recognized, and in our experience cesarean section is the route of delivery in at least three-fourths of breech cases.

Route of Delivery

Cesarean Section

An understanding of indications for cesarean section must be understood. These are listed in Table 9.2. An ultrasound examination to localize the placenta, rule out twins, and search for a fetal anomaly is useful before surgery.

Table 9.2
Indications for Cesarean Delivery of the Breech Fetus

Footling and complete breech presentations with EFW 750 g or more, or gestational age 26 weeks or more

Frank breech presentations with EFW less than 2000 g or more than 3800 g, or gestational age less than 36 weeks

Hyperextension of fetal head

Insulin-dependent diabetes mellitus

Floating presenting part

Pelvic contracture by x-ray or clinical pelvimetry

History of prior difficult or traumatic delivery or perinatal death

Any coexistent obstetric indication for cesarean section, whether or not patient receives oxytocin

A low transverse uterine incision is satisfactory if there is adequate room to avoid unnecessary trauma to the aftercoming fetal head. This incision is associated with decreased postoperative morbidity and will permit a trial of labor and attempt at vaginal delivery with any subsequent pregnancies. If the lower uterine segment is not well-developed, as is often seen in premature or low-birth-weight breech fetuses, a vertical uterine incision may be preferable to minimize entrapment of the fetal head.

Vaginal Delivery

Prerequisites for a trial of labor include the following findings: (*a*) no other indications for cesarean section, (*b*) frank breech presentation, (*c*) estimated fetal weight (EFW) 2500–3800 g by two examiners, (*d*) gestational age 36 weeks or more, (*e*) no space-occupying malformation or twins, (*f*) adequate medical personnel (another obstetrician, anesthesiologist/anesthetist, pediatrician), and (*g*) normal clinical or x-ray pelvimetry. Approximately half of these candidates will have inadequate pelvic measurements on x-ray examination. When all prerequisites are met, approximately half will safely deliver vaginally.

Anesthesia and neonatal personnel should be notified in advance. The patient's blood should be typed and screened. Internal FHR and uterine activity monitoring is essential. Progressive cervical dilation (1.5 cm/hour) and sufficient descent of the presenting part during the active phase of labor must occur. Oxytocin is either to be avoided or used very judiciously.

Compared with a total extraction, a controlled or partial breech extraction minimizes trauma. A well-controlled and properly-executed breech extraction is safer for both mother and fetus than a hastily-performed, difficult cesarean section. A second physician is necessary to assist in the extraction process. During any cesarean delivery after a trial of labor, another person may be necessary to push the presenting part up out of the maternal pelvis.

OPERATIVE VAGINAL DELIVERY

An arrest of fetal descent at the mid-pelvis is a common intrapartum complication. Accurate determination of the depth of fetal head descent into the pelvis is essential before midforceps or vacuum application is attempted. A cesarean section is necessary when a floating fetal head persists despite an adequate trial of la-

Table 9.3
Classification of Forceps Deliveries According to Station and Rotation

Type of Procedure	Classification
Outlet forceps	1) Scalp is visible at the introitus without separating labia 2) Fetal skull has reached pelvic floor 3) Sagittal suture is in anteroposterior position 4) Fetal head is at or on perineum 5) Rotation does not exceed 45°
Low forceps	Leading point of fetal skull is at station ≥+2 cm, and not on the pelvic floor a. Rotation ≤45° (left or right occiput anterior to occiput anterior, or left or right occiput posterior to occiput posterior) b. Rotation >45°
Midforceps	Station above +2 cm but head engaged
High forceps	Not included in classification

bor. Once the widest diameter of the presenting part has passed through the inlet (engagement), an abdominal operation with an assistant pushing the presenting part upward may not be necessary if forceps or a vacuum can be applied and used properly. If an abnormal FHR pattern occurs suddenly, an attempt at forceps or vacuum delivery may be undertaken with caution. Table 9.3 classifies forceps (or vacuum) deliveries according to station and rotation.

Forceps Application

Before application of the forceps, a staff physician should reassess the fetal position. Manual rotation should be attempted beforehand, since forceps delivery may be quite difficult if no rotation can be performed manually. The pediatricians should be notified in advance, before application of the forceps, and close monitoring of the FHR is necessary.

Forceps should be applied only after the cervix is completely dilated and if there is no evidence of cephalopelvic disproportion. Forceps may be applied only after the biparietal diameter has passed through the inlet, and the skull has passed below the ischial spines (station 0 to +2). A senior house officer or faculty member should check the forceps application before any rotation is undertaken. Traction on the fetal head should be along the least resistant pathway of the pelvis. Excess force should be avoided, especially in any incorrect line of access into the pelvis.

After delivery, the genital tract and infant should be examined carefully. Lacerations of the supporting pelvic tissues, tears of the cervix or uterus, or injury to the bladder and rectum should be sought. Injury to the fetus should also be sought and documented. These injuries include any intracranial hemorrhage (subdural, epidural, subarachnoid), linear or depressed skull fracture, brachial plexus injury, cephalhematoma formation, facial paralysis, clavicular fracture, or bruising.

Vacuum Extraction

The definitions, indications, and prerequisites for vacuum extraction of the fetus are the same as for forceps deliveries. Recent reports show little difference in injury between forceps and vacuum deliveries. The choice of instrument should be based primarily on the experience of the operator.

The principal extractors that are available consist of soft rubber or plastic rather than metal cups. Two vacuum extractors commonly used are the polymeric silicone cup and smaller disposable plastic cups. Advantages of the vacuum extractor include less force applied to the fetal vertex, reduced anesthesia requirements, ease of application, less perineal trauma, and the ability to permit the head to find its path out of the maternal pelvis. Disadvantages of the extractor include the application of traction only during contractions, its use limited to term infants, prolonged delivery when compared to forceps delivery, and the care required to maintain the vacuum. Morbidity and mortality are low, but caput formation for several hours is quite common.

The head must be engaged and the membranes must be ruptured. No vaginal mucosa or cervical tissue should be caught between the vacuum and the fetal head. Vacuum pressure of up to 50 cm Hg should be obtained and maintained during traction. When maintaining this pressure, it is easier for the cup to conform to the fetal head and allow proper traction. Traction should be applied during a contraction with the mother bearing down. Traction should be in a plane perpendicular to that of the cup application, since improper traction may cause scalp laceration or subgaleal hemorrhage. A safety feature of the vacuum cup is its inability to remain on the fetal head during excess traction. The vacuum pressure should be minimal between contractions. The operator's hand should be maintained on the cup, so that if the cup disengages inadvertently, it will not move freely through the vaginal canal and trap maternal tissue.

PROLAPSE OF THE UMBILICAL CORD

A prolapse of the umbilical cord occurs in 0.3–0.6% of all pregnancies. It is an obstetric emergency which is commonly associated with a breech presentation, polyhydramnios, premature delivery, early artificial rupture of the amniotic membranes, and malpresentation of the fetus. Perinatal mortality can be as high as 35% without immediate temporary therapy and prompt delivery. A prolapsed umbilical cord may be ignored when the fetus is either already dead, has a major malformation incompatible with life, or is so immature that survival is improbable.

Temporary Therapy

The examiner's hand should be placed in the vagina to ascertain the cervical dilation, station, and presenting part. The presenting part should be pushed up and away from the umbilical cord as the patient is placed in a knee-chest or Trendelenburg position.

The mother should be given oxygen by mask, and the FHR should be monitored continuously by auscultation or ultrasound imaging. Further assistance by a senior house officer or faculty member is necessary, and the anesthesia and neonatal staff should be notified promptly. Inserting a Foley catheter to distend the bladder and administering a beta-agonist (e.g., terbutaline 250 μg) intravenously may alleviate cord compression.

Delivery Considerations

Cervical dilation is perhaps the most important prognostic indicator. A cervix that is inadequately dilated and a delay of over 30 minutes increases fetal mortality significantly. Cesarean section is the best method of delivery, unless the cervix is dilated completely and the fetal head is low in the pelvis. Under these circumstances, fundal pressure and forceps should be applied to expedite vaginal delivery. If the cervix is incompletely dilated, manual dilation of the cervix is necessary as the cord is repositioned to avoid further compression.

In addition to FHR monitoring, the cord should be palpated for any pulsation while the mother is in the Trendelenburg position. Ultrasound visualization is also helpful, especially when the FHR is difficult to locate. The neonatal staff should be notified to be in attendance to institute immediate resuscitation of the newborn.

Postoperative febrile morbidity and signs of infection become evident invariably. Parenteral antimicrobial therapy with broad-spectrum antibiotics is recommended during the immediate postoperative period.

EMERGENCY CESAREAN SECTION

Between 20 and 25% of gravidas are now delivered by cesarean section. Approximately two-thirds of these procedures are performed after the onset of labor and are more likely to be considered emergency cesarean sections. It may be appropriate to subdivide this group into those requiring truly emergent surgery (intrapartum FHR abnormality, prolapsed cord, ruptured uterus, severe abruptio placentae, placenta previa with extensive hemorrhage) or urgent surgery (abnormal presentation and active labor, worrisome antepartum FHR testing, placenta previa with mild bleeding). Immediate delivery is required in the former category, whereas reasonably rapid intervention is required in the latter. It is important for the obstetric service at every hospital to have well-defined protocols for the performance of emergent and urgent cesarean sections.

Maternal Preparation

Blood samples should be sent routinely for a complete blood count and typing and screening. A platelet count, prothrombin time, partial thromboplastin time, fibrinogen, and fibrin split products should be determined in patients with excessive uterine bleeding.

Pulmonary aspiration of gastric contents remains the leading cause of anesthetic maternal mortality. Every gravida should receive oral antacid prophylaxis (such as sodium citrate) every 3 hours during labor. This therapy raises the pH of gastric contents (usually from 2.5 to 4) to decrease the severity of any aspiration during induction of general anesthesia.

The abdomen may be shaved with an electric shaver and a

Foley catheter inserted when the potential need for an emergency or urgent cesarean section is recognized. It may be prudent to move the patient and allow her to labor in the delivery room. Fetal monitoring should be continued in the delivery room.

Significant maternal metabolic disorders, hypoxia, and hypovolemia should be corrected. Maternal cardiopulmonary and neurologic function should be stable at induction of anesthesia.

Medical Personnel Preparation

Provisions for performing a cesarean section within 15 minutes should be available at any tertiary obstetric service. Each member of the surgical, anesthesia, and nursing team must understand his or her responsibilities. In less well-staffed hospitals, appropriate personnel should be notified when a potential problem is recognized, rather than when the actual decision is made to perform a cesarean section. Although there may be false alarms, this practice serves to avoid an unnecessary and potentially disastrous delay.

Primary and back-up scrub and circulating nurses should be clearly identified on each nursing shift. Anesthesia personnel responsible for cesarean sections should be notified of problems in advance if possible. Neonatal personnel should also be notified of potential problems, for they may also wish to interview the patient and evaluate her problem in the obstetrician's presence.

Technique

A rapid sequence induction with general anesthesia and endotracheal intubation is the preferred technique for most emergency cesarean sections. Although some highly experienced obstetric anesthesiologists prefer to inject a spinal block or to use an epidural catheter if it is already in place, preparation for administering general anesthesia is necessary if the spinal or epidural does not provide rapid anesthesia. There is usually sufficient time to administer a regional anesthetic in the case of an urgent cesarean section. While maximum surgical speed is necessary in emergency situations, maternal safety should never be sacrificed to haste.

Povidone-iodine (Betadine) spray to the abdomen and insertion of a Foley catheter are usually adequate for a truly emergent cesarean section. Operative delivery using local anesthesia is not considered to be faster than waiting for general anesthesia administration.

A vertical abdominal incision provides more rapid access to the uterus during emergency situations. There is usually no need to clamp minor bleeders or ligate major bleeders before delivery of the infant. Once the uterine incision has been made with a scalpel, it can be rapidly stretched in a transverse direction. A bladder injury should be sought, and if present should be repaired with two layers of continuous or interrupted 3–0 or 4–0 polyglycolic acid suture in an imbricating manner. Methylene blue or sterile formula may be injected above the clamped Foley catheter to determine the extent of any tear and to see if the repair is adequate.

Surgical techniques in performing a cesarean delivery have changed during the past decade. The surgeon is now more aware of the potential of HIV virus exposure and inclined to employ techniques to minimize contact with sharp objects during surgery. When possible, a low transverse uterine incision is attempted to allow an attempted trial of labor with any subsequent pregnancy. Spontaneous delivery of the placenta may decrease the chances of postoperative endometritis. Single-layer closure of the uterus without closure of the peritoneum is practical, time-efficient, and cost-effective. Wound disruption in obese patients can be decreased by reducing any large subcutaneous space by the placement of a drain with continuous suction.

Puerperal Hysterectomy

The most common contemporary indication for removal of the uterus at the time of a cesarean delivery is an abnormally adherent placenta. Other reasons include uterine atony that does not respond to medical management, uterine rupture, and laceration of major uterine vessels that is not controlled by suture ligation. There is arguably a role for scheduled cesarean hysterectomy for women with an indication for cesarean delivery and antecedent uterine bleeding, uterine leiomyomas, or high-grade cervical intraepithelial neoplasia. Morbidity from the procedure includes increased blood loss requiring transfusion, urologic injury, and pelvic cellulitis.

SHOULDER DYSTOCIA

True shoulder dystocia is uncommon but represents a very stressful intrapartum condition requiring vaginal delivery. It may be anticipated beforehand under the following circumstances: prolonged second stage of labor, fetal macrosomia, anencephaly, locked twins, enlargement of the fetal abdomen or thorax, and maternal diabetes.

Method of Delivery

A senior house officer or staff member and an anesthesiologist should be notified for further assistance. The mother's hips should be more fully flexed in the direction of her chest (McRoberts maneuver). An inhalation anesthetic such as halothane should be administered by an anesthesia staff member for complete muscle relaxation. An episiotomy, preferably large, should be made to provide more room, although this does not release the shoulders. In some instances a second episiotomy may be helpful.

Gentle upward traction on the delivered head should be performed as the patient is told to bear down. If this fails on one or two efforts, an attempt should be made either to deliver the anterior shoulder, to extract the posterior shoulder or arm, or to "corkscrew" the shoulders using the Wood's maneuver.

Delivery of Anterior Shoulder

The examiner's hand is placed behind the anterior shoulder, and the shoulder is rotated into the oblique diameter of the pelvis with the next uterine contraction. Suprapubic pressure is exerted by an assistant while the patient's hips are fully flexed. Firm, downward traction on the head is necessary to bring the anterior shoulder in and out of the pelvis. The obstetrician's forefinger may also be hooked under the axilla as early as possible during the extraction procedure.

Extraction of Posterior Shoulder and Arm

The examiner's hand may instead be placed behind the posterior shoulder with the arm being grasped and pushed forward over the front of the infant's abdomen. Once the hand is seized, it can be extracted with the arm to permit the anterior shoulder to be either delivered under the pubic arc or rotated 180° and delivered in the posterior position.

Corkscrew Rotation

Instead of grasping the posterior arm and delivering the hand, the front of the posterior shoulder is pressed so that the shoulder moves with force and with the back leading the way. It is rotated 180° until the posterior shoulder is delivered under the pubic arc. After delivering the posterior shoulder, the anterior shoulder is now posterior. Continued downward pressure on the fetus's buttocks by fundal pressure should permit another rotation of 180° in the same direction so that the shoulder is delivered under the pubic arc.

Other

Extraordinary measures may be needed: (*a*) deliberate fracture of the clavicle, (*b*) cephalic replacement (Zavanelli maneuver) followed by cesarean delivery, or (*c*) symphysiotomy (usually reserved for medically underserved areas).

PREPARATION FOR THE COMPROMISED INFANT

The quality of intrapartum care, resuscitation, and immediate neonatal care often determines whether a compromised infant will survive or suffer from extensive morbidity. Careful preparation is required. When a nonreassuring fetal status is present, precautions should be undertaken and the proper personnel notified.

Intrapartum Care

Unless there has been a prior antepartum complication, a compromised fetus is usually not anticipated until after the onset of labor. The presence of a fetal malpresentation, meconium staining, failure of descent, or abnormal FHR pattern suggests fetal compromise.

An abnormal FHR pattern (bradycardia, unexplained loss of beat-to-beat variability, or repetitive late or severe variable decelerations) warrants continued electronic monitoring, frequent pelvic examinations, reassessment of any underlying complication, and fetal acid-base status. Trauma to the fetus should be minimized, and oxygen should be given to the mother before and during any difficult delivery. Local or conduction anesthesia is preferred over excessive maternal sedation and prolonged inhalation anesthesia.

If a serious abnormality that arose during the delivery or any problem with the neonate persists after the first 5 minutes, blood from the umbilical cord should be drawn and sent to a laboratory for blood gases analysis. Umbilical blood should be sampled in a syringe (1–2 mL using 1000 U/mL heparin) and sent for pH and base excess determinations. Umbilical arterial blood best reflects the fetal condition, whereas venous blood reflects uteroplacental circulation. Moreover, it is possible to have a very low umbilical artery pH in a depressed fetus secondary to a cord prolapse and have a relatively normal umbilical vein pH. In difficult cases such as the very premature infant, an arterial sample from the chorionic surface of the placenta (the artery crosses over the vein) will provide accurate results.

Umbilical Blood Gas Interpretation

Although newborn acidemia has been classically defined as an umbilical artery pH of less than 7.2, it is now evident that this level is arbitrarily high. The umbilical artery level below which major neurologic morbidity occurs would appear to be closer to 7.00, and this is the cutoff currently recommended as one of the criteria necessary for defining birth "asphyxia" or hypoxia to a degree that might be associated with subsequent neurologic dysfunction. Interestingly, as many as two-thirds of term infants with an umbilical artery pH of less than 7.00 will be admitted to the normal nursery with no apparent morbidity.

Classifications of acidemia at birth are listed in Table 9.4. The pH of blood or tissue is directly related to the bicarbonate (HCO_3) metabolic buffer level and is inversely related to CO_2 levels. The two most important buffers in fetal blood that allow for a relatively constant pH are bicarbonate and hemoglobin. Base deficit refers to the amount of buffer below normal levels. Conditions that interrupt normal blood flow to the fetus from the placenta, such as umbilical cord occlusion, may cause a rapid rise in CO_2, resulting in respiratory acidosis. If reduced fetal perfusion persists, fetal hypoxia results and the products of anaerobic metabolism, the organic acids, accumulate. Since CO_2 diffuses very quickly, respiratory acidosis is rapidly corrected once the occlu-

Table 9.4
Classification of Fetal or Newborn Acidemia

Acidemia Type	pCO_2	HCO_3	Base Deficit
Respiratory	High	Normal	Normal
Metabolic	Normal	Low	High
Mixed	High	Low	High

sion is released. Metabolic acidosis takes longer to correct than does respiratory acidosis.

Newborn Care

After delivery, a potentially compromised infant should be handled gently, dried immediately, and kept warm in an area with properly controlled temperature and humidity. The upper airway should be cleared, and the head should be positioned down at an angle of 30° to horizontal. The upper airways should be suctioned of any mucus and debris.

Apgar scores should be assigned at 1 and 5 minutes after delivery using the scoring system shown in Table 9.5. Oxygen is the best therapy in the presence of a low Apgar score until the infant's respiratory center can maintain its regulatory function. Oxygen administered using a well-fitting mask may act as a physiologic stimulant to the anoxic respiratory center along with maintaining pulmonary ventilation. Direct endotracheal intubation with positive pressure ventilation is necessary when respiratory difficulties are encountered despite these initial measures.

Narcotic-induced depression of the newborn is uncommon, and proper resuscitation and adequate supportive care should diminish any need for a narcotic antagonist. Naloxone (Narcan), an almost pure opioid antagonist with minimal agonist action, is the drug of choice for narcotic-induced depression. The neonatal preparation (0.02 mg/mL) is recommended at a dose of 0.1 mg/mL intravenously. Less predictable absorption occurs with subcutaneous, intramuscular, and intralingual administration. To ensure lasting action, naloxone may be readministered within

Table 9.5
Apgar Scoring System

	0	1	2
Heart rate	Absent	Below 100 bpm	Over 100 bpm
Respiratory effort	Absent	Slow, irregular	Good crying
Muscle tone	Flaccid	Some flexion of extremities	Active motion; flexed extremities
Reflex irritability	No response	Grimace	Vigorous cry
Color	Blue; pale	Body pink; extremities blue	Completely pink

5 minutes of an initial positive response if rhythmic respirations are not sustained.

Established protocols for treatment of newborn brain edema, hypoperfusion, hypoxia, acidosis, anemia, and hypoglycemia are necessary. After resuscitation, it is necessary to monitor the infant closely for any signs of hypotonicity, irritability, jitteriness, seizures, or feeding problems. Potentially correctable metabolic disorders would include hypoglycemia, hyperbilirubinemia, and hypocalcemia. Antibiotics are often indicated when sepsis is suspected and are begun after appropriate cultures have been obtained. Signs of systemic hypotension in the neonate should be sought and corrected as quickly as possible. Since severe fetal-maternal hemorrhage may explain compromise or death in an anemic infant, a Kleihauer-Betke test of the mother's blood should be performed.

Subsequent Development

All stages of fetal and neonatal development influence normal neurologic outcome. Most neurologic disorders are not directly linked to a specific prenatal and perinatal event, and it cannot be said with any degree of certainty that mental retardation, cerebral palsy, and epilepsy are due to mild compromise at birth. Physician attitude is very important, however, since a given fetus assessed to be viable (at least 25 weeks or 600 grams) is more likely to survive with immediate attention. Improved obstetric techniques have reduced the number of cases of brain disease resulting from birth trauma from prolonged or difficult labor, difficult forceps delivery, or obstetric trauma. The nature, frequency, and severity of brain disorders are affected by such factors as race, socioeconomic status, lifestyle, and environmental influences both before and after birth. Social interaction of the infant and child with family, school acquaintances, and peers may play a role in the severity of an affliction.

The term "asphyxia" should be reserved for the clinical context of damaging acidemia, hypoxia, and metabolic acidosis. A neonate who has undergone hypoxia severe enough to result in encephalopathy will show other evidence of hypoxic damage, including all of the following: (*a*) profound metabolic or mixed acidemia (pH less than 7.00) on an umbilical cord arterial blood sample, (*b*) persistent Apgar score of 0–3 for longer than 5 minutes, and (*c*) evidence of neonatal neurologic sequelae and damage to one other end organ.

Pure mental retardation or grand mal seizures are rarely associated with intrapartum events. Birth trauma and "asphyxia" singly or together are infrequent causes of mental retardation, although they can cause brain disorders. Fewer than 15% of cases of severe mental retardation (IQ less than 50) can be attributed to perinatal events. Select termination of fetuses with certain malformations or with metabolic or chromosomal defects, and rapid intervention of neonates with metabolic disorders, can reduce the incidence and severity of the retardation. Social, economic, and cultural factors associated with prematurity and intrauterine growth retardation are related to mild mental retardation. Future preconception and prenatal counseling should include discussion of topics such as planned pregnancy, proper nutrition, avoidance of substance abuse, adequate prenatal care, and continuation of maternal education.

Although specific events within the intrapartum period are associated with a portion of infants later diagnosed with cerebral palsy, the illness is often linked with compounding factors such as low birth weight and prematurity. In the presence of neonatal seizures, there is a high risk of the later development of cerebral palsy and epilepsy. Severe "asphyxia" and prematurity are the only two major identifiable causes of cerebral palsy, but almost three-quarters of children with cerebral palsy have no evidence of such "asphyxia." Furthermore, at least three-quarters of severely "asphyxiated" infants who survive demonstrate no major handicap by the time they reach school age.

Suggested Readings

American College of Obstetricians and Gynecologists. Fetal and neonatal neurologic injury. ACOG Technical Bulletin 163. Washington, DC: ACOG, 1992.

American College of Obstetricians and Gynecologists. Umbilical artery blood acid-base analysis. ACOG Technical Bulletin 216. Washington, DC: ACOG, 1995.

American College of Obstetricians and Gynecologists. Operative vaginal delivery. ACOG Technical Bulletin 196. Washington, DC: ACOG, 1994.

Fishburne JI Jr, Greiss FC Jr, Hopkinson R, Rhyne AL. Response of the gravid uterine vasculature to arterial levels of local anesthetic agents. Am J Obstet Gynecol 1979;133:753.

Goldaber KG, Gilstrap LC 3d. Correlations between obstetric clinical events and umbilical cord blood acid-base and blood gas values. Clin Obstet Gynecol 1993;36:47–59.

Gross TL, Sokol RJ, Williams T, Thompson K. Shoulder dystocia: a fetal-physician risk. Am J Obstet Gynecol 1987;156:1408–1418.

Hagadorn-Freathy AS, Yeomans ER, Hankins GD. Validation of the 1988 ACOG forceps classification system. Obstet Gynecol 1991;77:356–360.

Myers SA, Gleicher N. A successful program to lower cesarean-section rates. N Engl J Med 1988;319:1511–1516.

Nocon JJ, McKenzie DK, Thomas LJ, Hansell RS. Shoulder dystocia: an analysis of risks and obstetric maneuvers. Am J Obstet Gynecol 1993;168:1732–1737; discussion 1737–1739.

Ophir E, Oettinger M, Yadoda A, Markovits Y, Rojansky N, Shapiro H. Breech presentation after cesarean section: always a section? Am J Obstet Gynecol 1989;161:25–28.

Rosen MG, Chik L. The effect of delivery route on outcome in breech presentation. Am J Obstet Gynecol 1984;148:909–914.

Rosen MG, Debanne SM, Thompson K, Dickinson JC. Abnormal labor and infant brain damage. Obstet Gynecol 1992;80:961–965.

Sanchez-Ramos L, Kaunitz AM, Peterson HB, Martinez-Schnell B, Thompson RJ. Reducing cesarean sections at a teaching hospital. Am J Obstet Gynecol 1990;163:1081–1088.

Sandberg EC. The Zavanelli maneuver: a potentially revolutionary method for the resolution of shoulder dystocia. Am J Obstet Gynecol 1985;152:479–484.

Socol ML, Garcia PM, Peaceman AM, Dooley SL. Reducing cesarean births at a primarily private university hospital. Am J Obstet Gynecol 1993;168:1748–1754; discussion 1754–1758.

Williams MC, Knuppel RA, O'Brien WF, Weiss A, Kanarek KS. A randomized comparison of assisted vaginal delivery by obstetric forceps and polyethylene vacuum cup. Obstet Gynecol 1991;78:789–794.

Yancey MK, Harlass FE, Benson W, Brady K. The perioperative morbidity of scheduled cesarean hysterectomy. Obstet Gynecol 1993;81:206–210.

Yeomans ER, Hankins GD. Operative vaginal delivery in the 1990s. Clin Obstet Gynecol 1992;35:487–493.

Zelop CM, Harlow BL, Frigoletto FD Jr, Safon LE, Saltzman DH. Emergency peripartum hysterectomy. Am J Obstet Gynecol 1993;168:1443–1448.

Chapter 10

Postpartum Care

POSTPARTUM HEMORRHAGE

The most commonly accepted definition of postpartum hemorrhage is a blood loss in excess of 500 mL in the immediate postpartum period. However, when blood loss has been measured carefully, the following findings have been observed consistently: (*a*) the average blood loss with vaginal delivery is approximately 600 mL; (*b*) only about 5% of women hemorrhage more than 1000 mL; and (*c*) the estimated blood loss is often approximately half of the carefully measured blood loss. An awareness of risk factors enumerated in Table 10.1 should allow anticipation of most cases of postpartum hemorrhage. Table 10.2 lists causes of postpartum hemorrhage.

All hospitalized patients should have their blood typed and screened before delivery. Early and aggressive management prevents hemorrhage from becoming life-threatening and decreases the likelihood of complications from anemia. The personal contact with blood bank personnel is to be encouraged.

Prophylaxis

1. A hematocrit level should be determined during labor, and blood should be sent for typing and screening.
2. When hemorrhage is anticipated, 2 units of blood should be cross-matched and available. A red-topped tube of blood should be tested for a prolonged clotting time (beyond 5 minutes) for possible transfusion.
3. Fibrinogen levels should be determined in cases of a large placental abruption, retained dead fetus, severe preeclampsia, or eclampsia.

Table 10.1
Conditions Predisposing to Postpartum Hemorrhage

Multiparity of more than five babies	Prolonged labor
Previous postpartum hemorrhage or manual removal of the placenta	Precipitous labor
	Difficult forceps delivery
Abruptio placentae	Version and extraction
Placenta previa	Chorioamnionitis
Excessive inhalation anesthesia	Breech extraction
Multiple pregnancy	Cesarean section
Polyhydramnios	Excessive or prolonged
Prolonged retention of dead fetus	oxytocin administration

Table 10.2
Causes of Postpartum Hemorrhage

Uterine atony
Retained placental fragment
Cervical or vaginal tear
Paravaginal, vulvar, or broad ligament hematoma
Intraperitoneal bleeding from a ruptured uterus
Afibrinogenemia, hypofibrinogenemia, thrombocytopenia, or inadequate
   platelet aggregation
Septic shock
Uterine inversion

4. Unless rapid delivery is imperative, the fetus and placenta should be delivered slowly to allow the uterus to contract sufficiently.

5. In cases where uterine atony is anticipated, intravenous oxytocin (10–40 units/liter intravenous fluid) added after delivery is continued for at least 1 hour postpartum.

6. Careful postpartum observation is necessary, and the uterine fundus should be massaged frequently for at least 1 hour postpartum.

Supportive Measures

1. In the presence of excessive bleeding, manual removal of the placenta should be carried out promptly, rather than waiting for spontaneous delivery. Voluntary pushing by the mother to expel the placenta may be helpful. Another physician should assist, while blood is set up for possible transfusion.

2. Careful inspection of the genital tract is necessary with adequate lighting. An assistant is an invaluable asset.
3. Any general anesthesia should be discontinued, and oxygen should be given by face mask.
4. Until blood is available, plasma expanders such as lactated Ringer's solution or normal saline are used. A minimum of 1 liter packed red blood cells or whole blood should be transfused.
5. Current estimates of risks of transfusing blood components are shown in Table 10.3.
6. If the blood pressure is falling, the foot of the table should be elevated.
7. Uterine atony is the most common reason for persistent postpartum bleeding. Uterine massage and compression of the aorta are recommended. Other causes of hemorrhage (listed in Table 10.2) should also be considered.
8. Transfusion with platelets, cryoprecipitate, or fresh frozen plasma is rarely necessary. Coagulation studies (PTT, PT, platelet count) should be performed after administration of every 5–10 units of blood. If hypofibrinogenemia is present, fibrinogen in cryoprecipitate (usually 10–20 packs) or fresh frozen plasma (usually 4 units) should be administered intravenously. If severe thrombocytopenia ($20,000/mm^3$ or less) is present, 6–10 packs of platelets should be infused to raise the platelet count by $15,000–60,000/mm^3$.
9. An ultrasound examination of the uterine cavity to look for retained placental fragments may be useful during immediate or delayed postpartum hemorrhage.
10. Autologous transfusion is the collection and reinfusion of

Table 10.3
Current Estimates of Transfusion Risks

Complication	Risk/Unit Transfused
Infection	
Hepatitis B	1:50,000
Hepatitis C	1:3,300
HIV-1, -2	1:150,000–1:1,000,000
HTLV-I, -II	1:50,000
Hemolytic reaction	1:6,000
Fatal transfusion reaction	1:100,000

the patient's own blood. Blood should be donated at least 2 weeks prior to surgery or delivery, and the patient must have an adequate red blood cell mass (the minimum criteria for donation are a hemoglobin level of 11 g/dL or more and a hematocrit level of 34% or greater). A placenta previa is the most common obstetric condition for which autologous donation may be appropriate. Another method of autologous transfusion is intraoperative blood salvage by the sterile collection and reinfusion of shed blood. Its safety during repair of a ruptured ectopic pregnancy and cesarean delivery has yet to be established.

Blood Component Replacement

Packed Red Blood Cells

Red blood cells provide a source of oxygen-carrying erythrocytes and mass for volume replacement. All units of blood are routinely screened for hepatitis B antigen and HIV antibody. Side effects and hazards (immunization, febrile reaction, iron overload, allergic reaction, hemolysis) of packed cell transfusion are similar to but less severe than from whole blood, since plasma, metabolites, and antibodies are removed. The typical red blood cell unit contains 200 mL of erythrocytes (hematocrit 70–80%), which should raise the recipient's hematocrit by 1–3%. When combined with isotonic saline, the transfusion of a unit should not exceed 4 hours. Infrequent side effects or hazards include hypokalemia with massive transfusion and microaggregates of fibrin, platelets, and white blood cells that would not be retained in the ordinary blood filter.

Platelets

Platelet concentrates derived from donor blood are used in patients with thrombocytopenia unless rapid platelet destruction is evident. Immunization to red blood cell antigens is possible because of the presence of a small number of red blood cells in the platelet packs. Therefore, prevention of $Rh_O(D)$ sensitization may require Rh immune globulin when an Rh-negative woman is transfused by an Rh-positive donor.

One unit of platelets usually increases the platelet count by 5,000–10,000/mm^3. The usual dose of a 10-unit pack is given when bleeding symptoms are evident or a platelet count is below 20,000/mm^3. Transfusion may also be indicated for platelet counts of 10,000–50,000/mm^3 if an operative procedure is planned, bleeding is active, or massive transfusions are anticipated. Repeat transfusion may be required because the half-life of platelets is only 3–4 days.

Fresh Frozen Plasma

Fresh frozen plasma is an excellent source of the clotting factors V, VII, IX, X, and fibrinogen. As with cryoprecipitate, donor compatibility is unimportant, but antibodies within the plasma can react to the recipient cells. It should not be used prophylactically with massive blood transfusion. If a coagulopathy is present and laboratory studies are not yet available, fresh frozen plasma should be used empirically.

Cryoprecipitate

Cryoprecipitate, a source of the coagulation factors VIII, XIII, and fibrinogen, is used for hemophilia A, hypofibrinogenemia, and von Willebrand's disease. As with other plasma products, viral hepatitis may be transmitted and febrile allergic reactions may occur. The quantity of these factors required for adequate coagulation is not easily predictable and varies with the clinical situation. Like fresh frozen plasma, cryoprecipitate is usually transported from a community facility, then thawed and kept at room temperature for up to 6 hours before use.

Treatment of Uterine Atony

Along with vigorous uterine massage and aortic compression, the following measures may be taken to control excess bleeding from presumed uterine atony.

Ergonovine	Ergonovine maleate (Methergine) 0.2 mg is given intravenously or intramuscularly (unless hypertension is already present).
Oxytocin	20–40 units oxytocin in 1 liter intravenous fluids at a speed sufficient to keep the uterus contracted.
Uterine exploration	Blood clots and placental fragments are removed.
Lacerations	The cervix, vagina, and vulva are examined and repaired under proper lighting and exposure by an assistant.

Prostaglandins	The vaginal insertion of a prostaglandin E_2 suppository (20 mg) with a vaginal pack or the intramuscular (in the buttock) or myometrial injection of prostaglandin $F_{2\alpha}$ (1 mL) may be useful if treatment using oxytocin or ergonovine is unsuccessful. Additional doses may be necessary.
Uterine packing or warm saline lavage	Most authorities condemn its use, since these procedures are not physiologic.
Intrauterine curettage	Unless placental fragments are palpable, curetting using a "banjo" curette is not usually beneficial.
Ligation of uterine arteries	The abdomen is opened, the uterus is elevated by the surgeon's hand, and the area of the uterine vessels in the lower broad ligament is exposed. Using a large needle and No. 1 chromic catgut or vicryl suture, a stitch is placed through a substantial part of the lower segment of the myometrium, 2–3 cm medial to the vessels. The vessels are ligated but not divided. Subsequent menstruation and pregnancy are usually unaffected.
Ligation of hypogastric arteries	The common iliac artery and its bifurcation into the external and internal iliac (hypogastric) arteries are palpated and visualized through the posterior peritoneum. The ureter crosses anterior to the bifurcation of the common iliac artery, and it must be identified to prevent potential damage. The posterior peritoneum is tented and incised in a longitudinal direction at the level of the origin of the internal iliac artery, lateral to the ureter and medial to the internal iliac artery. Two No. 2-0 silk sutures are placed around the internal iliac artery 1 cm apart and then tied on each side.
Angiographic embolization	A competent angiographer may be able to selectively embolize the uterine or hypogastric arteries with Gelfoam fragments.

Hysterectomy

Subsequent menstruation, fertility, and pregnancy are usually unaffected.

If the above procedures are ineffective or if time will not allow them, a hysterectomy should be performed (see Chapter 9). Deaths following and during hysterectomy usually result from delaying the operation until the patient is nearly moribund.

POSTPARTUM INFECTION

Postpartum infectious morbidity is present when a parturient experiences a fever of at least 38°C (100.4°F) on two occasions or more during the first 10 postpartum days, exclusive of the first 24 hours. The incidence of febrile morbidity varies widely, ranging from approximately 1% for nonindigent women delivering vaginally to as high as 87% for indigent women delivering by cesarean section. Factors definitely identified as increasing the risk of infection include emergency cesarean section, labor, ruptured membranes for 6 hours or more, and low socioeconomic status. Other factors such as anemia, general anesthesia, poor nutrition, obesity, and multiple vaginal exams may influence the risk of infection, but the correlation is less firmly established. All other factors being equal, the use of internal fetal monitoring does not appear to influence the risk of uterine infection.

The differential diagnosis for postpartum infection should include the seven W's: womb, wound, wind (atelectasis, pneumonia), water (urinary tract), wonder drug (drug allergy), walk (thrombophlebitis), and woman's breasts (bacterial and noninfectious mastitis). Most febrile morbidity results from an infection of the genital tract which is usually polymicrobial and frequently involves anaerobic organisms (*Bacteroides fragilis, Peptostreptococcus*). It is difficult to assess the role of transcervical cultures, because the normal resident flora of the genital tract makes interpretation of culture results difficult. The use of a double or triple-lumen lavage catheter may help to avoid vaginal or cervical contamination when collecting uterine specimens.

Wound and urinary tract infections are also relatively common. During evaluation of the febrile parturient, a diligent effort should be made to determine the site of infection and eliminate the less common causes of infection. Antibiotic regimens recommended to eradicate causative organisms in certain postpartum infections are shown in Table 10.4. Cure rates of endomy-ometritis using these regimens are expected to be 70–95%. Sequestered infections (abscess, hematoma, septic pelvic thrombophlebitis) or resistant organisms (*Klebsiella, Enterococcus,* nosocomial *Staphylococcus aureus*) may not respond well to these regimens.

INVASIVE HEMODYNAMIC MONITORING

The need for invasive hemodynamic monitoring is fortunately rare but occurs most often after delivery. Clinical impressions can quickly be either reinforced or refuted with accurate hemodynamic measurements in critically ill patients. The combination of peripheral arterial and pulmonary arterial lines provides sufficient information to assess the cardiac and pulmonary status of the patient. Although initial management of most acute events may not warrant invasive monitoring, failure to achieve the predicted clinical response to initial empirical therapy warrants consideration of invasive monitoring to collect additional information to guide and evaluate further therapeutic manipulations.

Clinical conditions for which invasive hemodynamic monitoring may assist in the management of obstetric-gynecologic patients include: (*a*) sepsis with oliguria, (*b*) unexplained or refractory pulmonary edema, heart failure, or oliguria, (*c*) severe pregnancy-induced hypertension with pulmonary edema or persistent oliguria, (*d*) intraoperative or intrapartum cardiovascular decompensation, (*e*) massive blood and volume loss or replacement, (*f*) adult respiratory distress syndrome, (*g*) shock of undefined etiology, and (*h*) some chronic conditions, particularly when associated with labor or major surgery.

Listed in Table 10.5 are hemodynamic values in healthy pregnant and postpartum patients. In the patient with acute and unexpected pulmonary edema, a primary lung injury (normal or low pulmonary capillary wedge pressure [PCWP]) can quickly be differentiated from heart failure (high PCWP), and specific targeted therapy may be administered. Volume status of the patient can be assessed by ventricular preload or filling pressures, which can be adjusted to optimize cardiac output.

CONTRACEPTIVE COUNSELING

Contraceptive counseling during the postpartum period is essential to educate the new mother about forms of contraception,

Table 10.4
Antibiotic Therapy for Certain Postpartum Infections

Infection/Common Isolates	Antibiotic Regimen	Alternate Regimen
Bacteriuria *Escherichia coli* *Proteus mirabilis* *Klebsiella* species	Amoxicillin 500 mg orally 4 times a day, 7–10 days Nitrofurantoin 50 mg orally 4 times a day, 7–10 days	Based on bacterial susceptibility testing
Endomyometritis and postpartum sepsis Group A or B β-hemolytic streptococcus	Penicillin G 1 10⁶ units i.v. every 4–6 hours until afebrile for 3 days, then oral penicillin to complete 10-day course	Cefazolin 50 mg/kg/day every 6 hours
Escherichia coli	Gentamicin 5 mg/kg/day i.v. every 8 hours **or** ampicillin	Cefazolin 50 mg/kg/day i.v. every 6 hours
Bacteroides fragilis	Clindamycin 20–25 mg/kg/day every 6 hours orally or i.v. every 6 hours **or** cefoxitin 2 g i.v. every 8 hours	Chloramphenicol 50–75 mg/kg/day
Undetermined	Cefoxitin 2 g i.v. every 8 hours, **or** clindamycin 600 mg i.v. every 6 hours **and** gentamicin 1 mg/kg i.v. every 8 hours	Piperacillin, ticarcillin, metronidazole
Postinstrumentation Mixed flora	Ampicillin 150–200 mg/kg/day i.v. every 4 hours **and** gentamicin 5 mg/kg/day i.v. every 8 hours	Based on bacterial susceptibility testing

Table 10.4—*continued*
Antibiotic Therapy for Certain Postpartum Infections

Infection/Common Isolates	Antibiotic Regimen	Alternate Regimen
Pelvic abscess Mixed aerobic and anaerobic flora	Ampicillin 150–200 mg/kg/day i.v. every 4 hours, gentamicin 5 mg/kg/day i.v. every 8 hr, and clindamycin 20–25 mg/kg/day i.v.every 6 hours	Based on bacterial susceptibility testing
Pelvic thrombophlebitis *Bacteroides* species	Ampicillin, gentamicin, and clindamycin (along with heparin)	Cefoxitin, piperacillin, metronidazole, or ticarcillin
Pneumonia *Streptococcus pneumoniae*	Benzyl penicillin 1×10^6 units i.v. every 6 hours **or** procaine penicillin 600,000 units i.m. every 12 hours	Erythromycin 0.5 g orally every 6 hours
Mycoplasma pneumoniae	Erythromycin 0.5 g orally every 6 hours	Tetracycline 500 mg orally or i.v.
Haemophilus influenzae	Ampicillin 150–200 mg/kg/day i.v. every 6 hours	Cefamandole 500 mg orally or i.v.

Staphylococcus aureus	Nafcillin 150–200 mg/kg/day i.v. every 4 hours	Cefazolin 1 g i.v. every 6 hours **or** clindamycin 300 mg orally or i.v. every 6 hours
Gram-negative enteric bacilli	Gentamicin or tobramycin 5 mg/kg/day i.v. every 8 hours	Based on bacterial susceptibility testing
Pseudomonas aeruginosa	Ticarcillin 200–300 mg/kg/day i.v. every 4 hours **and** tobramycin 5 mg/kg/day i.v. every 8 hours	Based on bacterial susceptibility testing
Cellulitis		
Staphylococcus aureus	Nafcillin 150–200 mg/kg/day i.v. every 4 hours	Based on bacterial susceptibility testing
β-hemolytic streptococcus	Aqueous penicillin G 1×10^6 units i.v. every 4 hours	Cefazolin 50 mg/kg/day i.v. every 6 hours

Table 10.5
Hemodynamic Values in Healthy Pregnant and Postpartum Subjects

Parameter (Units)	36–38 Weeks of gestation	Postpartum
Heart rate (beat/min)	83 ± 10	71 ± 10
Central venous pressure (mm Hg)	3.6 ± 2.5	3.7 ± 2.6
Pulmonary capillary wedge pressure (mm Hg)	7.5 ± 1.8	6.3 ± 2.1
Mean arterial pressure (mm Hg)	90.3 ± 5.8	86.4 ± 7.5
Cardiac output (L/min)	6.2 ± 1.0	4.3 ± 0.9
Stroke volume (mL/beat)	74.7	60.6
Systemic vascular resistance (dyne sec cm^{-5})	1210 ± 266	1530 ± 520
Pulmonary vascular resistance (dyne sec cm^{-5})	78 ± 22	119 ± 47

as well as when she may safely become sexually active. The proper contraceptive choice requires a knowledge of the patient's motivation and the effectiveness, safety, and convenience of the various contraceptives. First-year contraceptive failure rates are shown in Table 10.6. Hormonal contraception is the most effective nonpermanent form of birth control; however, if oral contraceptives are likely to be used improperly, barrier techniques may provide better protection.

Initiation of low-dose oral contraceptives depends on the time of delivery. An oral contraceptive may be started immediately after pregnancy termination at 12 weeks or less. Because of the added risk of thrombus formation in the postpartum period, a patient who delivers after 12 weeks should usually wait at least 3 weeks before beginning oral contraceptives. If she wishes to nurse while taking oral contraceptives, the pills should be started several days after delivery so as not to interfere with milk production or quality. The first choice of oral contraceptive should contain a low-dose estrogen component to minimize risks. The preparation may be changed to a more intermediate dose if menstrual problems (spotting, etc.) are not resolved after a usual three-month trial. A combination pill with a mildly androgenic progestin component is also desirable.

Table 10.6
First-Year Contraceptive Failure Rates

Form of Contraception	Pregnancies/Year/100 Users
Sterilization	0.1–0.4
Injectable progestins	0.4
Oral contraceptives	2
Condoms	10
Diaphragm	13
Foam, cream, jelly	15
Rhythm	19

Ovulation may occur as soon as 2 weeks after abortion and 4 weeks after a term delivery. Foam and condoms are often recommended as a "temporary" form of contraception before the postpartum office visit. The spermicidal agent in all vaginal foams, suppositories, and creams is nonoxynol-9 in sufficient concentration to effectively kill sperm and to act as a barrier between the sperm and the cervical canal.

Depot-medroxyprogesterone acetate is an aqueous suspension of microcrystals that is given in doses of 150 mg by intramuscular injection every 12 weeks. Nonlactating mothers may start the progestin within 5 days after delivery. Breast-feeding mothers should delay an injection until lactation is established. Contraceptive protection is immediate. Depot-medroxyprogesterone acetate does not decrease the volume of breast milk or adversely affect its composition. Patients who have spontaneous or induced abortions should receive their first injection immediately after the pregnancy termination. The general clinical approach is to repeat the injections every 12 weeks. About one-third of new starters will have increased numbers of episodes of bleeding and spotting. With continued use of the method, however, 50% of users will have amenorrhea by 1 year.

An unwanted teenage pregnancy is associated with multiple psychologic and medical sequelae which include an increased rate of therapeutic abortion, medical complications of pregnancy, enrollment in the welfare system, failure to complete high school, divorce, child abuse or neglect, and suicide. Hormonal contraception is often preferred, since barrier techniques require patient motivation and education. A low-dose oral contraceptive is recommended with the progestin component being other than norgestrel (too androgenic). Most side effects from oral contraceptive use are related directly to the estrogen dosage, so the lower-dose preparations are less likely to cause breast discomfort, breakthrough bleeding, nausea, or fluid retention. The 28-pill packet may be preferred to improve patient compliance. Ideally, the teenager should not begin oral contraceptives until well after her delivery and only after spontaneous menstrual cycles with predicted intervals have been reestablished.

POSTPARTUM HYPERTENSION

Elevations in blood pressure values among patients with pregnancy-induced hypertension will usually return to a normotensive range within a few days after delivery. The likelihood of developing essential hypertension later in adulthood is highly variable and is influenced by any renal impairment or preexisting hypertension. A search for signs of central nervous system irritability is also important, since eclampsia can occur as long as one week postpartum.

If blood pressure values remain elevated after the second postpartum day, the following measures may be taken: (a) consider the family dynamics, especially the patient's reaction to her newborn infant; (b) begin to evaluate renal function (creatinine clearance, urine protein); (c) instruct the patient on self blood pressure monitoring; (d) if blood pressures are borderline (140–150/90–100 mm Hg), sedate with phenobarbital 30 mg 2 to 4 times a day. If diastolic values are more than 100 mm Hg, begin drug therapy (e.g. nifedipine 10 mg twice daily). Although less commonly used, therapy with beta-blockers such as atenolol or labetalol has also been successful.

Unless normotensive within a few days after delivery, the patient should be reexamined in the clinic within 2 weeks. If the blood pressure remains elevated, an appointment should be made with an internist for diagnostic evaluation and continued antihypertensive therapy. A low-dose oral contraceptive or progestin may be prescribed at the 6-week postpartum visit if the patient is normotensive and other contraceptive methods do not fit the patient's needs. Blood pressure levels should continue to be monitored on a regular basis.

BREAST-FEEDING

Despite certain advantages to formula feeding, the benefits of breast-feeding are greater for the newborn infant. The mother will probably fare as well under one regimen as the other. Breast-feeding has numerous merits: (*a*) human milk is the most ideal food for the newborn; (*b*) breast milk is normally free of impurities; (*c*) human milk contains more calories per ounce than is usually possible in a formula; (*d*) fewer infections are found in breast-fed infants, because of passive immunization; (*e*) breast-feeding hastens involution of the uterus, so that the mother's reproductive organs return to normal more rapidly; (*f*) breast-feeding is at times more convenient for the mother; (*g*) breast-feeding is more economical, both for the mother and for society; and (*h*) intelligence quotients have been reported to be higher in premature infants who were breast-fed than in those who were not.

Milk production is related to prolactin stimulation. Although plasma prolactin falls after delivery to lower levels than during late pregnancy, each act of suckling triggers a rise in prolactin. The maintenance of high prolactin levels during the early postpartum period is proportional to the frequency, duration, and intensity of suckling. The peak production of breast milk is usually not before hospital discharge, since it increases gradually until reaching a plateau of approximately 400 mL per day by the fifth postpartum day.

It is important to be aware that breast milk can be a significant source of infant drug exposure, and as a precaution the decision to wean requires accurate information about the drug level in breast milk and its potential effect on the infant. Under most circumstances, the quantity of a drug or chemical excreted in the milk is quite low, with milk levels being less than maternal serum levels. Any effect on the infant is usually not significant unless maternal therapy is prolonged or in higher-than-therapeutic doses, or if the infant is premature. Unacceptably high drug concentrations may be found in milk when isoniazid, metronidazole, nitrofurantoin, and sulfa preparations are prescribed.

Despite many advantages to breast-feeding, a significant number of women choose not to nurse or are unable to do so, due to a variety of maternal or neonatal factors (e.g., hepatitis B, HIV). In a recent survey in the United States, more than one-third of women were found not to breast-feed their one-week-old infant. Nearly half of patients who do not breast-feed their infant or who cease breast-feeding will encounter breast engorgement and pain for 24 to 48 hours. Mounting concerns about bromocriptine (Parlodel) and rare cardiovascular and cerebrovascular accidents have prompted the manufacturers to remove the drug from the market for postpartum lactation suppression. No drug is available now or is likely to be in the foreseeable future for this indication. Lactation suppression can best be achieved by wearing a tight-fitting bra or wrap, avoiding stimulation (touch or warm shower), and applying ice or cold compression.

PARENT EDUCATION

Proper nutrition and continuing the iron or prenatal vitamins are necessary for the first 2 months after delivery. Exercises to promote support of the abdominal muscles may begin immediately after a vaginal delivery. Overly strenuous exercise is to be discouraged, however, during the initial 2 weeks. After a cesarean section, exercises are to be avoided until the patient sees her doctor 2 weeks after delivery.

Family visits at home should be well-planned, with the intent especially of allowing the patient to relax. Even though this is an exciting time, the new parents may have an emotional letdown because of a disruption of the normal routine, a lack of sleep, or reduced attention from the spouse.

Sexual intercourse may be resumed before the 6-week postpartum visit. Vaginal pain may be present in breast-feeding mothers or from an episiotomy. Birth control should be discussed again before discharge. A diaphragm cannot be fitted until the uterus has returned to normal size (usually 6 or more weeks after delivery). Although ovulation does not occur in the first month, it is possible to become pregnant before the next clinic visit, so foam and condoms should be used. Women who are breast-feeding require contraception also.

Mood swings are common. Postpartum "blues" in either parent is a transient disturbance occurring in 50–80% of puerperal women, starting within 2–3 days of delivery and remitting within a few days to 2–3 weeks. Postpartum depression is a major depressive disorder occurring in the first postdelivery weeks (occasionally starting during pregnancy) in about 10–12% of women. Parents with mental illness such as a bipolar disorder, and patients who must cope with stillbirths, neonatal deaths, and infants born with congenital anomalies require a special sensitivity, compassion, and guidance from the medical care team.

Before departure from the hospital, the parents should be aware of the infant's diet, safety (avoiding sleep on abdomen), sleep, elimination habits, growth and development, and signs of illness. Infants should see their primary care physician at the second postnatal week. A history and physical examination, body measurements, and hepatitis B immunization will be performed. The parents should be provided, before hospital discharge, with a telephone number or the name of a person to contact if there are problems with the neonate.

Suggested Readings

American College of Obstetricians and Gynecologists. Diagnosis and management of postpartum hemorrhage. ACOG Technical Bulletin 143. Washington, DC: ACOG, 1990.

American College of Obstetricians and Gynecologists. Invasive hemodynamic monitoring in obstetrics and gynecology. ACOG Technical Bulletin 175. Washington, DC: ACOG, 1992.

Bowes WA. The puerperium. Clin Obstet Gynecol 1980;23:971–983.

Clark SL, Phelan JP. Surgical control of obstetric hemorrhage. Contemp Ob Gyn 1984;24(2):70–84.

Clark SL, Yeh SY, Phelan JP, Bruce S, Paul RH. Emergency hysterectomy for obstetric hemorrhage. Obstet Gynecol 1984;64:376–380.

Dinsmoor MJ, Newton ER, Gibbs RS. A randomized, double-blind placebo-controlled trial of oral antibiotic therapy following IV antibiotic therapy for postpartum endometritis. Obstet Gynecol 1991;77:60–68.

diZerega G, Yonekura L, Roy S, Nakamura RM, Ledger WJ. A comparison of clindamycin-gentamicin and penicillin-gentamicin in the treatment of post–cesarean section endomyometritis. Am J Obstet Gynecol 1979;134:238–242.

Duff P. Pathophysiology and management of postcesarean endomyometritis. Obstet Gynecol 1986;67:269–276.

Gonsoulin W, Kennedy RT, Guidry KH. Elective versus emergency cesarean hysterectomy cases in a residency program setting: a review of 129 cases from 1984 to 1988. Am J Obstet Gynecol 1991;165:91–94.

Greenwood LH, Glickman MG, Schwartz PE, Morse SS, Denny DF. Obstetric and nonmalignant gynecologic bleeding: treatment with angiographic embolization. Radiology 1987;164:155–159.

Lucas A, Morley R, Cole TJ, Lister G, Leeson-Payne C. Breast milk and subsequent intelligence quotient in children born preterm. Lancet 1992;329:26–30.

Nelson KB, Ellenberg JH. Antecedents of cerebral palsy: multivariate analysis of risk. N Engl J Med 1986;315:81–86.

Osathanondh R. Conception control. In: Ryan KJ, Berkowitz R, Barbieri R, eds. Kistner's gynecology: principles and practice. 5th ed. St. Louis: Mosby-Year Book, 1990:480–529.

Plauche WC. Peripartal hysterectomy. Obstet Gynecol Clin North Am 1988;15:783–795.

Rosen MG, Hobel CJ. Prenatal and perinatal factors associated with brain disorders. Obstet Gynecol 1986;68:416–421.

Rulin MC, Davidson AR, Philliber SG, Graves WL, Cushman LF. Changes in menstrual symptoms among sterilized and comparison women: a prospective study. Obstet Gynecol 1989;74:149–154.

Shain RN, Miller WB, Holden AE, Rosenthal M. Impact of tubal sterilization and vasectomy on female marital sexuality: results of a controlled longitudinal study. Am J Obstet Gynecol 1991;164:763–771.

Stanco LM, Schrimmer DB, Paul RH, Mishell DR Jr. Emergency peripartum hysterectomy and associated risk factors. Am J Obstet Gynecol 1993;168:879–883.

Tucker HA. Endocrinology of lactation. Semin Perinatal 1979;3:199–223.

Wilcox LS, Martinez-Schnell B, Peterson HB, Ware JH, Hughes JM. Menstrual function after tubal sterilization. Am J Epidemiol 1992;135:1368–1381.

Gynecology

Chapter 11

Primary Care

Gynecologists function as primary health care providers for women (Appendix 11.1). Gynecologists provide the majority of general medical examinations for reproductive-age women, and many women see only a gynecologist for periodic screening. Gynecologists spend the majority of their time in office practice. It is important for gynecologists to recognize their role as primary care physicians and to be comfortable in that role.

A primary care physician is not the same thing as a generalist physician. A primary care physician is the first physician the patient sees in the evaluation of a problem. A primary care physician should be able to diagnose and manage the majority of problems with which patients present and recognize and refer other problems. The primary care physician should coordinate care given by referring physicians and serve as the patient's advocate, explaining care and diagnosis plans to the patient and making certain the patient understands these plans. The primary care physician is responsible for the integration of the patient's care into a coordinated whole. The obstetrician-gynecologist fulfills this role for the majority of reproductive-age females and for virtually all pregnant women.

BREAST DISEASE

Women expect their gynecologist to be responsible for education, screening, counseling, and treatment of disorders of the breast. The gynecologist is in an ideal position to diagnose and manage benign diseases of the breast and to screen for breast cancer. The gynecologist should be aware of the natural history, diagnosis, and treatment of both benign and malignant conditions of the breast. The gynecologist should be aware of screening protocols for breast disease as well as risk factors for breast cancer.

Benign Breast Disease

Puerperal Mastitis

The most common infectious disease of the breast is puerperal mastitis. True infections of the breast are rare in nonlactating women. Puerperal mastitis is usually due to Gram-positive aerobic organisms. Prompt therapy with antibiotics active against staphylococcal and streptococcal species is essential to reduce the risk of abscess formation. If an abscess is suspected, prompt incision and drainage is essential to prevent spread of the abscess and sinus formation. Ultrasound examination of the breast may be helpful to confirm an abscess, but the diagnosis is usually made by palpation. The mother with puerperal mastitis should be allowed to nurse during therapy.

Galactoceles

Galactoceles result from obstruction of the lactiferous ducts. They present as a painful mass in a woman who has recently stopped breast-feeding. Sometimes a galactocele can be "milked" toward the nipple and drained, but they usually resolve with time.

Duct Ectasia

Duct ectasia presents with a mass and a tender red breast, usually in a perimenopausal woman. The patient typically has a thick, gray, green, or black nipple discharge. Microscopically the lesions are dilated terminal collecting ducts obstructed by secretions. There is an intense periductal plasma cell response. The lesions resolve over time but are often treated by excision biopsy to distinguish them from carcinoma.

Fat Necrosis

Fat necrosis presents with a hard, tender mass that is mobile and indurated. It rarely enlarges after it is first noted. Fat necrosis is often secondary to trauma but may occur spontaneously. These lesions are often treated by excision biopsy because of their worrisome clinical appearance. If the diagnosis is strongly suspected on clinical grounds, a period of one to two weeks of observation is indicated. The lesions should resolve in this time period.

Mondor's Disease

Mondor's disease is superficial thrombophlebitis of the breast. The patient complains of pain with a unilateral, erythematous, tender, hard cord in or near the breast. The diagnosis is usually made by physical examination. Warm compresses and analgesics result in resolution in 2–8 weeks. Anticoagulants are not indicated.

Fibrocystic Changes

Fibrocystic changes of the breast occur in at least 50% of women. These patients may have symptoms of breast pain, tenderness, and nodularity which worsens before menses. Fibrocystic change is clinically manifested by an ill-defined thickness or palpable lumpiness. Fibrocystic changes are usually bilateral and more pronounced in the upper outer quadrants. Painful breasts associated with fibrocystic changes are the most common breast complaint.

The patient with fibrocystic change should have a careful examination and evaluation to exclude other breast conditions. Reassurance is often all that is needed for management. Medical management is directed toward symptomatic relief. Reduction of caffeine is often prescribed, but there is little evidence to support this therapy. Vitamin E therapy has been reported to be efficacious in uncontrolled trials, but controlled trials have shown vitamin E to be no more effective than placebo. Oral contraceptives appear to reduce the symptoms associated with fibrocystic changes, and a trial of oral contraceptives may be warranted depending on the patient's desire for fertility. Danazol (Danocrine sulfate) is approved for the treatment of severe fibrocystic change of the breast. With danazol therapy, symptoms are improved by 60–100%. Symptoms recur in 30–65% of women following discontinuation of therapy. Danazol is given in dosages of 100–400 mg/day in two divided doses. The dose should be tapered to the lowest effective dose. Danazol has androgenic side effects which may not be reversible when the drug is discontinued.

Tamoxifen appears to be useful in decreasing symptoms of fibrocystic breast changes. Approximately 70% of women report symptom relief with tamoxifen therapy. Tamoxifen acts as a stimulant to the endometrium and is associated with an increased risk of endometrial carcinoma. Bromocriptine has been reported to be useful even in women who do not have elevated prolactin levels, although some investigators have not found it to be effective. Its use is limited by side effects of nausea and vomiting.

Breast Carcinoma

Risk factors for breast cancer are shown in Table 11.1. Conditions which result in prolonged exposure to estrogen such as late menopause, early menarche, delayed childbearing, and obesity appear to increase the risk of breast cancer. A positive family history is the single greatest risk factor for breast cancer. Women with one first-degree relative (mother or sister) with breast cancer have a twofold increased risk of developing breast cancer, and women who have two first-degree relatives with breast cancer have a 14-fold increased risk of developing breast cancer. However, only 20% of women with breast cancer have even a remote family history of breast cancer. Two-thirds of women with breast cancer cannot be identified as high-risk by epidemiologic criteria.

Gynecologists perform the majority of breast screening examinations and need to be familiar with physical signs associated with breast cancer (Table 11.2). These signs do not establish the diagnosis, but they should alert the physician to the need for further evaluation. Mammography, ultrasonography, or fine-needle aspiration should be considered.

If a dominant mass is present, breast aspiration is indicated. A dominant mass is a mass that can be localized in three dimensions and held between the fingers; it is usually at least one centimeter in diameter. Aspiration of the mass is performed with a 22-gauge needle with a clear plastic hub. The mass is stabilized between the fingers, preferably over a rib, and the needle is in-

Table 11.1
Risk Factors for Breast Cancer

Increased age
Prior breast cancer
Nulliparity
Delayed childbearing (>30 years of age)
Early menarche (<12 years)
Late menopause (>53 years)
Family history of breast cancer
Ductal or lobal hyperplasia on biopsy
High socioeconomic status
Obesity

Table 11.2
Physical Signs Associated with Breast Cancer

Asymmetry
Skin thickening
Dimpling or retraction of the skin
Nipple retraction, inversion, or excoriation
Nipple discharge
Erythema
Excoriation
Mass

troduced into the mass. Suction is applied using a syringe after the needle is in the mass. If clear or cloudy fluid is aspirated and the mass disappears, the patient can be followed. A residual mass requires repeat fine-needle aspiration or open biopsy. Bloody fluid should be sent for cytology. A guaiac card may be useful in determining microscopic blood. Malignant cells on cytology require an oncology workup. Atypical cells require an open biopsy. If there are only benign cells found, the patient can be followed.

If no fluid is obtained, the needle is moved through the mass ten times while suction is applied. Suction should be immediately released if blood is seen in the hub and the needle removed. If not, suction is then released while the needle is in the mass. The needle is removed and the syringe removed from the needle. Air is aspirated into the syringe and the needle replaced. The air is then used to expel the tissue from the needle onto a clean glass slide. Pressure is applied to the site and a bandage placed.

The slide is smeared and immediately fixed for cytology using the technique preferred by the cytopathologist. The presence of malignant cells requires an oncology evaluation. Atypical cells require an open biopsy. If the cells are benign and the remainder of the evaluation is not suspicious for carcinoma, the patient can be followed. If there is any suspicion of malignancy, biopsy is indicated.

All women with a dominant mass should have a bilateral mammogram to determine the characteristics of the mass and to examine the other breast for occult malignancy. Ultrasonography may help in distinguishing cystic from solid lesions and in select cases can obviate the need for aspiration.

Pregnant women with a dominant mass should be evaluated in the same way as nonpregnant women. The evaluation of a mass is more difficult in pregnancy because a mass is more difficult to palpate and mammography and ultrasonography are more difficult to interpret. However, pregnancy must not delay the evaluation of a dominant mass. Pregnancy does not appear to worsen the prognosis for breast cancer matched stage for stage. Pregnancy may delay the diagnosis of breast cancer.

Screening mammography has been shown to permit early diagnosis of breast cancer and to reduce deaths from breast cancer when used in large populations. There is general consensus that all women over the age of 50 should have annual mammography. In women under the age of 35, the utility of screening mammography is limited due to dense breast tissue and a relatively low risk of breast cancer. Screening mammography is therefore not indicated in women under 35, unless the patient has a strong family history of early breast cancer or a personal history of breast cancer.

There is no general consensus on the use of screening mammography between the ages of 35 and 50. The American Cancer Society and the American College of Radiology recommend a baseline mammogram between the ages of 35 and 40, with annual or biennial mammography from ages 40 to 50. The National Cancer Institute recommend that a baseline mammogram be obtained from ages 35 to 50 and that the use of screening mammography in that period be determined by each woman's physician.

The controversy over the utility of screening mammography in this age group is related to several issues. One-third of breast cancers arise in women under the age of fifty, so it would seem reasonable to screen this group. However, there is no compelling evidence to show that screening mammography reduces cancer death rates in women under 50. Dense breast tissue found in younger women reduces the utility of screening mammography, and breast cancer may behave differently in premenopausal than postmenopausal women. The resolution of this dilemma awaits further study.

COLON CANCER

Colorectal cancer is the third leading cause of cancer deaths in women in the United States, after lung cancer and breast cancer. In the U.S. an individual has about a 1 in 20 lifetime risk of developing colorectal cancer. Gynecologists are in a unique position to screen for colorectal cancer because so many women see gynecologists for annual examination and because screening techniques can be easily incorporated into gynecologic practice.

The largest risk factors for colon cancer are age and diet. Only about 3% of colon cancers occur in individuals under 40 years of age. The risk increases sharply after age 65. Diets high in fat, particularly animal fat, are associated with a higher risk of colorectal cancer, and diets high in fiber are associated with a lower risk. Dietary fiber may mitigate the risk of animal fat. Alcohol consumption increases the risk for colorectal cancer.

Adenomatous polyps of the large bowel are precursors of colorectal cancer. An untreated adenoma greater than 1 cm has a 2.5% risk of progression to cancer in 5 years, 8% in 10 years, and 24% in 20 years. The presence and degree of atypia in the polyp also affects the risk of progression to cancer. Endoscopic removal of polyps decreases the risk of colon cancer.

About 15% of colorectal cancer patients have a family history of colorectal cancer in a first-degree relative. About 1% have familial adenomatous polyposis (FAP), an autosomal dominant condition. Individuals with FAP develop hundreds of polyps, usually at a young age. Left untreated, most patients with FAP develop colorectal cancer by age 40.

The American Cancer Society, the National Cancer Institute, and the American College of Surgeons recommend that asymptomatic individuals have a sigmoidoscopic examination every three to five years and an annual rectal exam with a fecal occult blood test beginning at age 50. The American College of Obstetricians and Gynecologists recommends an annual rectal examination and fecal occult blood test beginning at age 40 and sigmoidoscopy every three to five years beginning at age 50. These recommendations have not been uniformly accepted because colorectal screening has not been shown to reduce mortality from colorectal cancer. Rigid sigmoidoscopy detects about 28% of colorectal cancers, but flexible sigmoidoscopy can detect about 60% of colorectal cancers. Flexible sigmoidoscopy is more comfortable for the patient and is preferred by many physicians. Widespread use of flexible sigmoidoscopy is deterred by expense and patient acceptance.

The peroxidase (Hemoccult) test has a false-positive rate of 2% and may miss 20–30% of cancers. Nevertheless, annual rectal examination with screening for occult blood will detect some cancers early. A positive test for fecal occult blood requires a thorough evaluation including sigmoidoscopy and barium enema. If no cause of bleeding is found, an investigation of the upper tract may be necessary. Repeat screening for occult blood is not indicated because the test has a 20–30% false-negative rate. Rectal bleeding in a patient over the age of 40, no matter how bright-red, cannot be dismissed as hemorrhoidal without appropriate endoscopy or radiologic evaluation.

CORONARY AND VASCULAR DISEASE

Coronary artery disease (CAD) is the leading cause of death in women. Heart disease causes approximately 35% of all deaths at all ages in females. The incidence of coronary artery disease begins to increase about ten years later in women than in men. Women with a myocardial infarction (MI) are twice as likely to die in the first 60 days as men. Half of women and one-fourth of men die with their first MI. Women are twice as likely as men to have a second MI. Women are more likely to have an unrecognized MI than are men. A woman is less likely to be referred for angioplasty or coronary bypass surgery than a man.

Lipid profiles differ in women and men. Triglyceride levels greater than 190 mg/dL are predictive of CAD in women but not in men. Increased LDL (low density lipoprotein) is not as predictive in women as in men. There is a dramatic increase in CAD when the total cholesterol level is greater than 260 mg/dL in women, compared to 240 mg/dL in men.

Smoking places a patient at high risk for heart disease. More women than men start smoking, and fewer women stop. In the U.S., about 25% of women smoke, with smoking rates much higher in some regions of the country. More teenage girls are smoking now than in prior years.

Gynecologists can screen for risk factors for heart disease. All patients should be counseled not to smoke. Patients aged 19 years and older should have their cholesterol level checked every five years if it is normal. Abnormal values should prompt a referral to an internist. Annual weight and blood pressure checks can identify women at risk for cardiovascular disease.

HYPERTENSION

Hypertension is found in 15% of the population aged 18–74, and the incidence increases with age. Blacks have twice the incidence of whites at any age. Hypertension is defined as a blood pressure level greater than 140/90 mm Hg on two separate occasions.

Studies on hypertension in women are lacking, as most studies have been done on men. However, actuarial tables show that men and women who were treated for blood pressure levels greater than 140/90 mm Hg have normal survival over a 10 to 20 year period. It seems reasonable to institute therapy for women if sustained blood pressure levels exceed 140/90 mm Hg. Patients should have their blood pressure level recorded at an annual examination by their gynecologist.

Minimal laboratory evaluation for the patient with uncomplicated hypertension consists of a dipstick urinalysis, determinations of hemoglobin or hematocrit, creatinine, potassium, fasting glucose, total cholesterol, HDL (high density lipoprotein), and triglycerides, and an electrocardiogram. Abnormalities of any of these, or blood pressure levels greater than 180/120 mm Hg, should prompt a referral to an internist or cardiologist.

Treatment of uncomplicated hypertension can be safely begun by a gynecologist. "Lifestyle modifications" are the first line of therapy unless the diastolic pressure is greater than 110 mm Hg. Weight loss in obese patients and decreased sodium intake may be the only therapy needed. Cholesterol and fat intake should be limited. Patients who smoke should be counseled to stop.

If these modifications are not successful in lowering the blood pressure into a normal range, pharmacologic therapy is indicated. Thiazide diuretics have been utilized as first-line therapy for many years but may cause hypokalemia. It appears that 25 mg per day of a thiazide diuretic is as effective as the more commonly prescribed 50 mg. Potassium-sparing diuretics such as spironolactone, triamterene, or amiloride may be used to prevent hypokalemia.

Patients who do not respond adequately to diuretics are candidates for treatment with beta-blockers. The newer formulations (such as atenolol) are water soluble and have longer half-lives, resulting in once daily dosing in some formulations. Beta-blockers should not be used in asthmatics. They increase triglyceride levels, decrease HDL levels, and blunt the adrenergic response to hypoglycemia. These effects reduce their usefulness in diabetics. Other contraindications include chronic obstructive pulmonary disease (COPD), congestive heart failure, and sick sinus syndrome. Beta-blockers may worsen symptoms of depression.

Angiotensin-converting enzyme inhibitors are often used as first-line therapy. These agents have few side effects and are relatively safe. They are contraindicated in pregnancy and should not be used in women who are at risk for pregnancy. They can be used in patients with asthma, COPD, diabetes, and depression.

Calcium channel blockers can be used in patients with concomitant coronary artery disease. They are especially useful in elderly patients and in those with migraines or angina.

Each class of drugs has multiple drugs. It is advisable for the physician to become familiar with one or two drugs of each class and limit use to those drugs.

DEPRESSION IN WOMEN

The lifetime risk of developing depression is 20% for women, compared to 10% for men. Depression is most common in women of reproductive age, with a prevalence of 8–10%. It is estimated that only about one-fourth of patients with criteria for major depression receive appropriate therapy. Depressed women often see gynecologists, both for annual examination and for complaints related to depression such as abdominal or pelvic pain; chronic, clinically unconfirmed vaginitis; premenstrual syndrome; or multiple somatic complaints. Patients may also present to the gynecologist with complaints of depression. The gynecologist must be able to distinguish the patient with depression from the patient with other causes for these symptoms or with transient emotional disturbances.

Depression may present in a variety of ways. Depressive disorders are a group of clinical conditions characterized by a disturbance of mood, a loss of sense of control, and intense mental, physical, and emotional pain. Depression may be unipolar with episodes lasting at least two weeks, or bipolar with episodes of depression, mania, and normal mental state. A sad mood does not necessarily indicate depression. A sad mood may be a normal reaction to disappointment or loss. Depressed patients may or may not have a sad mood.

Specific criteria for depression are shown in Table 11.3. At least five of these symptoms must have been present during the same two-week period and represent a change from previous functioning. At least one of the symptoms is either a depressed mood or a loss of interest or pleasure. Symptoms that are clearly due to a physical condition, mood-incongruent delusions, and marked loosening of associations should not be included.

Table 11.3
Diagnostic Criteria for Major Depression

1. Depressed mood most of the day, nearly every day, as indicated by subjective account or by observation of others
2. Markedly diminished interest or pleasure in all or almost all activities most of the day, nearly every day, as indicated by subjective account or by observation of others
3. Significant weight loss or weight gain when not dieting (more than 5% body weight in a month) or decrease or increase in appetite nearly every day
4. Insomnia or hypersomnia nearly every day
5. Psychomotor retardation or agitation nearly every day (observable by others, not merely feelings of restlessness or being slowed down)
6. Fatigue or loss of energy nearly every day
7. Feelings of worthlessness or excessive or inappropriate guilt (which may be delusional) nearly every day
8. Diminished ability to think or concentrate, or indecisiveness, nearly every day (as indicated by subjective account or by observation of others)
9. Recurrent thoughts of death (not just fear of dying), recurrent suicidal ideation without a specific plan, or a suicide attempt, or a specific plan for committing suicide

Patients with depression often do not receive therapy because their symptoms are not recognized or because depression is perceived as a personal weakness. Patients should be counseled that depression is due to an alteration in the serotonin pathways in the brain and not due to any character flaw or weakness. Depression can be compared to thyroid disease for patient education. If the thyroid does not make enough hormone, the treatment is thyroid replacement. If the brain does not make enough serotonin, medical treatment is needed.

Treatment of depression requires an understanding of social, predisposing childhood, family, and gender factors in the individual patient. Generally, any medical illness or substance abuse must be treated. Psychotherapy can be used for patients with mild to moderate depression and those who have had an incomplete response to medication. Psychotherapy and medical therapy appear to be equally effective in treating mild to moderate depression.

Medical therapy should be considered for patients with severe, chronic, or recurrent depression. Categories of drugs used to treat depression include the tricyclic and heterocyclic antidepressants, selective serotonin reuptake inhibitors, and monoamine oxidase

(MAO) inhibitors. The serotonin reuptake inhibitors are quite effective, have a better side effect profile than the older drugs, and are commonly used as first-line therapy.

THE BATTERED WOMAN

Domestic violence and spouse abuse refer to violence occurring between partners in an ongoing relationship, regardless of whether they are married. A battered woman is any woman who has suffered physical abuse on at least one occasion at the hands of a male partner. Although abuse is most commonly thought of as physical violence, in most violent relationships there is also an element of mental abuse and intimidation. As domestic violence is probably underreported, it is difficult to calculate its incidence. It has been estimated that there are as many as 1.5 million cases each year in the United States, so domestic violence has a large public health impact. There is a strong correlation between domestic violence and child abuse, with both the abusive spouse and the abused spouse more likely to abuse children.

Gynecologists play a vital role in the detection of the battered woman, and the ability to do so depends on the degree of the physician's suspicion. These women have frequent visits to the physician with a variety of somatic complaints including headache, insomnia, hyperventilation, gastrointestinal upset, and chest, pelvic, or back pain. Women who were abused as children are more likely to have been abused as adults. Patients who were raised in a single-parent home, married as a teenager, or became pregnant prior to marriage are also at risk. The patient may appear frightened, evasive, embarrassed, anxious, or passive, and may cry easily. The abusive spouse often accompanies the patient to the physician and stays close at hand to monitor the patient's disclosures to the physician.

Physical examination may show evidence of trauma of varying ages. "Defensive" wounds or bruises over the forearms are often seen. Bruises over the breasts, buttocks, or abdomen are suspicious. If the patient is wearing sunglasses it is important to ask the patient to remove them to examine the eyes.

Battering acts seem to occur in a cycle consisting of three phases. First there is a gradual building of tension, with gradual escalation of name-calling, intimidating remarks, meanness, and mild physical abuse. The woman tries to placate the batterer and frequently withdraws. She believes that she can control his actions by not provoking him.

The second phase is the hostile act of acute battering. There is an uncontrollable discharge of tensions culminating in a verbal and physical attack which often leaves the woman injured. Approximately two-thirds of batterers abuse alcohol, and the violent event often occurs during a bout of heavy drinking. The battered woman often believes that the drinking is the cause of the beating, rather than the excuse.

In the third phase, the batterer apologizes profusely and asks for forgiveness. He often performs acts of atonement and remorse, showering the victim with gifts and promises. The battered woman may believe that the problem is resolved and that the relationship can be saved.

Efforts at counseling must take into account the dynamics of the relationship. The patient may not wish to leave the relationship or resort to legal authorities because of the fear of severe economic consequences, the fear that the batterer will inflict even more punishment, the belief that the situation will resolve itself, or the belief that the courts will minimize her accusations. If she does not wish to leave the home she should be given telephone numbers of support services available in the community such as shelters and agencies that can inform her of her legal rights. It is reasonable to discuss an exit plan with the woman, including access to a change of clothes, cash, identification papers, and financial records if available.

Some patients will deny the existence of an abusive relationship even if directly asked. Pamphlets available in the waiting room that explain domestic violence and contain telephone numbers of community resources may allow some women an opportunity for intervention.

SEXUAL ASSAULT

Sexual assault can be defined as any sexual act performed by one person on another without that person's consent. Sexual assault accounts for about 6% of all reported violent crimes, but it is probable that many sexual assaults are unreported. It has been estimated that as many as 44% of women have been victims of actual or attempted sexual assault in their lifetimes.

The physician who evaluates a victim of sexual assault has both legal and medical responsibilities and must be aware of statutory obligations in the jurisdiction. Many jurisdictions require specific evidence kits to be collected and handled in specified ways to establish an evidentiary trail. The physician has an obligation to obtain specific information (Table 11.4). The physician's first obligation is to the patient. Treatment of serious injuries is the first priority and takes precedence over evidence collection. After acute injuries have been determined and stabilized, a careful history and physical examination is performed (Table 11.4). It is essential that a chaperone be present during the examination to provide reassurance and support. In many areas, specially trained rape crisis counselors are available to provide support.

If not already done, the police should be notified. The patient should state in her own words what happened to her. If the assailant is not known to her, a detailed description of the assailant may be helpful. The patient should describe the specific acts performed and whether the attacker used a condom. A history of the last consensual sexual activity can help to distinguish whether sperm or secretions came from the attacker or someone else. A contraceptive and menstrual history can distinguish whether or not the patient might be already pregnant. If any possibility exists of current pregnancy, a sensitive pregnancy test must be per-

Table 11.4
Physician's Responsibilities in a Sexual Assault Case

History
    Menstrual history
    Contraceptive history
    Sexual history to include time of last unforced intercourse
    Accurate history of details of assault including oral or anal sodomy and
        other injuries
Physical examination
    Survey for injuries—cuts, bruises, bites
    Oral cavity
        Secretions, injuries due to oral sodomy, culture for gonorrhea
    Genitalia
        Hair combing
        Hair sample
        Vaginal secretions
        Air-dried smear for spermatozoa
        Wet mount to confirm motile spermatozoa
        Culture for gonorrhea and chlamydia
        Examination for pathology, trauma, foreign bodies
    Rectal for trauma, gonorrhea culture

formed. This information may be critical to determine whether a pregnancy arose from the assault.

A careful examination of the entire body is performed. Photographs or drawings of any bruises, injuries, or bite marks should be obtained. In some jurisdictions photographs must be obtained by a police photographer. Superficial or extensive lacerations of the vulva, vagina, or hymen may be present but the absence of obvious trauma does not exclude a sexual assault. Colposcopy of the vulva and staining with toluidine blue dye may reveal microscopic evidence of trauma to the vulva and vestibule. Illumination with a Wood's lamp may show semen stains on skin or clothing.

A pelvic examination is performed to obtain vaginal secretions for motile sperm, acid phosphatase, and secretions. Motile sperm may be found in the vagina for up to 8 hours and in the cervix for as long as 2 to 3 days. Nonmotile sperm may be found in the vagina for up to 24 hours and in the cervix for up to 17 days. Acid phosphatase may be found in the vagina even if the attacker has had a vasectomy. Secretions from the attacker may contain blood types and possibly DNA. Approximately 80% of people secrete major blood groups in their body secretions. Although DNA "fingerprinting" is not available in all jurisdictions, its availability is growing rapidly. Hairs from the attacker may be obtained by combing the victim's pubic hair. Hairs can be used to positively identify the attacker. At least 10 to 20 pubic and head hairs should be plucked from the victim and submitted as evidence. Finding the victim's hair on the assailant's body or clothing may be essential evidence. Fingernail scrapings should be obtained if the victim scratched the assailant.

The risk of acquiring syphilis from a sexual assault has been estimated to be up to 3%; for gonorrhea the risk is 6–12%, and for chlamydia it is probably equal or greater. Patients should be offered prophylactic antibiotics to cover these infections. Ceftriaxone 250 mg intramuscularly plus doxycycline 100 mg orally twice daily for 7 days is appropriate. Azithromycin 1 gram orally may be substituted for the doxycycline. If the patient is pregnant, erythromycin may be substituted for the doxycycline. Serological tests for syphilis, hepatitis B, and HIV can be useful in further counseling.

If the patient is not pregnant and pregnancy is a possibility, postcoital contraception should be offered. Two Ovral tablets every 12 hours for a total of 4 tablets is approved for postcoital contraception. Other contraceptives containing 50 μg estrogen may be substituted. Alternate regimens of high-dose estrogen (5 mg ethinyl estradiol or 20 mg conjugated estrogens) for 5 days may be substituted. An IUD can be placed up to 7 days postcoitus to prevent implantation. If the patient is found to be pregnant after these therapies, she should be counseled on all options, including keeping the pregnancy, adoption, and abortion.

After the examination, the physician should discuss the degree of injury and the probability of infection and pregnancy. The physician should outline the general course of follow-up and how follow-up will be obtained. The patient should be allowed to express her concerns and understanding of what has happened and what will occur. Any misconceptions should be addressed. Persons trained in rape crisis counseling should be consulted to aid in counseling and follow-up. Many patients will be more comfortable with a female counselor. A follow-up visit should be scheduled in 1–2 weeks to evaluate medical and psychological well-being and in 3–4 weeks to determine the possibility of pregnancy.

Suggested Readings

American College of Obstetricians and Gynecologists. The battered woman. Technical Bulletin 124. Washington, DC: ACOG, 1989.

American College of Obstetricians and Gynecologists. Depression in women. Technical Bulletin 182. Washington, DC: ACOG, 1993.

American College of Obstetricians and Gynecologists. Nonmalignant conditions of the breast. Technical Bulletin 156. Washington, DC: ACOG, 1991.

American College of Obstetricians and Gynecologists. Precis V, pp. 1–111. Washington, DC: ACOG, 1994.

American College of Obstetricians and Gynecologists. The role of the obstetrician-gynecologist in the diagnosis of breast disease. ACOG Committee Opinion 67. Washington, DC: ACOG, 1989.

American College of Obstetricians and Gynecologists. Sexual assault. Technical Bulletin 172. Washington, DC: ACOG, 1992.

Anastos K, Charney P, Charon A. Hypertension in women: what is really known? Ann Intern Med 1991;115:287–293.

DeCosse JJ, Tsioulias GJ, Jacobsen JS. Colorectal cancer: detection, treatment, and rehabilitation. CA 1994;44:27–42.

Drukker BH, DeModonca W. Benign disease of the breast. In: Sciarra JW, ed. Gynecology and obstetrics. Philadelphia: Harper & Row, 1988.

The Fifth Report of the Joint National Committee on the Detection, Evaluation, and Treatment of High Blood Pressure. Arch Intern Med 1993;153:154–183.

Hindle WH, ed. Breast disease for gynecologists. Englewood Cliffs, NJ: Appleton & Lange, 1990.

Levin B, Murphy GP. Revision in American Cancer Society recommendations for the early detection of colorectal cancer. CA 1992;42:296–299.

Noland TE. Evaluation and treatment of uncomplicated hypertension. Clin Obstet Gynecol 1995;38:156–165.

Seltzer V, ed. The role of the obstetrician gynecologist in diagnosing and treating breast disease. Clin Obstet Gynecol 1994;37:877–1018.

U.S. Department of Health and Human Services, Agency for Health Care Policy and Research. Depression in primary care: volume 1. Detection and diagnosis. Rockville, MD, 1993.

Primary Health Care in Gynecology

AGES 13–18

Screening

Periodic History
Reason for visit
Health status: medical, surgical, family
Dietary/nutritional assessment
Physical activity
Tobacco, alcohol, other drugs
Abuse/neglect
Sexual practices

Periodic Physical
Height
Weight
Blood pressure
Secondary sexual characteristics (Tanner staging)
Pelvic examination
   Yearly when sexually active or by age 18
Skin (HR1)

Laboratory Tests
Periodic
Pap test
   Yearly when sexually active or by age 18

Evaluation and Counseling

Sexuality
Development
High-risk behaviors
Contraceptive options
   Genetic counseling
   Prevention of unwanted pregnancy
Sexually transmitted diseases
   Partner selection
   Barrier protection

Fitness
Hygiene (including dental)
Dietary/nutritional assessment
Exercise: discussion of program

Psychosocial Evaluation
Interpersonal/family relationships
Sexual identity
Personal goal development
Behavioral/learning disorders
Abuse/neglect

Immunizations

Periodic
Tetanus-diphtheria booster
   Once between ages 14–16

High-Risk Groups
Measles, mumps, rubella (MMR) (HR7)
Hepatitis B vaccine (HR10)
Fluoride supplement (HR11)

Leading Causes of Death
Motor vehicle accidents
Homicide
Suicide
Leukemia

AGES 13–18—*Continued*

Screening

High-Risk Groups
Hemoglobin (HR2)
Bacteriuria testing
(HR3)
Sexually transmitted
disease testing
(HR4)
Human immunodefi-
ciency virus test-
ing (HR5)
Genetic testing/coun-
seling (HR6)
Rubella titer (HR7)
Tuberculosis skin test
(HR8)
Lipid profile (HR9)

**Evaluation and
Counseling**

**Cardiovascular Risk
Factors**
Family history
Hypertension
Hyperlipidemia
Obesity/diabetes mel-
litus

Health/Risk Behaviors
Injury prevention
  Safety belts and
    helmets
  Recreational haz-
    ards
  Firearms
  Hearing
Skin exposure to ultra-
  violet rays
Suicide: depressive
  symptoms
Tobacco, alcohol,
  other drugs

Immunizations

**Leading Causes of
  Morbidity**
Nose, throat, and up-
  per respiratory
  conditions
Viral, bacterial, and
  parasitic
  infections
Sexual abuse
Injuries (musculoskele-
  tal and soft tissue)
Acute ear infections
Digestive system condi-
  tions
Acute urinary tract
  conditions

AGES 19–39

Screening

Periodic History
Reason for visit
Health status: medical,
  surgical, family
Dietary/nutritional
  assessment
Physical activity
Tobacco, alcohol, other
  drugs
Abuse/neglect
Sexual practices

Periodic Physical
Height
Weight
Blood pressure
Neck: adenopathy,
  thyroid

**Evaluation and
Counseling**

Sexuality
High-risk behaviors
Contraceptive options
  Genetic counseling
  Prevention of un-
    wanted pregnancy
Sexually transmitted
  diseases
  Partner selection
  Barrier protection
Sexual functioning

Fitness
Hygiene (including
  dental)
Dietary/nutritional as-
  sessment
Exercise: discussion of
  program

Immunizations

Periodic
Tetanus-diphtheria
  booster
  Every 10 years

High-Risk Groups
Measles, mumps,
  rubella (MMR)
  (HR7)
Hepatitis B vaccine
  (HR10)
Influenza vaccine
  (HR15)
Pneumococcal vaccine
  (HR16)

**Leading Causes of
  Death**
Motor vehicle accidents
Cardiovascular disease

AGES 19–39—*Continued*

Screening

Breasts
Abdomen
Pelvic examination
Skin (HR1)

Laboratory Tests
Periodic
Pap test
  *Physician and patient
  discretion after 3 con-
  secutive normal tests*
Cholesterol
  Every 5 years

High-Risk Groups
Hemoglobin (HR2)
Mammography
  (HR12)
Fasting glucose test
  (HR13)
Sexually transmitted
  disease testing
  (HR4)
Human immunodefi-
  ciency virus test-
  ing (HR5)
Genetic testing/coun-
  seling (HR6)
Rubella titer (HR7)
Tuberculosis skin test
  (HR8)
Lipid profile (HR9)
Thyroid-stimulating
  hormone (HR14)

**Evaluation and
Counseling**

**Psychosocial Evalua-
tion**
Interpersonal/family
  relationships
Domestic violence
Job satisfaction
Lifestyle/stress
Sleep disorders

**Cardiovascular Risk
Factors**
Family hypertension
Hyperlipidemia
Obesity/diabetes mel-
  litus
Lifestyle

Health/Risk Behaviors
Injury prevention
  Safety belts and hel-
    mets
  Occupational haz-
    ards
  Recreational haz-
    ards
  Firearms
  Hearing
Breast self-examina-
  tion
Skin exposure to ultra-
  violet rays
Suicide: depressive
  symptoms
Tobacco, alcohol,
  other drugs

Immunications

Homicide
Coronary artery
  disease
Acquired immunodefi-
  ciency syndrome
  (AIDS)
Breast cancer
Cerebrovascular dis-
  ease
Uterine cancer

**Leading Causes of
Morbidity**
Nose, throat, and up-
  per respiratory
  conditions
Injuries (musculo-
  skeletal and soft
  tissue, including
  back and upper
  and lower extrem-
  ities)
Viral, bacterial, and
  parasitic
  infections
Acute urinary tract
  conditions

AGES 40–64

Screening

Periodic History
Reason for visit
Health status: medical,
  surgical, family
Dietary/nutritional as-
  sessment
Physical activity

**Evaluation and
Counseling**

Sexuality
High-risk behaviors
Contraception options
  Genetic counseling
  Prevention of un-
    wanted pregnancy

Immunizations

Periodic
Tetanus-diphtheria
  booster
  Every 10 years
Influenza vaccine
  *Annually beginning at
  age 55*

AGES 40–64—*Continued*

Screening

Periodic History
Tobacco, alcohol,
    other drugs
Abuse/neglect
Sexual practices

Periodic Physical
Height
Weight
Blood pressure
Oral cavity
Neck: adenopathy, thy-
    roid
Breasts, axillae
Abdomen
Pelvic and rectovaginal
    examination
Skin (HR1)

Laboratory Tests
Periodic
Pap test
    *Physician and patient
    discretion after 3
    consecutive normal
    tests*
Mammography
    *Every 1–2 years until
    age 50, yearly begin-
    ning at 50*
Cholesterol
    Every 5 years
Fecal occult blood test
Sigmoidoscopy
    *Every 3–5 years after
    age 50*

High-Risk Groups
Hemoglobin (HR2)
Bacteriuria testing
    (HR3)
Mammography
    (HR12)
Fasting glucose test
    (HR13)

**Evaluation and
Counseling**

Sexuality
Sexually transmitted
    diseases
    Partner selection
    Barrier protection
Sexual functioning

Fitness
Hygiene (including
    dental)
Dietary/nutritional as-
    sessment
Exercise: discussion of
    program

**Psychosocial
    Evaluation**
Family relationships
Domestic violence
Job/work satisfaction
Retirement planning
Lifestyle/stress
Sleep disorders

**Cardiovascular Risk
    Factors**
Family history
Hypertension
Hyperlipidemia
Obesity/diabetes mel-
    litus
Lifestyle

Health/Risk Behaviors
Hormone replacement
    therapy
Injury prevention
    Safety belts and
    helmets
    Occupational
    hazards
    Recreational hazards
    Sports involvement
    Firearms
    Hearing

Immunizations

Periodic
High-Risk Groups
Mumps, measles,
    rubella (MMR)
    (HR7)
Hepatitis B vaccine
    (HR10)
Influenza vaccine
    (HR15)
Pneumococcal vaccine
    (HR16)

**Leading Causes of
    Death**
Cardiovascular disease
Coronary artery
    disease
Breast cancer
Lung cancer
Cerebrovascular dis-
    ease
Colorectal cancer
Obstructive pulmonary
    disease
Ovarian cancer

**Leading Causes of
    Morbidity**
Nose, throat, and up-
    per respiratory
    conditions
Osteoporosis/arthritis
Hypertension

AGES 40–64—*Continued*

Screening	Evaluation and Counseling	Immunizations
High-Risk Groups	**Health/Risk Behaviors**	**Leading Causes of Morbidity**
Sexually transmitted disease testing (HR4)	Breast self-examination	Orthopaedic deformities and impairments (including back and upper and lower extremities)
Human immunodeficiency virus testing (HR5)	Skin exposure to ultraviolet rays	
	Suicide: depressive symptoms	
Tuberculosis skin test (HR8)	Tobacco, alcohol, other drugs	Heart disease
Lipid profile (HR9)		Hearing and vision impairments
Thyroid-stimulating hormone (HR14)		
Colonoscopy (HR17)		

65 YEARS AND OLDER

Screening	Evaluation and Counseling	Immunizations
Period History	**Sexuality**	**Periodic**
Reason for visit	Sexual functioning	Tetanus-diphtheria booster
Health status: medical, surgical, family	Sexual behaviors	*Every 10 years*
	Sexually transmitted diseases	Influenza vaccine
Dietary/nutritional assessment		*Annually*
Physical activity	**Fitness**	Pneumococcal vaccine
Tobacco, alcohol, other drugs, polypharmacy	Hygiene (general and dental)	*Once*
	Dietary/nutritional assessment	**High-Risk Groups**
Abuse/neglect	Exercise: discussion of program	Hepatitis B vaccine (HR10)
Sexual practices		
	Psychosocial Evaluation	**Leading Causes of Death**
Period Physical	Neglect/abuse	Cardiovascular disease
Height	Lifestyle/stress	Coronary artery disease
Weight	Depression/sleep disorders	Cerebrovascular disease
Blood pressure	Family relationships	Pneumonia/influenza
Oral cavity	Job/work/retirement satisfaction	Obstructive lung disease
Neck: adenopathy, thyroid		
Breasts, axillae	**Cardiovascular Risk Factors**	Colorectal cancer
Abdomen	Hypertension	Breast cancer
Pelvic and rectovaginal examination		Lung cancer
Skin (HR1)		Accidents

65 YEARS AND OLDER—*Continued*

Screening

Laboratory Tests

Periodic

Pap test
Physician and patient discretion after 3 consecutive normal tests
Urinalysis/dipstick
Mammography
Cholesterol
Every 3–5 years
Fecal occult blood test
Sigmoidoscopy
Every 3–5 years
Thyroid-stimulating hormone test
Every 3–5 years

High-Risk Groups

Hemoglobin (HR2)
Fasting glucose test (HR13)
Sexually transmitted disease testing (HR4)
Tuberculosis skin test (HR8)
Lipid profile (HR9)
Colonoscopy (HR17)

Evaluation and Counseling

Cardiovascular Risk

Hypercholesterolemia
Obesity/diabetes mellitus
Sedentary lifestyle

Health/Risk Behaviors

Hormone replacement therapy
Injury prevention
Safety belts and helmets
Occupational hazards
Recreational hazards
Hearing
Firearms
Visual acuity/glaucoma
Hearing
Breast self-examination
Skin exposure to ultraviolet rays
Suicide: depressive symptoms
Tobacco, alcohol, other drugs

Immunizations

Leading Causes of Morbidity

Nose, throat, and upper respiratory conditions
Osteoporosis/arthritis
Hypertension
Urinary incontinence
Heart disease
Injuries (musculoskeletal and soft tissue)
Hearing and vision impairments

Chapter 12

Sexual Medicine

SEXUAL DIFFERENTIATION

Normal Development

The gender of a person is dependent on multiple factors including genetic, hormonal, morphological, and core identity. Gender identity is distinct from gender roles and from gender sex object preference. The gender identity of a patient is the gender as perceived by the patient. Gender roles are the ways in which people behave. Most gender roles are learned behavior. Gender sex object preference is the gender to which an individual is sexually attracted.

The determination of gender begins at conception with the establishment of genetic sex. Most individuals have either a 46,XX (female) or 46,XY (male) karyotype. Under the control of the genetic sex, the gonads develop and differentiate, which determines the hormonal environment of the embryo and the development of internal duct systems and the external genitalia. The embryonic brain is also sexually differentiated, probably under hormonal influence.

Development of the indifferent gonad begins about the fifth week of gestation as protuberances overlying the mesonephric ducts. At the sixth week the migration of primordial germ cells to the gonadal ridge is complete. Germ cells do not induce gonadal development but take the form of the gonad in which they arrive. If germ cells do not migrate, gonads do not develop, and streak gonads result. At seven weeks, the gonads are undifferentiated and bipotential. Further development is under genetic control, with a single gene determinant on the Y chromosome (testes determinant factor—TDF) necessary for testicular development. The TDF gene acts as a "master control switch" for male differentiation. It interacts with the H-Y locus to induce a surface antigen, the H-Y antigen, which is universally present in individuals with testes and absent in those without testes. The H-Y antigen is not induced by androgen.

The development of testes is the earliest sexual development in the embryo. Testicular development begins around 7 weeks with spermatogenic cords followed by seminiferous tubules and then Leydig cell formation. Human chorionic gonadotropin (hCG) causes Leydig cell hypertrophy and testosterone formation. Fetal testosterone levels reach their peak at 12 weeks. The development of the wolffian duct into epididymis, vas deferens, and seminal vesicles, and the development of male external genitalia, are dependent on androgen stimulation. Regression of the müllerian system in the male is not dependent on androgen but rather on another substance known as müllerian inhibiting factor (MIF).

In the absence of a Y chromosome and TDF, ovarian development begins about two weeks later than testicular development (at about 9 weeks). In the absence of testosterone, the wolffian duct does not develop. In the absence of MIF, the müllerian system develops. In the absence of testosterone, female external genitalia develop. Male and female developmental homologues and their embryological precursors are shown in Table 12.1.

Abnormal Sexual Development

Abnormalities may occur at any point in the process of sexual development. Chromosomal abnormalities may be due either to loss of sex chromosome DNA from deletions or missing chromosomes, or from duplications of sex chromosomes. A missing sex chromosome (45,XO) leads to Turner's syndrome, characterized by short stature, lymphedema of the hands and feet, webbed neck, and streak gonads. A deletion of any part of an X chromosome leads to streak gonads. Similarly, deletion of the short arm of the Y chromosome leads to short stature and streak gonads.

Duplication of sex chromosomes leads to a variety of abnormalities. Individuals with 47,XYY are phenotypic males who are taller, have increased acne, and may be more aggressive. They have a normal range of intelligence and are not more likely to have antisocial tendencies than other males. Males with more than one additional Y chromosome (48,XYYY) or an additional X and Y (48,XXYY) have significant mental retardation and a variety of physical abnormalities. Individuals with 47,XXY (Klinefelter's syndrome) have a feminized affect with small testes and infertility.

Table 12.1
Embryologic Sources of Genital Structures

Female	Embryonic Structure	Male
ovary	genital ridge (undifferentiated gonad)	testis
ovarian ligament round ligament	gubernaculum	gubernaculum testis
epoöphoron paroöphoron Gartner's duct appendix of ovary	mesonephric ridge (tubules) mesonephric duct	epididymis paradidymis ductus deferens seminal vesicles appendix of epididymis
renal collecting system	metanephric duct	renal collecting system
fallopian tube uterus upper vagina hydatid cyst of Morgagni	paramesonephric duct (müllerian duct)	prostatic utricle appendix of testis
lower vagina vaginal vestibule urinary bladder urethra urethral and paraurethral glands greater vestibular glands hymen	urogenital sinus	urinary bladder prostate prostatic utricle bulbourethral glands urethra (nonglandular) seminal collicle
clitoris corpora cavernosa clitoridis bulb of vestibule	genital tubercle	glans of penis corpora cavernosa and spongiosum of penis
labia minora vestibular bulbs	urethral plate	cavernous urethra
labia minora	urogenital folds	ventral portion of penis
labia majora	labioscrotal swellings	scrotum

Females with one additional X (47,XXX) may be indistinguishable from those with normal karyotypes although infertility is more common. Females with more than three X chromosomes exhibit varying degrees of mental retardation and physical abnormalities.

In males, failure of formation of MIF leads to development of the müllerian system (hernia uteri inguinale). A small uterus develops in the inguinal canal and may be mistaken for a hernia. It is inherited as a recessive trait, either X-linked or autosomal. Failure of the testes to respond to gonadotropins leads to male pseudohermaphroditism with female external genitalia or incompletely masculinized male external genitalia. Lack of androgen receptors (androgen insensitivity, testicular feminization) leads to male pseudohermaphroditism. Incomplete androgen insensitivity may present only with azoospermia. Androgen insensitivity is an X-linked recessive characteristic.

Females who are exposed to excessive androgen during the period of genital development present as incompletely masculinized males (female pseudohermaphroditism). Most cases are due to congenital adrenal hyperplasia. The most common defect is 21-hydroxylase deficiency, followed by 11β-hydroxylase deficiency and 3β-hydroxysteroid dehydrogenase deficiency.

HUMAN SEXUALITY

Sexual dysfunctions are common problems. About one couple in five suffers from some sexual dysfunction. The most common presentation for a sexual dysfunction is to a gynecologist. Patients may present with an overt complaint of sexual dysfunction or may present with a hidden complaint. The complaint may only be found on review of systems, and every review of systems should include questions about sexual health.

Concepts and Precepts

Most physicians approach clinical problems using a medical model. In a medical model, we traditionally look at an alteration of normal physiology to explain a disease state. We endeavor to find the cause of the pathophysiology and alter or remove the cause. The approach consists of history, physical examination, laboratory evaluation, diagnosis, and therapy. Each physician decides, on the basis of experience and ability, what problems to evaluate and treat, or to refer. Sexual problems can be addressed using a traditional medical model. The sexual response is a normal physiologic response, similar to other physiologic responses. As such, it cannot be learned and is present in all people. Like other physiologic responses, it can be altered by disease states and by psychological changes. Sexual dysfunctions result from alterations in normal physiology. The medical model depends on identification of the alteration in normal physiology and removal or alteration of the factor or factors responsible for it.

In order to apply this medical model to the management of sexual dysfunctions, it is first necessary to understand normal sexual physiology. The sexual response cycle was described by Masters and Johnson as consisting of four phases: excitement, plateau, orgasm, and resolution. Kaplan has described a fifth phase, the desire phase. Desire for intercourse is a primary desire like that for food, water, or air. Some degree of sexual desire is always present. Like all appetites, sexual desire can be whetted or inhibited by circumstances. Sexual desire is not lust.

The excitement phase is the second phase of the cycle and the first phase that has measurable physiologic responses. These consist of vasocongestion of the pelvis, caused by a shift in blood flow away from gut and skeletal muscle to the pelvis. There is an increase in heart rate and respiration. Skin "mottling" and a feeling of warmth results from increased blood flow to the skin. Nipple erection occurs in both sexes. In the male, penile erection is caused by distension of the corpus callosum with blood. Scrotal shortening occurs late in the excitement phase.

In the female, vaginal lubrication and expansion both result from increased blood flow to the pelvis. Clitoral vasocongestion leads to increase in clitoral size. Vaginal lubrication results from direct transudation across the vaginal wall and not from secretion of any glands.

The plateau phase is essentially a more advanced stage of arousal. Physiology remains unchanged for some time with no further increase in heart rate and respiration, and no blood flow shifts.

Orgasm is accompanied by a series of rhythmic contractions of the perineal muscles occurring every 0.8 seconds. In the male it is accompanied by 3 to 7 ejaculatory spurts of seminal fluid. In the female it is accompanied by elevation of the "orgasmic platform." In both sexes there are involuntary contractions of skeletal muscles and EEG changes.

The resolution phase is the last phase of the cycle. In males, orgasm is followed by an obligatory resolution phase in which physiologic changes return to baseline and further stimulation cannot produce excitement. The length of the resolution phase varies with age, ranging from less than 5 minutes in adolescents to 24 hours or longer in elderly men. In females resolution is not always obligatory—women may have repeated orgasm without resolution to a basal state, but some women do have an obligatory resolution phase.

Sexual Dysfunctions

Dysfunctions are manifested by an alteration in normal physiologic response. These alterations may be due to psychological, physical, or pharmacologic factors. Sexual dysfunctions always have anxiety as an essential component. Abnormal sexual physiology results from "blocks" in normal physiology. "Blocks" to the normal response can come from a variety of sources. Pain is a potent modifier of behavior and is a strong inhibitor of the sexual response. "Spectatoring" often occurs in people with a sexual dysfunction. Rather than participating in the sexual response, these patients watch to see what will happen. As a result, they have an interruption of the response. Patients with a dysfunction often wonder "what's wrong with me?" This anxiety leads to interruption of the sexual response. Drugs such as alcohol inhibit the sexual response.

Disorders of the desire phase are the most common dysfunctions. Inhibited sexual desire results from pain associated with intercourse, severe negative conditioning, anxiety over another dysfunction, or anger or boredom. Inhibited sexual desire is not the same as lack of desire. Many patients complain that they have no desire for intercourse. Careful history reveals that most of these patients have an inhibited desire for intercourse. Most will admit to a desire, but find that in a sexual situation they have an averse reaction to intercourse. The most common etiology is pain, physical or psychic. True lack of desire is often associated with a chronic disease state such as depression, hyperprolactinemia, hypogonadism, malignancies or other chronic illnesses, or substance abuse. Inhibited desire is a learned behavior or a conditioned response. It may be secondary to another dysfunction, pain, boredom, anger, or marital discord.

Excitement Phase Dysfunctions

In men, erectile dysfunctions are manifested by failure of penile engorgement, resulting in insufficient penile erection to begin or maintain penetration. They may be a result of vascular disease or performance anxiety. They may also result from vasoactive drugs such as beta-blockers and other antihypertensives.

Premature ejaculation is a failure of excitement. Most men with premature ejaculation believe that they are too excited and try to limit excitement, which has the effect of making the problem worse.

Vaginismus is an involuntary spasm of the muscles around the lower third of the vagina. It may make penetration impossible. Vaginismus may be global or situational, and may be primary or secondary. The etiology is pain, either physical or psychological. Severe negative parenting about sexuality is often found.

Dyspareunia is pain with intercourse. Dyspareunia may be due to physical causes such as vaginitis, endometriosis, or chronic pelvic inflammatory disease. It may be due to failure of excitement with failure of lubrication and vaginal expansion. Failure of lubrication may occasionally be related to drugs such as antihypertensives or decongestants. Dyspareunia may result from failure of excitement due to psychic pain from abuse, marital strife, or boredom.

Plateau Phase Disorders

Orgasmic dysfunction may be defined as the inability to achieve orgasm (anorgasmia). It may be situational or constant, primary or secondary. The etiology is usually performance anxiety, although it may be due to inadequate clitoral stimulation, boredom, or fear of loss of control.

Delayed ejaculation is the male equivalent of anorgasmia. It is usually due to performance anxiety but has also been reported in association with the use of serotonin reuptake inhibitors used to treat depression.

Orgasm

Pain with orgasm is a rare condition that may be due to pelvic adhesions or tears in the endopelvic fascia. In males it may be associated with urethritis.

Resolution

Prolonged resolution phases may lead to a false diagnosis of erectile dysfunction. In elderly men, the resolution phase may be prolonged enough to interfere with erection at a subsequent sexual encounter.

Diagnosis of Sexual Dysfunctions

History

A careful history is the first step in diagnosis. The history should determine exactly what happens when the patient has intercourse or is in a sexual situation. Often it is helpful to describe to patients the normal sexual response and then ask what happens to them. A description of "spectatoring" and performance anxiety may help patients to recognize the problem on their own.

The complaint of a sexual problem may be hidden and only found by a review of symptoms. A sexual review of systems should include the following questions:

1. How often do you have intercourse?
2. Do you have pain with intercourse?
3. How often do you have orgasms with intercourse? (females)
4. Do you ever have orgasm before you want to? (males)
5. Do you ever have trouble getting or keeping an erection? (males)
6. Are you generally satisfied with your sex life?

These few questions will uncover virtually all sexual dysfunctions.

Physical Examination

A general physical examination with particular attention to signs of hypogonadism should be performed. Pelvic examination is particularly important to document vaginismus and to determine if there are anatomic reasons that might cause dyspareunia.

Determination of "Internal Theory"

All patients have an internal theory of the cause and often treatment of their problem. Everything we tell them is filtered through this theory. We must discover this internal theory and if it is correct (we agree with it!) then fine. If not, we must educate the patient about our theory or at least persuade the patient to try our theory and therapy.

Sex Therapy

Therapy is derived from the diagnosis. All physicians must decide what they are willing to treat and what they wish to refer. The PLISSIT model is helpful in making these decisions. PLISSIT stands for Permission, Limited Information, Specific Suggestions, Intensive Therapy. Many sexual problems can be managed with permission. Examples: "It is okay to touch your clitoris during intercourse." "It is normal to want to try intercourse in different positions." The physician can "give permission" for patients to experiment with solutions to their problems.

Limited Information and education can resolve many problems. Examples: "It is normal to have an erection every 90 minutes at night." "You don't have to be 'in the mood' to have intercourse." "Many couples do not achieve simultaneous orgasm." "Many women enjoy oral intercourse."

Some problems may respond to specific suggestions. Examples: "Try a lubricant." "Try touching your clitoris." "Tell your partner what you like or don't like."

Many dysfunctions will only respond to intensive therapy. Traditional sex therapy takes from 12 to 16 visits, and is based on sensate focus. Each physician must decide what therapies to undertake and what to refer. As always, accurate diagnosis is the key to successful therapy.

CONTRACEPTION

Of the approximately 58 million women of reproductive age in the United States, some 60% use some form of contraception. Of the 40% who do not, only about one in six are at risk for pregnancy. Thus about 90% of the women at risk for pregnancy are using some form of contraception. The most popular methods of contraception are shown in Table 12.2. Overall, sterilization (female and male combined) is the most common method used in the United States.

Choice of a contraceptive method depends on the risks and benefits of the method. No one method is ideal, and each patient

Table 12.2
Methods of Contraception Used in the United States

Method	Number Using
Oral contraceptives	10.7 million
Female sterilization	9.6 million
Condoms	5.1 million
Male sterilization	4.1 million

Table 12.3
Summary of Contraceptive Methods

	Condoms	Diaphragm	Sponge	Female Condom	Cervical Cap
			A. Barrier Methods		
Description/ Name	Sheath of latex of animal tissue that covers the penis to collect the semen	Dome-shaped rubber disk in various sizes	Today Sponge, disk-shaped sponge containing nonoxynol-9	Vaginal pouch, polyurethane sheath to cover femal reproductive tract	Rubber cap
Mechanism of action	Forms a barrier that prevents sperm from entering the female reproductive tract	Covers cervix to block sperm entry into upper female reproductive tract, used with a spermicide	Barrier to sperm entering the female reproductive tract, used with a spermicide	A barrier that prevents sperm entry into female reproductive tract	Covers cervix to block sperm entry into female reproductive tract, used with a spermicide
Advantages	Over-the-counter, protect against STDs, inexpensive	Non-hormonal, STD protection, reusable, decreased dysplasia	Over-the-counter, can be placed hours before intercourse, some STD protection, effective up to 24 hours	Over-the-counter, STD protection, more variety of placement time, no latex allergy	Non-hormonal, STD protection, reusable

Disadvantages (side effects)	Allergic reaction, decreased male sensation	May need to interrupt sexual activity to place, may dislodge during sex, allergy to rubber, inability to insert/remove, increased risk of bladder infections, requires fitting by health care professional, must remain in place 6–8 hours	Allergic reaction, may dislodge during sex, infection risk if not removed in 24 hours (such as toxic shock syndrome)	Insertion difficulty, may dislodge during sex, vaginal irritation, tear or break	May need to interrupt foreplay, may dislodge during sex, allergy to rubber, inability to insert/ remove, requires fitting by health care professional
Contraindications	None	None	None	None	Cervical dysplasia
Typical user failure rates	5–15%, as low as 2% if used with spermicide	10–20%, as low as 2% with spermicide	10–25%	10–15%	10–20%; as low as 2% with spermicide
Cost	$0.25–$2.00 per use	$10–$25, plus spermicide and office visit	$1.00–$2.50 each	$1.00–$2.50 each	$20–$25, plus spermicide and office visit

Table 12.3—*continued*

		B. Spermicides		
Type:	Suppositories	Foam	Jelly or Cream	Film
Description/Name	Spermicide	Spermicide	Spermicide	Vaginal contraceptive film containing spermicide
Mechanism of action	Chemical (nonoxynol-9 or octoxynol) to destroy the sperm cell membrane so no viable sperm reach ovum	Chemical (nonoxynol-9 or octoxynol) to destroy the sperm cell membrane so no viable sperm reach ovum	Chemical (nonoxynol-9 or octoxynol) to destroy the sperm cell membrane so no viable sperm reach ovum	Chemical (nonoxynol-9) to destroy the sperm cell membrane so no viable sperm reach ovum; place over cervix and wait to melt
Advantages	Over-the-counter, some STD protection, easy to insert, adds lubrication, use alone or with condom, good for a backup method if other method in question	Over-the-counter, some STD protection, easy to insert, adds lubrication, use alone or with condom, good for a backup method if other method in question	Over-the-counter, some STD protection, easy to insert, adds lubrication, usually used with a diaphragm, good for a backup method if other method in question	Over-the-counter, some STD protection, easy to insert, adds lubrication, use alone or with condom, good for a backup method if other method in question
Disadvantages (side effects)	Sensitivity to chemical, messy, short time of effectiveness so must replace with each act of	Sensitivity to chemical, messy, short time of effectiveness so must replace with each act	Sensitivity to chemical, messy, short time of effectiveness so must replace with each act	Sensitivity to chemical, messy, short time of effectiveness so must replace with each act

intercourse, short time to wait for dispersion	of intercourse, short time to wait for dispersion	of intercourse, short time to wait for dispersion	of intercourse, short time to wait for dispersion
Contraindications	Allergy, inability to place correctly	Allergy, inability to place correctly	Allergy, inability to place correctly	Allergy, inability to place correctly
Typical user failure rates	3–20%, decreased with condom use	3–25%, decreased with condom use	3–25%, decreased with condom use	3–25%, decreased with condom use
Cost	$4–$10/package	$4–$10/package	$4–$10/package	$4–$10/package

C. Hormonal

Types:	Oral Contraceptive	Depot Medroxyprogesterone Acetate	Norplant
Description/Name	Combinations of estrogen (usually ethinyl estradiol) and progestins, dosages vary, progestin-only pills available also	Depo-Provera, intramuscular progesterone injection	Levonorgestrel subepidermal implants in silicone capsules
Mechanism of action	Prevent ovulation by suppression of gonadotropins, thicken cervical mucus, alter endometrium to prevent implantation	Slow release to prevent ovulation, thicken cervical mucus, create thin, atrophic endometrium	Slow release of progestin to suppress ovulation and thicken cervical mucus, keeps endometrium thin and atrophic

Table 12.3—*continued*

Types:	Oral Contraceptive	Depot Medroxyprogesterone Acetate	Norplant
Advantages	Does not interrupt sex, highly effective, decreases flow and cramps, regulates menses, protective against ovarian and endometrial cancer, may improve PMS, decreased PID, may suppress ovarian cyst formation, decrease benign breast tumors, premenopausal hormone replacement, easily reversible, may improve cholesterol profile	Injection of 150 mg good for 3 months, already in place for sexual activity, decreased menses and cramps	Always in place for sexual activity, long-lasting—up to 5 years, rapid return to fertility after removal, no estrogen side effects, may have decreased cramps and menses
Disadvantages (side effects)	Must be remembered daily, no STD protection, minor side effects (nausea, weight gain, breast tenderness, breakthrough bleeding, etc.), circulatory complications/increased blood clots, benign liver tumors	Repeated injections, irregular bleeding, headaches, depression, nausea, breast tenderness, delayed return to fertility, no STD protection	Irregular menses, weight gain, no STD protection, trained professional for insertion and removal
Contraindications	Over 35 and a smoker, known clotting disorder/CVA/CAD, known estrogen-dependent tumor, liver disease, pregnancy, unexplained vaginal bleeding, hypertension	Sensitivity to medication, unexplained vaginal bleeding	Sensitivity to levonorgestrel, liver disease, unexplained vaginal bleeding, thrombotic or coronary artery disease, pregnancy

Typical user failure rates	1–3%	0.3%	0.1%
Cost	$20–$30/month, plus annual exam fee	$50–$100/shot, plus office visit	$350 for device, plus office visit with insertion fee

D. Intrauterine Device

	Intrauterine Device
Description/Name	Plastic device placed in the uterine cavity; Paraguard and Progestasert only ones available in the United States
Mechanism of action	Interferes with ova and sperm activity, fertilization and implantation, creates local sterile inflammatory reaction. Exact mechanisms poorly understood, hormonal effects of progesterone in Progestasert
Advantages	Already in place without interrupting sexual activity, may decrease menses if contains progesterone
Disadvantages (side effects)	Possible increased menstrual flow and cramps, risk of pelvic infections, increase of ectopic pregnancy if pregnancy occurs, risk of displacement/spontaneous expulsion, uterine perforation, no STD protection
Contraindications	High risk factors for PID, desired fertility, anomalous uterine cavity, pregnancy, unexplained vaginal bleeding
Typical user failure rates	1–2%
Cost	$150–$400 including examination with insertion

Table 12.3—*continued*

E. Rhythm/Natural Family Planning

Types:	Rhythm
Description/Name	Natural family planning, fertility awareness, periodic abstinence
Mechanism of action	Avoid sex during fertile time in natural cycle, identified by basal body temperature (BBT) elevation, cervical mucus thinning, and calendar identification of individual's ovulatory time
Advantages	No medications or devices involved, compatible with some religious beliefs
Disadvantages (side effects)	Requires dedication of patient to accurate record keeping, not good if natural cycles are not regular especially early and late in reproductive years, no STD protection
Contraindications	None
Typical user failure rates	10–20%
Cost	Nothing unless BBT thermometer brought

F. Abortion

Types:	Abortion
Description/Name	Removal of the products of conception
Mechanism of action	Surgically performed as a dilation and suction curettage, dilation and evacuation, hysterotomy, or hysterectomy. Medically performed with prostaglandin E2, hypertonic saline, or urea

Advantages	Useful for implanted pregnancy up to 24 weeks	
Disadvantages (side effects)	Surgical risks of infection, injury, bleeding, complications for future fertility; requires trained personnel	
Contraindications	Pregnancy 24 weeks or greater	
Typical user failure rates	<1%	
Cost	Varies—$250 and up	

	G. Postcoital	
Types:	Hormonal	Mechanical
Description/Name	"Morning After Pill," (Ovral 2 tablets every 12 hours times 2 doses)	IUD placement
Mechanism of action	Luteolytic effect, out-of-phase endometrium, disordered tubal transport	Prevent implantation
Advantages	Useful if other method fails, after rape	Have 5–7 days to place, nonhormonal, can remain for continued contraception
Disadvantages (side effects)	Nausea, must be taken within 72 hours	All IUD complications, requires health care professional, not good method for anyone with infection risk
Contraindications	Similar to oral contraceptive	Desired pregnancy, abnormal uterine cavity
Typical user failure rates	1%	<1%
Cost	$20–$30	$150–$400 for IUD and insertion

should be counseled about available methods. Patients need accurate information from their physicians about effectiveness and risks of contraception. Many patients receive their information from the lay press and from friends; they may have a distorted view of risks and effectiveness.

Contraceptive failure should be distinguished from contraceptive effectiveness. If 3% of women using oral contraceptives become pregnant in a year, the contraceptive failure rate is 3%. It does not follow, however, that the oral contraceptive is 97% effective, because not all women would have conceived if they had not used contraception. User failure rates are different from theoretical failure rates. It is best to discuss typical user failure rates with patients in a way the patient can understand—i.e., "Of 100 women who use an IUD for one year, about two will get pregnant."

Contraceptives may have health benefits other than contraception and may have health risks associated with them. All of these should be discussed with the patient. Because the costs of contraception can vary widely, patients need to know the relative costs. Table 12.3 summarizes the risks, contraindications, benefits, effectiveness, and costs of various contraceptive methods.

Suggested Readings

American College of Obstetricians and Gynecologists. Hormonal contraception. Technical Bulletin 198. Washington, DC: ACOG, 1994.

American College of Obstetricians and Gynecologists. The intrauterine device. Technical Bulletin 164. Washington, DC: ACOG, 1992.

Hatcher RA, ed. Contraceptive technology: 16th revised edition. New York: Irvington Publishers, 1994.

LoPiccolo J, LoPiccolo L, eds. Handbook of sex therapy. New York: Plenum Press, 1978.

Masters WH, Johnson VE. Human sexual inadequacy. Boston: Little, Brown, 1970.

Speroff L, Glass RH, Kase NG. Clinical gynecologic endocrinology and infertility. 5th ed. Baltimore: Williams & Wilkins, 1994.

Chapter 13

Infections

VAGINITIS

Vaginitis is a common complaint, leading to approximately 5 million office visits per year. Vaginitis is among the top 25 reasons for physician visits. Vaginal itching and burning may be from a variety of causes, which may be infectious or noninfectious. Vaginitis may be confused with urinary complaints or gastrointestinal complaints. "Vaginitis" or "yeast infection" may be the only term a patient knows for genital symptoms. Vulvovaginal complaints require a careful evaluation.

Normal Vaginal Flora

Normally there are 10^5–10^7 organisms per square centimeter of vaginal wall. The predominant microbe is usually *Lactobacillus*. Three to eight other species can usually be isolated by careful microbiology. Normal bacterial flora are listed in Table 13.1.

Normal vaginal secretions are composed primarily of desquamated epithelial cells. They are not visible at the introitus. Normal secretions are flocculent, white, and nonmalodorous, with a pH of 3.8–4.4.

Evaluation of a Patient with Vaginitis

The history should include any itching, burning, or pain, and the amount, color, and odor of any discharge. The duration of symptoms, any prior therapy including self-therapy, and any underlying medical conditions such as diabetes, pregnancy, or immune suppression are documented. A history of antibiotic use for other conditions must be documented. The location (introital, vaginal, pelvic, or lower abdomen) and severity of dyspareunia is important. Sexual history should include the number of sexual partners

Table 13.1
Flora Isolated from Normal Vaginas

Lactobacilli	60–80%
Group B streptococci	10–20%
Mycoplasma hominis	20–35%
Ureaplasma urealyticum	35–85%
Gardnerella vaginalis	40–60%
Bacteroides species	10–20%
Peptococcus/Peptostreptococcus	6–10%
Anaerobic Gram-positive rods	4–10%
Gram-negative aerobes	1–2%

and whether there have been any recent new partners. Physical examination includes a search for vulvar lesions or inflammation, the presence of discharge at the introitus, and the character of the vaginal discharge. Laboratory evaluation always includes a saline mount to evaluate for trichomonads, "clue" cells, white blood cells, and squamous cells. A potassium hydroxide preparation using 10% KOH is used to evaluate for fungal forms.

The vaginal pH is normally between 3.8 and 4.5. A pH greater than 4.5 indicates bacterial vaginosis or trichomoniasis. A pH less than 3.8 accompanied by evidence of cytolysis indicates cytolytic vaginosis. The whiff test relies on the odor released on addition of 10% KOH. A foul or fishy odor indicates bacterial vaginosis, and a "yeasty" odor indicates fungal infection. Gram stain of a direct smear from the vagina will indicate the predominant bacterial species and is the most reliable way to diagnose bacterial vaginosis (Table 13.2).

Vaginal cultures are rarely indicated except in difficult or recurrent cases. If they are done, they MUST be done in a quantitative manner to be meaningful. They MUST be done separately for anaerobes, aerobes, fungi, and trichomonads, with appropriate transfer media. The laboratory must be capable of isolating and identifying aerobes, anaerobes, trichomonads, and fungi.

Common Types of Vaginitis

Bacterial Vaginosis

Bacterial vaginosis is an alteration in the normal flora. There is a decline in numbers of lactobacilli and an overgrowth of *Gardnerella*, anaerobes, and mycoplasma species. The symptoms are of

Table 13.2
Gram Stain Score for Bacterial Vaginosis

Organism	Quantity	Score
Lactobacilli	0	4
	< 1	3
	1–4	2
	5–30	1
	> 30	0
G. vaginalis/Bacteroides	0	0
	< 1	1
	1–4	2
	5–30	3
	> 30	4
Mobiluncus	0	0
	< 1–4	1
	5– > 30	2

The average of three oil immersion fields is used. A score of 0–3 is normal. A score of 7–10 and a pH > 4.5 indicates bacterial vaginosis. A score of 4–6 is intermediate and is often found with trichomoniasis.

an increased, malodorous discharge. The discharge is usually not associated with itching or burning. The diagnosis is made by wet mount with "clue" cells and minimal white blood cells. A Gram stain will have a score of 7–10. The pH is greater than 4.5, and a whiff test is usually positive.

Bacterial vaginosis causes approximately 40–50% of symptomatic vaginitis. It is found in approximately 15–25% of asymptomatic women, and at least 50% of those with laboratory signs are asymptomatic. Therapy of bacterial vaginosis is by oral or vaginal metronidazole or clindamycin, which appear to be equally effective (Table 13.3).

Fungal Vaginitis

Approximately 80% of fungal vaginitis is due to *Candida albicans*. The remainder are due to other *Candida* species, *Torulopsis,* or other species. Symptoms are of itching and burning with an increased discharge. Diagnosis is by identification of the fungus by KOH preparation or special cultures. Therapy is with vaginal imidazoles, all of which appear to be equally effective. Boric acid vaginal tablets are effective against many strains that are resistant to imidazoles. Oral antifungal preparations such as ketoconazole

Table 13.3
Therapies for Bacterial Vaginosis

Medication	Dose	Duration
Metronidazole	250 mg 3 times daily	5–7 days
	500 mg twice daily	5–7 days
	2 g	one dose
	2 g	day 1 and 3
	Vaginal gel	7 days
Clindamycin	300 mg twice daily	7 days
	Vaginal cream	5 days

or fluconazole should be reserved for those who fail therapy with vaginal preparations.

Lactobacilli are almost always found in the vagina of women with fungal infections, and the pH is usually less than 4.5. Many women report that they develop a fungal infection after using broad-spectrum antibiotics. Although the vaginal flora is changed by these antibiotics, it does not appear that elimination of lactobacilli is responsible for the fungal infection.

Trichomonas

Trichomonas vaginalis is a flagellated protozoan that is sexually transmitted. It produces a yellow-green discharge and inflammation, erythema, and edema of the vagina. Itching, pain, and odor are usually present. The diagnosis is made by wet mount. Cultures for trichomonads must be transported and incubated in Diamond's media, and most clinical laboratories are not equipped to perform these cultures. When cultures are done on asymptomatic women, up to 10% are found to carry trichomonads in the vagina. Women may carry the organism for years without developing symptoms.

Metronidazole is the only drug approved for the therapy of trichomoniasis. A 2-g single dose is as effective as 250 mg 3 times daily for 7 days. It is essential to treat all sexual partners as well to prevent re-exposure.

VULVITIS

Evaluation of a Patient with Vulvitis

The history should include the nature, duration, and location of symptoms, as well as any previous diagnosis and therapy. If the

patient has had prior biopsies, these should be obtained to be reviewed. Physical examination includes a gross examination of the
vulva for lesions. Colposcopy may be helpful if dystrophies are
suggested. A wash with dilute acetic acid (3–5%) to find hyperkeratotic lesions, and a stain with toluidine blue to find hyperplasia, are helpful. Laboratory evaluation consists of cultures of
ulcers for herpes virus and biopsy of suspected lesions.

Common Types of Vulvitis

Fungal infections are the most common etiology. Vulvar dystrophies such as lichen sclerosis, hyperplastic dystrophy, and vulvar
intraepithelial neoplasia are common. Atrophic vulvitis is due to
lack of estrogen. It is characterized by thin, atrophic skin with
symptoms of itching and burning. Allergic and irritant vulvitis is
due to contact with chemicals. Fabric softeners, deodorants,
soaps, and perfumes may be the cause.

Vestibular adenitis or vulvar vestibulitis is a rare syndrome
characterized by intense tenderness and burning of the vulvar
vestibule. Physical findings are limited to vestibular erythema of
varying degree. The symptoms are limited to the vestibule, and
the area of tenderness can be sharply delimited. Biopsy shows
nonspecific chronic inflammation. Paget's disease of the vulva
causes an erythematous, scaly lesion that can be very tender.

Pudendal neuralgia may be due to sacral nerve root compression or obstetric or other trauma. The symptom is of unre-
lenting pain. Physical examination of the vulva is usually normal,
but there may be decreased sensation over sacral nerve roots.

Most episodes of vaginitis or vulvitis respond to therapy with
no sequelae. However, if there is a recurrent or persistent problem, sexual dysfunction is common. Inhibited sexual desire is the
most common dysfunction. Vaginismus may also result. Treatment of the vaginitis may or may not resolve a sexual dysfunction.

SEXUALLY TRANSMITTED DISEASES

Gonorrhea

An estimated 1 million new cases of gonorrhea occur each year.
Many females with gonorrhea are asymptomatic, causing them to
delay diagnosis and treatment. Untreated gonorrhea can lead to
pelvic inflammatory disease or disseminated gonorrhea infections. A presumptive diagnosis can be made on the basis of a cer-

vical Gram stain, identification of gonococcal enzymes in the cervix, or endocervical culture. Culture remains the mainstay of diagnosis. The sensitivity of a cervical culture ranges from 80–90%.

Gonorrhea can be treated by a variety of antimicrobial agents. The selection of an antibiotic depends on the anatomic site of infection, the potential resistance of *Neisseria gonorrhoeae* to antimicrobials, concurrent infection with *Chlamydia trachomatis,* side effects and costs, and any recent antibiotic treatment. Recommended treatment regimens for gonorrhea are listed in Table 13.4.

In most states, the presence of a gonococcal infection must be reported to the health department. All sexual contacts should be referred for treatment.

Chlamydial Infections

All sexually active adolescents and young adults should be screened for chlamydia. Chlamydia is approximately twice as common as gonorrhea, and there is an approximately 50% co-infection between the two organisms. Chlamydia is usually asymptomatic in women and leads to an upper tract infection that is more indolent than that caused by gonorrhea. Tubal damage is a common sequela of chlamydial infection.

Chlamydia can be cultured using human cells in cell culture. This process is expensive and time-consuming, so most clinics use an enzyme-linked immunosorbent assay or a monoclonal antibody test to detect the organism. Polymerase chain reaction is a new modality for diagnosis that is being used in some clinics. These nonculture techniques have sensitivities from 80–95% and specificity of 90–95%. The specificity is excellent in a high prevalence population such as an STD clinic. However, in a low prevalence population the specificity of these tests can lead to a high

Table 13.4
Treatment Regimens for Gonorrhea

A single dose of:
    Ceftriaxone 125 mg i.m., **or**
    Cefixime 400 mg orally, **or**
    Ciprofloxacin 500 mg orally, **or**
    Ofloxacin 400 mg orally
PLUS
    A regimen effective against chlamydia such as doxycycline 100 mg twice daily for 7 days, or azithromycin 1 g orally in a single dose

number of false positives. For example, assume a population that has a true positive rate for chlamydial infection of 5% and that 100 women were screened. A test with a sensitivity of 90% would probably detect all 5 true positives. A test with a specificity of 95% would also have 4 false positives. Therefore, almost half of the positives would be false positives. A diagnosis of a sexually transmitted disease may have a profound effect on a relationship that was presumed to be monogamous. Careful judgment must be used in deciding whether to accept the diagnosis of chlamydia from nonculture techniques. It is reasonable to confirm all positive results in a low prevalence population.

Recommended regimens are doxycycline 100 mg orally twice daily for 7 days or azithromycin 1 gram as a single oral dose. Alternative regimens include ofloxacin 300 mg orally twice daily for 7 days; erythromycin base 500 mg orally 4 times daily for 7 days; or sulfisoxazole 500 mg orally 4 times daily for 10 days. Doxycycline and ofloxacin are contraindicated in pregnancy. The sex partners of patients with chlamydia should be referred for treatment.

Syphilis

Syphilis is caused by a spirochete, *Treponema pallidum.* The disease can be transmitted sexually or through the placenta. The number of reported cases has risen steadily each year since 1986, and the current incidence is estimated to be 15/100,000.

The disease progresses through four stages if not treated. Primary syphilis is characterized by a chancre. It is typically a raised, painless ulcer, although it may be painful, particularly if secondarily infected. The chancre appears from 10 to 90 days after exposure to the organism. Painless lymphadenopathy may or may not be present.

Secondary syphilis is characterized by a bacteremia with involvement of all organ systems. It occurs 6 weeks to 6 months after the chancre and persists for 2 to 6 weeks. The hallmark symptom is a diffuse rash involving the entire body, including the soles and palms. Generalized lymphadenopathy accompanies the rash. Hepatitis, glomerulonephritis, and arthritis may be found.

Latent syphilis lasts from 1 to 20 years before the onset of tertiary syphilis. Tertiary syphilis occurs in one-third of untreated patients. Involvement of the cardiovascular system, central nervous system, and musculoskeletal system causes the majority of morbidity.

A darkfield examination of a slide prepared from a chancre may show spirochetes. The mainstay of diagnosis is serological testing. Nontreponemal antibody tests include the Venereal Disease Research Laboratory Test (VDRL), the rapid plasma reagin (RPR), and the automated reagin test (ART). These tests become positive 4–5 weeks after onset of infection or about 1 week after the appearance of a chancre. False-positive results may occur in pregnancy or in patients with autoimmune diseases. The fluorescent treponemal antibody absorbed with nonpallidum treponema (FTA-ABS) is a very sensitive and specific test for syphilis and should be used to confirm the diagnosis.

Penicillin is the only proven effective therapy. Patients with primary, secondary, or latent syphilis of less than one year's duration are treated with benzathine penicillin 2.4 million units intramuscularly in a single dose. Patients with latent syphilis of more than one year's duration or uncertain duration should receive benzathine penicillin 2.4 million units weekly for 3 weeks. Patients with a documented penicillin allergy should be hospitalized and undergo rapid desensitization.

PELVIC INFLAMMATORY DISEASE

Pelvic inflammatory disease (PID) incorporates a wide range of clinical entities, including any combination of endometritis, salpingitis, tubo-ovarian abscess, or pelvic peritonitis. Symptomatic PID accounts for 2.5 million outpatient visits each year, as well as 275,000 hospitalizations. Early diagnosis and therapy can prevent sequelae such as infertility, ectopic pregnancy, and chronic pelvic pain. The majority of PID is associated with STDs such as gonorrhea or chlamydia. However, anaerobic organisms can cause PID alone or in combination with a sexually transmitted disease.

The diagnosis of PID is difficult. Empiric diagnosis of PID can be made if all three of the following criteria are met: lower abdominal tenderness, adnexal tenderness, and cervical motion tenderness. The presence of one or more of the following increases the specificity of the diagnosis: oral temperature greater than 38°C, abnormal cervical or vaginal discharge, elevated sedimentation rate, elevated C-reactive protein, or laboratory evidence of infection with *N. gonorrhoeae* or *C. trachomatis*. The presence of endometritis on an endometrial biopsy, tubo-ovarian abscess on ultrasonography, or laparoscopic abnormalities consistent with PID is definite evidence of PID.

Inpatient regimens for PID include cefoxitin 2 g intravenously every 6 hours or cefotetan 2 g intravenously every 12 hours, plus doxycycline 100 mg intravenously or orally every 12 hours. An alternate regimen is clindamycin 900 mg intravenously every 8 hours plus gentamicin 2 mg/kg as a loading dose plus 1.5 mg/kg every 8 hours. These regimens must be given for 48–72 hours to allow for clinical improvement and continued for at least 48 hours after the patient shows improvement.

Outpatient regimens include cefoxitin 2 g intramuscularly plus probenecid 1 g orally in a single dose plus doxycycline 100 mg twice daily for 7 days; or ofloxacin 400 mg orally twice daily for 14 days plus either clindamycin 450 mg 4 times daily or metronidazole 500 mg twice daily for 14 days.

Suggested Readings

American College of Obstetricians and Gynecologists. Antimicrobial therapy for gynecologic infections. Technical Bulletin 153. Washington, DC: ACOG, 1991.

American College of Obstetricians and Gynecologists. Gonorrhea and chlamydial infections. Technical Bulletin 190. Washington, DC: ACOG, 1994.

American College of Obstetricians and Gynecologists. Vulvovaginitis. Technical Bulletin 135. Washington, DC: ACOG, 1989.

Biswas MK. Bacterial vaginosis. Clin Obstet Gynecol 1993;36:166–176.

Centers for Disease Control and Prevention. Sexually transmitted diseases treatment guidelines. MMWR 1993;42(RR-14):1–102.

Ernest JM. Topical antifungal agents. Obstet Gynecol Clin North Am 1992;19:587–607.

Graves A, Gardner WA Jr. Pathogenicity of Trichomonas vaginalis. Clin Obstet Gynecol 1993;36:145–152.

Kaufman RH, Faro S, eds. Benign diseases of the vulva and vagina. 4th ed. St. Louis: Mosby, 1994.

Lugo-Miro VI, Green M, Mazur L. Comparison of different metronidazole therapeutic regimens for bacterial vaginosis. JAMA 1992;268:92–95.

Pastorek J, ed. Obstetric and gynecologic infectious disease. New York: Raven Press, 1994.

Chapter 14

Common Gynecologic Problems

LEIOMYOMATA

Leiomyomata, sometimes called fibroids or myomas, are benign tumors originating from smooth muscle cells. They contain varying amounts of fibrous tissue that is probably comprised of degenerated smooth muscle cells. Most fibroids are diagnosed during the fourth or fifth decade of life. They are the most frequent pelvic tumor. Myomas are usually multiple. Growth of myomas is stimulated by estrogen. Myomas grow by pushing borders with a pseudocapsule, and they may grow to be quite large. The most common pelvic site is in the uterine corpus. Leiomyomas are found in 25% of white women and 50% of black women.

Leiomyomas may be found in several locations. Subserosal myomas are located under the outer serosal surface of the uterus. Intramural (interstitial) myomas are within the muscular wall of the uterus. Submucous myomas are under the endometrium and may prolapse through the cervix. Intraligamentary myomas are within the broad ligament and may be confused with adnexal masses. Pedunculated myomas are attached by a pedicle and may originate from serosal or mucosal locations. Parasitic myomas usually begin as pedunculated myomas that obtain an alternative blood supply, other than from the uterus. Cervical myomas are located in the cervix and may protrude or prolapse into the vagina.

On gross inspection the uterus may appear grossly nodular or smooth but enlarged. The cut surface is pearl-white and glistening. The base of a pedicle has the major blood supply. The histologic appearance is of proliferation of smooth muscle cells in bundles. Fibrous connective tissue is seen between bundles.

Leiomyomas may be asymptomatic. Symptoms can include pelvic pressure and urinary frequency due to a mass effect. The pelvic mass can lead to ureteral obstruction and a hydroureter. Pain may be manifested as dysmenorrhea, dyspareunia, or chronic pelvic pain. An infarcted fibroid may cause acute pelvic pain and an acute abdomen.

Abnormal uterine bleeding is common with submucous fibroids and can occur with interstitial fibroids. Abnormal bleeding occurs through two mechanisms. Submucous myomas have a thin endometrium over the surface that may not respond normally to hormonal influences. Submucous myomas may ulcerate or necrose and bleed directly. Interstitial fibroids may cause an increase in the surface area of the endometrium as the uterus increases in size, leading to hypermenorrhea. Anemia can result from the hypermenorrhea.

Infertility can result from repeated spontaneous abortions or from occlusion of the cornual portion of the uterine tube. Pregnancy complications can include preterm labor, abortion, abruptio placentae, and dystocia. Fibroids may grow rapidly during pregnancy and infarct. An infarcted fibroid can cause severe pain and can be a very difficult complication of pregnancy to manage.

The diagnosis is suggested by history. Bimanual examination is often confirmatory. Pelvic ultrasound examination may be useful to confirm the pelvic examination and to differentiate between fibroids and adnexal masses. Ultrasound may also be useful to diagnose small submucous fibroids that cause abnormal bleeding or may be asymptomatic. Laparoscopy may be needed to differentiate a myoma in the broad ligament from a solid adnexal mass. Abdominal x-ray may identify a myoma with calcifications.

Degeneration occurs from ischemia when the blood supply can no longer reach the center of a myoma. Hyaline degeneration is the most common form, occurring in 65% of cases. It is an acellular change that occurs slowly. Myxomatous change accounts for 15% of cases of degeneration. Calcific change causes 10% of cases of degeneration and is more common in larger myomas and in older women. Cystic degeneration probably results from infarction. Fatty degeneration is rare. "Red," or necrotic or carneous, degeneration is an acute form of degeneration that often occurs in pregnancy due to rapid growth beyond the blood supply. Infarcted fibroids may become secondarily infected. Sarcomatous or malignant degeneration is rare. It has been commonly believed that rapidly growing fibroids were at greater risk of being malignant. In a recent study, however, no relationship was found between the rapidity of growth and the risk of sarcoma.

Treatment

Progestin therapy can be administered to reduce estrogen levels and to decrease bleeding. Gonadotropin-releasing hormone (GnRH) agonists mimic menopause by stopping gonadotropin stimulation of the ovary. This decreases estrogen production and stimulation of tumor growth. Myomas will decrease in size when estrogen stimulation is decreased. GnRH agonists are often used preoperatively to decrease myoma size. They may also be used in selected cases to treat myomas that cause infertility. When GnRH agonists are stopped, myomas begin to grow again.

Myomectomy is the removal of individual fibroids with preservation of the uterus. It is usually performed with plans to preserve fertility. The risk of recurrence of myomas is as high as 40% and the risk of infertility after the myomectomy is as high as 40%. Myomectomy is often performed by laparotomy but can be accomplished by laparoscopy in selected patients. Submucous myomas can be removed by hysteroscopy. Myomectomy by any route can relieve symptoms and preserve fertility, but patients should be counseled that symptom recurrence and infertility may occur.

Hysterectomy is the usual treatment when fertility is no longer desired. Hysterectomy is indicated when symptoms are severe enough to justify the risk of surgery. It is often performed when the uterus attains the size of a 14-week pregnancy because it is difficult to detect adnexal masses in the presence of an enlarged uterus and because further growth is likely to result in compression of urinary structures.

If fibroids are asymptomatic or only mildly symptomatic and smaller in size than a 14-week pregnancy, they may be followed with observation. Myomas will usually shrink at menopause as estrogen stimulation diminishes. Any presumed myoma that grows after menopause should be evaluated carefully because the patient may actually have an ovarian cancer.

PELVIC RELAXATION

Pelvic relaxation is a disorder of pelvic support structures. The term includes cases of cystocele, rectocele, enterocele, urethrocele, and uterine prolapse. The cause of pelvic relaxation is a defect in the endopelvic fascia.

In order to manage patients with pelvic relaxation, it is essential to have a clear understanding of the anatomy of the pelvic support structures. The uterus, vagina, bladder, and anterior rectum are supported by the endopelvic fascia. The endopelvic fascia is a sheet of connective tissue that wraps around the vagina. It is attached laterally to the arcus tendineus where the obturator internus and the levator ani join, and posteriorly and superiorly to the sacrum and the lateral pelvic side wall. The uterosacral ligaments and the cardinal ligaments are condensations of this tissue and are not separate structures. Tears in the endopelvic fascia cause pelvic relaxation.

There are a number of factors that increase the risk of pelvic relaxation. Obesity increases the risk of pelvic relaxation by increasing the intraabdominal pressure. Childbirth can lead to injuries to the endopelvic fascia. Smoking results in lower estrogen levels and in chronic cough. Estrogen deficiency associated with menopause leads to weakening of the pelvic support. Repeated and long-term lifting increases intraabdominal pressure. Nonobstetric trauma can also damage the endopelvic fascia.

Symptoms

Pelvic or vaginal pressure or fullness and the sensation of "things falling out" (pelvic instability) are common symptoms. Stress urinary incontinence is a particularly bothersome complaint. Straining or digitalization with bowel movement is a common symptom of a rectocele. Backache and chronic pelvic pain are often overlooked complaints. Low back pain can be due to a variety of causes and may not respond to treatment for pelvic relaxation. Dyspareunia is common. Occasional urinary urgency and a feeling of incomplete voiding are commonly seen with a cystocele.

Examination

The examination of a patient with suspected pelvic relaxation should be directed toward identifying defects in the pelvic support. It is often helpful to disassemble a speculum to create a retractor. Use of the posterior blade as a retractor allows examination of the anterior and posterior vaginal walls separately.

A urethrocele is a bulge in the lower third of the anterior vaginal wall underlying the urethra. Pressure applied may cause a small amount of urine to be expelled. It is caused by a tear in the endopelvic fascia centrally and distally. Isolated urethroceles are rare and usually result from a laceration of the lower anterior vaginal wall. Most presumed urethroceles are due to lateral tears in the endopelvic fascia at the arcus tendineus. The bladder and urethra may rotate with strain or cough with a lateral tear. The anterior vagina has normal rugae and typically does not have a defined bulge.

A cystocele is a bulge of varying degrees in the anterior vaginal wall and is caused by a tear in the central anterior endopelvic fascia. The bladder then herniates into the anterior vagina. On examination, the cystocele will typically have smooth vaginal mucosa with loss of rugae. The lateral vaginal supports are intact and do not move with strain or cough.

A rectocele is a bulge of the posterior vaginal wall into the vagina. It is most evident with a Valsalva maneuver. Rectovaginal exam can help confirm its extent. It is caused by a central tear in the posterior endopelvic fascia.

An enterocele is a hernia of the vaginal apex through the rectouterine pouch (pouch of Douglas or cul-de-sac). It includes peritoneum and small bowel. Enteroceles are most common after hysterectomy. They are caused by a herniation of the endopelvic fascia at the site of the cervicovaginal junction, usually between the uterosacral ligaments.

Procidentia uteri is prolapse or descent of the uterus. It is described by degrees. First degree procidentia is prolapse into the upper vagina; second degree is from the lower vagina to introitus; third degree is a prolapse through the introitus. Procidentia is caused by tears in the upper endopelvic fascia at the uterosacral and cardinal ligaments.

Pelvic relaxation defects may occur alone but usually occur in combinations. Thus it is rare, for example, to see a cystocele without associated rectocele. Failure to repair all defects at the initial surgery leads to failure of therapy and the need for further surgery.

Nonsurgical Treatments

Pessaries

The type of pessary needed depends on the type of anatomic defect. Usually a Smith-Hodge pessary is best for lateral defects without a great deal of descent. A donut or inflatable pessary is best for descent. Pessaries can be used for all types of relaxation.

Kegel exercises strengthen the levator ani muscles. They may be performed with the aid of weighted vaginal cones but are usually done without artificial devices. Kegel exercises are of most benefit in the woman with mild stress incontinence who has minimal descent. Estrogen can help to improve the integrity of vaginal tissues in women who are estrogen-deprived, leading to increased vascularity in the pelvis and reduced atrophy. Either systemic or vaginal estrogen can be used.

Surgical Therapies

Successful surgical therapy must be directed toward correction of the anatomic defect. Urethroceles and cystoceles that are due to a central defect with good lateral support are repaired by anterior colporrhaphy that includes a Kelly plication stitch. Sutures are placed in the endopelvic fascia at the level of the urethrovesical junction (bladder neck) and continued along the urethra where the urethrocele is present.

Rectoceles are repaired by a posterior colporrhaphy to approximate the perirectal fascia, which includes portions of the levator ani muscles, over the rectum. Often a perineorrhaphy is also performed to correct vaginal outlet relaxation. Perineorrhaphy is a separate procedure from posterior colporrhaphy. The goal of perineorrhaphy is to reapproximate the transverse perineal muscles, the bulbocavernosus, and the distal levator ani.

Enterocele repair may be performed abdominally or vaginally, usually in conjunction with other reparative procedures. The peritoneal sac is separated from other tissue and ligated at its neck. Obliteration of the cul-de-sac may be accomplished by plicating the uterosacral ligaments or by purse-string sutures of the endopelvic fascia. This procedure will help to prevent recurrence of enterocele.

Uterine prolapse repair is usually accompanied by vaginal or abdominal hysterectomy. An anterior and posterior colporrhaphy is also usually needed. Resuspension of the vaginal apex can be accomplished by shortening of the uterosacral ligaments, abdominal mesh colposacropexy, or vaginal sacrospinous ligament suspension.

A colpocleisis may be done, which adheres the anterior and posterior vaginal walls with or without a uterus present above the closure. Colpocleisis can be performed rapidly under local anesthesia and should be reserved for women with procidentia who are poor surgical risks and do not wish to preserve vaginal function. Vaginal intercourse is impossible following colpocleisis.

URINARY INCONTINENCE

Urinary incontinence is involuntary loss of urine that can be objectively demonstrated. Approximately 10% of women complain of urinary incontinence. These are three types of incontinence: Stress, urge, and extraurethral.

Stress Incontinence

Stress or anatomic incontinence is an involuntary and immediate loss of urine when intravesical pressure exceeds urethral pressure. It occurs with increased intraabdominal pressure in the absence of detrusor activity. Stress incontinence may include 75–80% of incontinence problems.

Predisposing factors include pregnancy and delivery, obesity, chronic cough, and heavy lifting and frequent straining (similar to the causes of pelvic relaxation). There appears to be a genetic predisposition in certain patients. Symptoms of stress incontinence include urine leakage with cough, sneeze, laugh, lifting, and often certain exercise activities.

The anatomic defect is lowered urethral resistance due to displacement of the urethra and urethrovesical junction away from the pubic bone and out of the abdominal cavity with increased intraabdominal pressure. Under normal circumstances, an increase in abdominal pressure is accompanied by a reflex contraction of the levator ani and an elevation of the posterior urethrovesical junction. When the pelvic supports are damaged, contracture of the levator ani does not elevate the urethra and the urethra rotates out of position. Pressure is then transmitted directly from the bladder through the urethra and urine loss occurs. Lateral detachments of the endopelvic fascia (at the arcus tendineus) are associated with the greatest degree of stress incontinence.

Nonsurgical therapy can be attempted by Kegel exercises. Biofeedback and bladder training (voiding schedule) are helpful in some cases. Estrogen therapy is helpful if the patient is estrogen-deprived. Medications that can decrease intravesicular pressure such as oxybutynin chloride (Ditropan) or imipramine may be effective. Phenylpropanolamine increases intraurethral pressure and may be helpful.

Surgical therapy has the goal of returning the proximal urethra to an intraabdominal position and supporting the bladder base. Surgical therapy is most successful when it is directed toward a specific anatomic defect. Anterior colporrhaphy with Kelly plication is the treatment of choice for the patient with a large central defect and good lateral support. Kelly plication is unsuccessful if there is a significant lateral defect or if the endopelvic fascia is not reapproximated. In skilled hands with proper patient selection the Kelly plication has been shown to have five-year success rates equal to those of the retropubic procedures.

The Burch procedure resuspends the anterior and lateral vaginal wall to the pectineal ligament (Cooper's ligament) and results in high retropubic placement of the urethra. It is best performed on a patient with a lateral defect. The Burch procedure may result in an increased risk of enterocele due to the anterior displacement of the vagina.

The Marshall-Marchetti-Krantz (MMK) procedure suspends the anterior vaginal wall to the posterior pubis. Possible postoperative complications include the temporary inability to void spontaneously and osteitis pubis in approximately 1% of patients following retropubic urethropexies. Retropubic needle suspension procedures including the Pereyra, Stamey, and Raz procedures, all suspend the anterior vaginal wall and periurethral endocervical fascia to the insertion of the rectus abdominis at the superior pubis. The needle suspension procedures can easily be combined with an anterior and posterior colporrhaphy. They are best performed on a patient with a lateral defect.

Sling procedures are reserved for patients with previously failed procedures and for patients with low-pressure urethras. Fascia taken from the fascia lata or the rectus abdominis is used to suspend the urethra to the rectus abdominis at the superior pubis. Use of synthetic grafts for the sling is not recommended due the risk of erosion of the base of the urethra.

Urge Incontinence

Urge incontinence is defined as an inappropriate contraction of the detrusor resulting in urinary incontinence. Urge incontinence is also called detrusor dyssynergia or unstable bladder. Urge incontinence causes 10–30% of incontinence problems, but the percentage increases with age. The majority of patients (90%) are otherwise neurologically normal.

Normal bladder function depends on a sensory neuronal pathway and a motor neuron pathway. The sensory arc begins with stretch receptors in the detrusor muscle and proceeds along the pelvic parasympathetic nerves to the spinal cord. Urge incontinence may result from uninhibited detrusor contractions without a strong sensory input (motor type) or from strong sensory input from the bladder (sensory type). The motor type is usually of unknown etiology, but it may be due to an upper motor neuron lesion. The sensory type is usually due to inflammation, mechanical irritation, neoplastic or hormonal epithelial changes, interstitial cystitis, or radiation.

Symptoms

Patients with the motor type have uninhibited loss of small amounts of urine, nocturia, and frequency. Patients with the sensory type can inhibit contractions and may have discomfort with bladder filling and dysuria. Symptoms are nonspecific and a definitive diagnosis cannot be made from the history. Anatomic defects are not present except bladder mucosal changes with some cases of sensory urge incontinence.

Diagnosis is confirmed by cystometry that reveals uninhibited bladder contractions at pressures greater than 15 cm H_2O and opening of the vesical neck with a detrusor contraction. Treatment consists of treatment of any identifiable cause such as a bladder infection, bladder stone, or estrogen deficiency. Otherwise, pharmacological therapy, such as anticholinergic agents, α-adrenergic agents, or imipramine, is used to reduce bladder contractions.

Overflow incontinence is caused by urinary retention (overdistension) with intravesical pressure exceeding maximum urethral pressure. It is not associated with detrusor activity. The postvoid residual urine volume is elevated. It is sometimes called neurogenic bladder.

Predisposing factors include neurologic disease, CNS trauma or tumors, medications that reduce bladder contractions, and peripheral neuropathies. Symptoms include voiding small amounts, the sensation of incomplete emptying, and leaking small amounts without awareness of urine loss. Anatomic defects may be present. If the patient has a detached urethra, surgical repair may leave the patient permanently unable to void.

Diagnosis is confirmed by a high residual urine volume and cystometry that shows a high-volume, low-pressure bladder. Therapy consists of treatment of any medical illnesses as much as possible, bladder training, and possibly intermittent self-catheterization.

Extraurethral Incontinence

Extraurethral incontinence is defined as loss of urine other than through the urethra. The loss is usually through a fistula. Predisposing factors include surgery, congenital anomalies, and radiation therapy. Symptoms are of constant small amounts of urine loss that may be confused with vaginal discharge. The anatomic defect can be a vesicovaginal fistula, ureterovaginal fistula, or ectopic ureter.

Diagnosis may be made by history and physical examination by visualization of a fistula or ectopic ureter. Cystoscopy, urethroscopy, or intravenous pyelogram (IVP) may help to visualize a fistula. Dye studies for leakage site can differentiate a vesicovaginal from a vesicourethral fistula. To perform a dye study, place three cotton balls or tampons in the vagina. Then fill the bladder with a solution of methylene blue or indigo carmine. If the most distal tampon is stained, it may be due to a urethrovaginal fistula or to urinary incontinence. If the upper tampons are stained, it is due to a vesicovaginal fistula. If the upper tampons are wet but not stained it is indicative of a ureterovaginal fistula. The diagnosis of ureterovaginal fistula can be confirmed by placing new tampons and then giving intravenous indigo carmine. If the upper tampon is then stained, the diagnosis is confirmed. Treatment is repair of the anatomic defect.

Evaluation of Urinary Incontinence

Genitourinary History

The specifics of incontinence must be detailed. The duration, frequency of occurrence, and precipitating factors are recorded. Any history of dysuria, hematuria, enuresis, urgency, or frequency is recorded. Medical diseases associated with neuropathy, medications, or surgery (particularly gynecologic or urologic) may be important.

Initial Examination

Pelvic examination should include evaluation of the pelvic support loss and estrogen status. Bimanual examination may aid in the evaluation of the pelvic supports and other pelvic pathology. Neuro-logic deficits of S2–S4 can be evaluated by the anal wink reflex and by evaluating sensation over these dermatomes. A urine culture is obtained at the first visit. Demonstration of urine leakage on a Valsalva maneuver and a full bladder may be seen in the upright position if not seen in the supine position. A "Q-tip" test will document urethrovesical junction mobility. The urethra is hypermobile if change greater than 35° is noted. A Smith-Hodge pessary elevates the urethrovesical junction without occlusion of the urethra. Continence with the pessary in place suggests stress incontinence.

Additional Testing

Cystourethroscopy allows visualization of the bladder mucosa, urethra, urethrovesical junction function and mobility, and any abnormalities at the urethrovesical junction such as inflammation, fistula, diverticula, or foreign body. Urodynamic testing measures the relationship between bladder pressure, volume, and sensations. It is especially useful for demonstration of uninhibited detrusor contractions. Urodynamics may be performed using a single or multichannel system. Use of a multichannel system allows simultaneous recording of intravesical, intraurethral, and intraabdominal (intrarectal or intravaginal) pressures. The bladder may be filled with sterile water, saline, CO_2, urine, or dye solutions. The fill rate should be between 10 and 100 mL/minute, often in appropriately timed 50-mL increments.

Pressures are recorded at rest and then either continuously or every 50 mL. The volume and pressure at first urge (usually at 150 mL), urgent need, maximum pressure (500 mL), and bladder capacity (300–500 mL) are recorded. The normal intraurethral pressure is 15–20 cm H_2O and the normal intravesicular pressure is less than 5 cm H_2O. The presence and frequency of detrusor contractions are noted. The residual volume after the patient empties her bladder is recorded.

Uroflowmetry measures the average urine flow rate. The normal rate is more than 20 mL/second. Normal voiding is complete in 20 seconds. Abnormal rates indicate bladder neck obstruction.

Interpretation of Cystometrograms

An increase in intravesical pressure with cough or a Valsalva maneuver that is greater than intraurethral pressure and is not accompanied by a bladder contraction is diagnostic of stress incontinence. If simultaneous urethroscopy is performed, the urethrovesical junction may be seen to gape open. An uninhibited contraction that is greater than urethral pressure or greater than 15 cm H_2O is diagnostic of urge incontinence. A postvoid residual greater than 50 mL with a low-pressure bladder and a bladder capacity greater than 500 mL without urge to void is diagnostic of overflow incontinence.

ENDOMETRIOSIS

Endometriosis is the presence of endometrial glands and stroma in locations outside the uterine cavity. It is found in up to 15% of reproductive-age women and in up to 30% of infertile women. Risk factors for endometriosis are listed in Table 14.1.

Theories for the etiology of endometriosis include retrograde menstruation, vascular or lymphatic dissemination, coelomic metaplasia, immunologic defects, and genetic predisposition. There is experimental evidence to support all of these theories and it is probable that all play a role in some patients. Endometriosis implants may be found in the ovaries, uterosacral ligaments, posterior cul-de-sac, round and broad ligaments, fallopian tubes, rectosigmoid, bladder, and in extraperitoneal sites such as the cervix, vagina, vulva, incision sites, umbilicus, lung, and lymph nodes.

The gross appearance may be new blood-filled, red or blue-black lesions appearing raised or cystic. With time lesions become flatter and dark-brown. Large cystic structures may remain filled with old blood and are called chocolate cysts. Old lesions may appear as pale, scarred areas puckering local tissue. Lesions can range from small lesions of less than 1 mm to cysts of greater than 10 cm. The histologic appearance is of ectopic endometrial glands, ectopic endometrial stroma, hemorrhage into adjacent tissue, and

Table 14.1
Risk Factors for Endometriosis

1. Nulliparity
2. Age 25–40
3. Infertility
4. First-degree relative with endometriosis
5. Improved with prior pregnancy

sometimes hemosiderin. Biopsy examination of grossly evident endometriosis sometimes fails to reveal pathologic changes.

Symptoms

The patient may present with pelvic pain, especially secondary dysmenorrhea, infertility, dyspareunia, abnormal uterine bleeding, or rectal or urinary pain or bleeding associated with menses. Endometriosis symptoms are usually cyclic and vary with menses but may be constant. Many patients with endometriosis are asymptomatic, and there is little correlation between the degree of symptoms and the severity of the disease.

Signs

Physical signs of endometriosis include a fixed retroverted uterus, nodularity of uterosacral ligaments and posterior cul-de-sac, asymmetric adnexal masses, and tenderness on bimanual examination. None of these signs is diagnostic and the patient may not exhibit any physical signs. Visible lesions on speculum or external examination are highly suggestive of endometriosis and, if present, should be examined by biopsy.

Diagnostic Evaluation

Visualization of endometriosis is required to confirm the diagnosis. Laparoscopy to visualize lesions and take biopsy specimens is the usual method of diagnosis. The American Fertility Society has devised a classification scheme to aid in the standardization of endometriosis severity (Figures 14.1 and 14.2). A biopsy examination of external or vaginal lesions can occasionally confirm the diagnosis. Pelvic ultrasound examination may be helpful to evaluate masses and can suggest endometriomas. Cancer antigen 125 (CA-125) levels are elevated in many patients with endometriosis. Cystoscopy, intravenous pyelogram (IVP), proctoscopy, and barium enema may help to evaluate bladder or bowel involvement.

Treatment

Medical Therapies

Therapy of endometriosis depends on the patient's reproductive plans and the degree of her symptoms. Medical therapy is indicated for patients who wish to retain fertility or have mild symptoms. Hor-

**THE AMERICAN FERTILITY SOCIETY
REVISED CLASSIFICATION OF ENDOMETRIOSIS**

Patient's Name _____ Date_____

Stage I   (Minimal) - 1-5
Stage II   (Mild)   - 6-15   Laparoscopy_____ Laparotomy_____ Photography_____
Stage III (Moderate) - 16-40   Recommended Treatment_____
Stage IV   (Severe)   - >40   _____
Total_____   Prognosis_____

	ENDOMETRIOSIS	<1cm	1-3cm	>3cm
PERITONEUM	Superficial	1	2	4
	Deep	2	4	6
OVARY	R Superficial	1	2	4
	Deep	4	16	20
	L Superficial	1	2	4
	Deep	4	16	20
	POSTERIOR CULDESAC OBLITERATION	**Partial**		**Complete**
		4		40
	ADHESIONS	<1/3 Enclosure	1/3-2/3 Enclosure	>2/3 Enclosure
OVARY	R Filmy	1	2	4
	Dense	4	8	16
	L Filmy	1	2	4
	Dense	4	8	16
TUBE	R Filmy	1	2	4
	Dense	4*	8*	16
	L Filmy	1	2	4
	Dense	4*	8*	16

*If the fimbriated end of the fallopian tube is completely enclosed, change the point assignment to 16.

Additional Endometriosis: _____ | Associated Pathology: _____
_____ | _____
_____ | _____

To Be Used with Normal | To Be Used with Abnormal
Tubes and Ovaries | Tubes and/or Ovaries
L   R | L   R

Figure 14.1

monal therapy can consist of oral contraceptives taken continuously to produce months of amenorrhea (pseudopregnancy). This therapy is best for the relief of symptoms in mild cases. Pseudopregnancy leads to a decidual-like reaction and atrophy of the endometrial implants. Medroxyprogesterone acetate can also be used

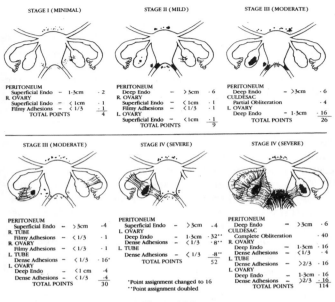

Figure 14.2

to create a pseudopregnancy, using 200 mg/month of a depot form.

GnRH analogues suppress the ovarian-pituitary axis and reduce levels of follicle-stimulating hormone (FSH), luteinizing hormone (LH), and estrogen, creating a pseudomenopause. GnRH analogues are useful in mild cases to treat infertility and provide relief of symptoms in many cases. The length of therapy is limited by the risk of osteoporosis. Therapy is usually limited to 6–9 months.

Danazol (Danocrine sulfate) is an androgen analogue that creates a pseudomenopause by acting on the hypothalamus to reduce GnRH release. Danazol is used for 6–9 months. Danazol has significant androgen side effects which may not be reversible. Its use has been largely supplanted by GnRH analogues.

Surgical Therapy

Conservative surgery can be accomplished by laparoscopy or laparotomy to remove cysts, lyse adhesions, and destroy implants by laser or electrocautery. The goal of conservative therapy is to restore fertility and relieve symptoms.

Extirpation therapy by hysterectomy and possible oophorectomy is the most effective for the relief of symptoms. Removal of any associated lesions is recommended. In rare cases, it may be necessary to remove sections of colon or bladder in order to remove all endometriosis implants.

ADENOMYOSIS

Adenomyosis is defined as the presence of endometrial glands and stroma within the myometrium of the uterus. Adenomyosis may be found in up to 60% of women.

Gross pathology shows enlargement of the uterus, either globally or focally. There is a spongy appearance with no cleavage plane. Histologically there is a direct extension of the basalis layer of endometrium into the myometrium. Adenomyosis may involve the uterus uniformly. Focal areas may have a pseudocapsule.

Secondary dysmenorrhea and menorrhagia are the most common symptoms. Dyspareunia may also occur. The majority of patients are asymptomatic.

Physical signs include an enlarged, tender uterus that is often 2–3 times the normal size. The uterus has a soft, "boggy" feel. The signs are often most evident just prior to and during menses.

Endometrial biopsy examination is used to rule out pathology for menorrhagia. Ultrasound examination may help to exclude leiomyoma. The diagnosis can only be confirmed by histologic evaluation of a hysterectomy specimen.

Trials of cyclic hormones and prostaglandin synthetase inhibitors may be helpful. However, the definitive treatment is by hysterectomy.

CHRONIC PELVIC PAIN

Chronic pelvic pain is defined as pain present for more than 6 months that interferes with daily functions and relationships. Diagnosis of the cause of pain is critical for successful management. Diagnosis begins with a careful history. The history of the present illness should include the duration, character, location, exacerbating or relieving factors, associated discomforts, severity, pain pattern, things that worsen or improve the pain, and whether the pain is incapacitating.

Past medical history of prior infections, treatments, surgeries, diagnostic procedures, diagnoses, other medical problems, as well as menstrual history, should be obtained. Psychological history of any prior diagnosis or treatments is important. In addition, the patient's current psychological status should be determined. A Beck Depression Inventory is a useful screen for depression (see Table 11.3).

Social history of family dynamics, financial status, job stress, children and spousal relationships, recent life or lifestyle changes, and sleep or diet changes may point to a cause or exacerbating factor. A sexual history is critical. The history should include any association of pain with intercourse, whether the patient is orgasmic, any prior counseling or therapy, any history of abuse or incest, inhibited desire, and frequency of intercourse. Marital or relationship distress may cause a patient to present with pain.

Every patient with chronic pelvic pain has an internal theory of the cause of her pain. All evaluations, therapies, and explanations of the pain will be filtered through this theory. In order for therapy to be successful, the patient's internal theory must be identified and addressed. The patient's theory may be correct. Often, if the physician listens to the patient, the patient will tell the physician what is wrong with her.

The patient's pain should not be minimized. Validation of the symptoms and sympathetic listening will often lead to the discussion of relationship issues or other stress factors and to amelioration of the pain. If the patient keeps a diary of her pain and associated symptoms or factors, then a pattern consistent with stress may emerge.

Examination

A general physical examination with abdominal examination directed toward point tenderness is the first step. Pelvic examination should include evaluation for external causes of superficial dyspareunia; evidence of pelvic relation; masses or tenderness of adnexa, uterus, or parametria; mobility, position, and size of the uterus; and evidence of infection such as discharge or cervicitis. Chlamydia and gonorrhea cultures, Pap smear, and stool guaiac are obtained at the initial exam.

Laboratory work may include a complete blood count, urinalysis with culture, β-hCG test (beta human chorionic go-nadotropin) if indicated by history, and a VDRL. An ultrasound examination may be helpful to confirm pelvic masses.

Possible etiologies for chronic pain may be gynecologic or nongynecologic. Gynecologic etiologies include pelvic inflammatory disease, pelvic adhesions, endometriosis, pelvic relaxation, adenomyosis, chronic ectopic or ovarian cystic growth or bleeding, or leiomyoma. Urinary causes include cystitis, bladder spasm, calculi, or tumors. Gastrointestinal (GI) causes include constipation, irritable bowel syndrome, inflammatory problems such as Crohn's disease, appendicitis, diverticulitis, and ulcerative colitis.

Psychological problems may present with chronic pelvic pain. Depression may present with somatization. Stress may lead to chronic GI upset. Musculoskeletal and neurologic causes of pain include pudendal neuralgia, myofascial pain, herpes zoster (shingles), and nerve root compression.

Systemic illnesses that can cause pelvic pain include hyperparathyroidism, acute intermittent porphyria, and mesenteric lymphadenitis.

Diagnostic Procedures

Pelvic ultrasonographic examination is useful to evaluate for masses. A hysterosalpingography study can demonstrate hydrosalpinx and tubal occlusions and may show tubal adhesions. Laparoscopy can help to evaluate for pelvic pathology and may provide tubal patency information. It can also allow for treatment attempts by laser or cautery of endometriosis, lysis of adhesions, aspiration of cysts, uterosacral nerve ablation, and myomectomy or oophorectomy if such procedures are indicated.

Psychiatric evaluation for depression is critical. Chronic pelvic pain is often a somatic manifestation of depression. A history of sexual abuse is often found in women with chronic pain when no organic etiology is found.

Colonoscopy or barium enema may be useful to diagnose irritable bowel syndrome or colitis. Urologic studies such as cystoscopy and intravenous pyelography are useful to confirm a suspicion of urethritis, urolithiasis, or interstitial cystitis.

Treatment

The treatment is started by performing studies as indicated by history and examination and having the patient keep a diary of pain and associated events. Validation of the pain and reassurance of normal findings can be therapeutic.

Medical therapy should be based on a suspected etiology. Nonsteroidal antiinflammatory drugs (NSAIDs) are useful for dysmenorrhea and mittelschmerz, and may be useful if the diagnosis is uncertain. Narcotics should be avoided for chronic use as the potential for dependence is high. Oral contraceptives are useful for mittelschmerz and dysmenorrhea. Tricyclic antidepressants are useful for depression but also are useful in the treatment of chronic pain that appears to be due to neuropathy. Tricyclics may also be of use in pain of uncertain etiology. The mechanism of action may be a direct effect on peripheral nerves.

Laparoscopy is indicated if other studies do not indicate a source of pain or if the history and physical examination are suggestive of gynecologic pathology. Tubal insufflation, lysis of adhesions, and laser or cautery ablation of endometriosis will often relieve pain if indicated.

If a normal pelvis is found at laparoscopy, continue NSAIDs or other therapy and offer counseling. Studies have shown that nondirected group therapy is the most effective approach to chronic pain in women who do not have an organic etiology documented. Counseling as indicated for family dynamics, sex therapy, depression, and stress management is also useful.

If all other therapy fails, a total abdominal hysterectomy and bilateral salpingo-oophorectomy (TAH/BSO) may be performed. Approximately 10% of all hysterectomies are performed for chronic pelvic pain. The recurrence rate of chronic pain may be 50% if no pathology is found.

PREMENSTRUAL SYNDROME

Premenstrual syndrome (PMS) is a group of symptoms that occur during the luteal phase of the menstrual cycle. The symptoms are relieved with the onset of menses or within 2–3 days of menses. There should be a symptom-free period of at least one week during the follicular phase. Symptoms often interfere with work and relationships. Symptoms should be present for 3 months. A severe form of PMS is classified by DSM-IV as a late luteal phase dysphoric disorder.

Up to 40% of reproductive-age women have PMS. Two to three percent of women have severe symptoms. The peak age of onset is in the mid-30s but PMS can occur anytime during the reproductive years.

Some symptoms of PMS are listed in Table 14.2. This list is not exhaustive, as patients may report other symptoms, but is useful to suggest some of the symptoms that the patient may have.

Pathophysiological Theories

There are many theories of the etiology of PMS, and there is no universally accepted theory of its etiology or pathophysiology. Increased estrogen has been proposed to be the cause. The fact that PMS symptoms are least during the follicular phase when estrogen effects are greatest, however, weakens this theory. A deficiency of vitamin B_6 has been proposed, and many patients with PMS are treated with vitamin B_6. Studies of other signs of vitamin

Table 14.2
Symptoms of Premenstrual Syndrome

Physical	
abdominal bloating	change in bowels
breast tenderness	acne
headache	backache
leg cramps/swelling	crave sweets/salt
pelvic pain	palpitations
incoordination	sensitivity to noise/light
increased appetite	rash/itching
nasal congestion	hot flash
Emotional	
depression	hostility
anxiety	anger
inability to cope	paranoia
fatigue	change in sex drive
tearfulness	poor concentration
aggression/violence	insecurity
forgetfulness	suicidal thoughts
insomnia	desire to be alone
tension	guilt feelings
irritability	weakness

B_6 deficiency, however, have not supported this hypothesis. Elevated prolactin and hypoglycemia, fluid retention, and thyroid deficiency have all been considered but not confirmed. Prostaglandin abnormalities may be responsible for some physical symptoms, and double-blind studies have shown NSAIDs to be more effective than placebo for the treatment of PMS. Endorphin withdrawal has been proposed as an etiology and remains a viable theory. Progesterone deficiency was an early theory that is no longer accepted, as double-blind studies have shown that progesterone is no more effective than placebo for the treatment of PMS. Although the specific etiology remains unclear, PMS appears to be a multifactorial psychoendocrine disorder.

Evaluation Methods

Patient History

The diagnosis of PMS can be suggested by a retrospective history but MUST be confirmed by a prospectively kept symptom diary. A typical symptom calendar is shown in Figure 14.3. Personality and psychological testing such as MMPI, Beck Depression Inventory, Hamilton Depression scale, or Zung's anxiety scale, may be useful to differentiate PMS from depression or chronic anxiety.

Therapy

Therapy for PMS falls into three categories. Symptomatic therapies are designed to relieve symptoms. Specific therapies are designed to treat a specific proposed etiology of PMS. Ablative therapies treat PMS by stopping menstruation.

Education about premenstrual syndrome is a key component of any therapy. Validation of symptoms and reassurance that the patient has a treatable condition are themselves therapeutic. Dietary therapy consists of small meals high in protein, vitamins, and complex carbohydrates that are low in fat and refined sugars. Alcohol, tobacco, and caffeine are to be avoided. Salt intake is limited. Vitamin B_6 supplements may be taken. Exercise consisting of 30 minutes of daily aerobics may increase endorphins. Stress management in the form of counseling or psychotherapy is designed to supplement other treatment. Psychotherapy may be individual or include support groups.

PNS CLINIC

MENSTRUAL SYMPTOMS DAILY LOG

CHART NO. _____

GRADING OF MENSES		GRADING OF SYMPTOMS (COMPLAINTS)
0-none 1-slight 2-moderate 3-heavy 4-heavy and clots		0-none 1-minimum 2-mild 3-moderate 4-severe 5-extreme

Cycle Day (indicate menses days)	1	2	3	4	5	6	7	8	9	10	11	12	13	14	15	16	17	18	19	20	21	22	23	24	25	26	27	28	29	30	31	32	33	34	35
Date																																			
Menses																																			
Basal Weight in lbs.																																			
Basal Body Temperature																																			
Restlessness																																			
Mood Swings																																			
Irritability																																			
Anxiety																																			
Headaches																																			
Sweets craving (caffeinated drinks or other foods)																																			
↑ or ↓ Appetite																																			
Fatigue																																			
Depression/ Sadness																																			
Forgetfulness																																			
Crying																																			
Confusion																																			
Insomnia																																			
Weight Gain																																			
Swelling of Extremities																																			
Breast Tenderness/ Pain																																			
Abdominal Bloating																																			
Avoid Activities/ People																																			
Poor Coordination More Accidents																																			
Angry																																			
Changed Sexual Desire ↑ or ↓																																			
Suicidal Feelings																																			
Increased Energy or Well-being																																			
Abdominal Cramps/Pain																																			
Pain in Muscles/ joints/Back																																			
Other (add your own comments)																																			

Figure 14.3

Therapies directed toward symptoms include diuretics (potassium sparing) for bloating, antidepressants and anxiolytics for mood swings and depression, bromocriptine for breast tenderness, and antiprostaglandins for breast tenderness, joint pain, and musculoskeletal pain.

Therapies directed toward specific proposed etiologies include natural progesterone to treat progesterone deficiency, although progesterone therapy has been shown to be no more effective than placebo. Vitamin B_6, a cofactor for serotonin, is proposed to treat serotonin deficiency.

Ablative therapies to stop menstruation include GnRH analogues, danazol, and progestins such as depot-medroxyprogesterone acetate. Cessation of menses is often effective, but all available methods have side effects. Oophorectomy is effective, but should only be considered if the patient has disabling symptoms not relieved by conservative therapy, has relief on GnRH analogues with recurrence of symptoms when GnRH analogues are discontinued, does not desire further fertility, and has at least 10 years of menstruation remaining. Hysterectomy without oophorectomy is ineffective.

Suggested Readings

American College of Obstetricians and Gynecologists. Chronic pelvic pain. Technical Bulletin 129. Washington, DC: ACOG, 1989.

American College of Obstetricians and Gynecologists. Endometriosis. Technical Bulletin 184. Washington, DC: ACOG, 1993.

American College of Obstetricians and Gynecologists. Precis V, pp. 230–245. Washington, DC: ACOG, 1994.

American College of Obstetricians and Gynecologists. Premenstrual syndrome. Committee Opinion 155. Washington, DC: ACOG, 1995.

American College of Obstetricians and Gynecologists. Urinary incontinence. Technical Bulletin 100. Washington, DC: ACOG, 1987.

American College of Obstetricians and Gynecologists. Uterine leiomyomata. Technical Bulletin 192. Washington, DC: ACOG, 1994.

Baden WF, Walker T. Surgical repair of vaginal defects. Philadelphia: JB Lippincott, 1992.

Barbieri RL. Etiology and epidemiology of endometriosis. Am J Obstet Gynecol 1990;162:565–567.

Buttram VC Jr, Reiter RC. Uterine leiomyomata: etiology, symptomatology, and management. Fertil Steril 1981;36:433–445.

Nichols DH, ed. Gynecologic and obstetric surgery. St. Louis: Mosby-Year Book, 1993.

U.S. Public Health Service. Urinary Incontinence Guideline Panel. Urinary incontinence in adults: clinical practice guidelines. Rockville, MD: Agency for Health Care Policy and Research, 1992.

Vollenhoven BJ, Lawrence AS, Healy DL. Uterine fibroids: a clinical review. Br J Obstet Gynaecol 1990;97:285–298.

Chapter 15

Common Postoperative Complications

ACUTE RENAL FAILURE

Acute renal failure is characterized by low urine output. Oliguria is a symptom, not a diagnosis, and it is critical to determine its cause prior to any therapeutic maneuvers. Prerenal oliguria is secondary to hypoperfusion of the kidneys. Causes include hypovolemia, pump failure (low cardiac output), and hypotension secondary to vasodilation. The treatment of prerenal oliguria is to identify the cause of renal hypoperfusion and to correct it—volume expansion or correction of pump failure.

Renal oliguria is caused by an acute decrease in glomerular filtration rate (GFR). There are several theories as to the cause of a decrease in GFR. The "back leak" theory is that the GFR remains normal but glomerular filtrate is reabsorbed secondary to the damage of tubular necrosis. This theory is supported by observations of tubular necrosis in acute renal failure. However, experiments utilizing single nephron canalization show a greater decrease in GFR and not an increase in glomerular filtrate reabsorption. The "tubular obstruction" theory is that debris and interstitial edema obstruct tubules. This theory is supported by the fact that early intervention with fluid or diuretics tends to correct acute renal failure. The "vascular" theory is that preglomerular vasoconstriction decreases GFR. Since most glomeruli are in the cortex, all blood may go through the medulla. However, the observed lack of efficacy of vasodilators in acute renal failure weakens this theory. Probably all three processes play some role in the pathophysiology of acute renal failure. The acute decrease in GFR leads to oliguria, azotemia, and electrolyte imbalances.

Postrenal oliguria is caused by obstruction. An obstructed catheter is a common cause. Obstruction of the urethra by surgical trauma, edema, or a pelvic mass or hematoma can cause a low urine output. Ureteral obstruction is a rare cause of oliguria and must be bilateral in order to cause oliguria or anuria.

The diagnosis of acute renal failure is made by exclusion of other causes and by studying the urinary findings, which are summarized in Table 15.1. It is critical to measure the urinary electrolytes prior to the administration of diuretics. Diuretics change the kidney's ability to retain sodium and can cause an iatrogenically high fractional excretion of sodium. If the kidney is functioning normally and is being hypoperfused, it will retain sodium and the urinary sodium and fractional excretion of sodium will be low.

Fluid restriction is important in the management of acute renal failure. Normally, fluid is restricted to 1 liter per day. Alternatively, fluid may be restricted to replacing insensible loss (500–750 mL/day) plus the daily urine output. Electrolyte management is to restrict potassium and sodium. Frequent determinations of urinary and serum electrolytes may be helpful.

Dialysis is indicated for uremic symptoms, hyperkalemia, or fluid overload. Controversy exists over the role of "prophylactic" dialysis. Some authorities recommend dialysis on a scheduled basis while others think that dialysis should only be done when indicated.

DEEP VEIN THROMBOSIS

Management of deep vein thrombosis depends on accurate diagnosis. Ascending venography is the most accurate test for diagnosis, but it is suboptimal in examining deep femoral and pelvic veins because they may be difficult to visualize. Doppler ul-

Table 15.1
Urinary Findings in Acute Renal Failure (ARF)

Urine Findings	Prerenal	ARF
Urine osmolality	> 500	< 400
Urine sodium	< 20	> 40
Urine/plasma creatinine	> 40	< 20
"Renal failure index"	< 1	> 2
Fractional excretion sodium	< 1	> 2

"Renal failure index" = (urinary Na/plasma Na)/(urinary creatinine/plasma creatinine) × 100.

trasound scanning is another modality that can be used to detect deep venous thrombosis. Normally, venous flow varies with respiration, Valsalva maneuver, squeezing muscles, and release of pressure over a distal vein. These changes can be detected by Doppler ultrasound shifts. Lack of Doppler shift indicates occlusion of the vein distally and is indicative of a deep venous thrombosis. This technique works best on calf veins and is suboptimal for femoral and pelvic veins.

Impedance plethysmography is a technique that measures the changes in electrical resistance to reflect blood volume in a limb. With inflation of a thigh cuff, blood is retained in the leg. In the absence of venous occlusion, deflation of the cuff results in blood outflow and a concomitant increase in electrical resistance. With venous occlusion, change in electrical resistance is much slower and indicates occlusion of the vein and deep venous thrombosis.

Iodine-125 (^{125}I) scanning is a very sensitive and specific test for deep venous thrombosis. ^{125}I is incorporated into developing thrombi, and sequential scans at 24, 48, and 72 hours show incorporation of ^{125}I into the thrombus. The major drawback of this technique is that it takes up to three days to establish the diagnosis, and the test depends on continuing thrombus formation.

Management of Deep Vein Thrombosis

Anticoagulation therapy is the primary management strategy. Heparin is usually the initial drug therapy. Heparin binds to antithrombin III. It facilitates neutralization of thrombin and factors XIIa, IXa, Xa, XIa. Small amounts of heparin can inhibit the initial clotting cascade. After a thrombus is formed, large amounts of heparin are needed to neutralize the larger amounts of already formed thrombin. The dose needed may vary with thrombin production, so it is essential to monitor the patient's response to the drug. The goal is to keep the aPTT (activated partial thromboplastin time) at 1.5–2.5 times the normal value. Typical doses of heparin are 10,000 units initially followed by 5,000–10,000 units every 4–6 hours intravenously, either undiluted or diluted in 50 mL isotonic saline. Heparin may be given by continuous infusion with an initial dose of 5,000 units followed by 20,000–40,000 units in 1,000 mL isotonic saline for daily infusion.

Warfarin inhibits regeneration of vitamin K and prevents activation of factors II, IV, IX, X, and protein C. Because warfarin crosses the placenta, it is contraindicated in pregnancy. Warfarin is secreted in breast milk in an inactive form and breast-fed infants whose mothers take warfarin show no change in PT (prothrombin time) or clotting abnormalities.

The dosage of warfarin should be adjusted by monitoring the patient's PT to keep it 1.5–2.5 times the control value. Typical starting doses of warfarin are 2–5 mg/day and daily doses may range from 2–15 mg/day. Warfarin is typically given for 6 weeks following deep vein thrombosis.

PULMONARY EMBOLISM

The diagnosis of pulmonary embolism (PE) can be very challenging. There are a variety of available tests that may be helpful. Arterial blood gases (ABG) are often drawn. Although PE is unlikely with a pO_2 greater than 85 mm Hg, it is not excluded. In one study, 14% of 43 patients with angiographically proven PE had a pO_2 greater than 85 mm Hg.

The chest x-ray is normal in 30% of patients with PE. Hemidiaphragm elevation (Hampton's hump), atelectasis, and pleural effusion are suggestive of PE. Focal oligemia occurs in 2% of cases. A chest x-ray is most useful to exclude other causes of hypoxemia and chest pain such as pneumonia.

The electrocardiogram typically shows tachycardia. Acute cor pulmonale is uncommon and is only seen with massive emboli. Right axis shift with $S_1 Q_3 T_3$ pattern and T wave inversion are often seen. The ECG is also useful to exclude other causes of chest pain such as myocardial infarction.

Swan-Ganz catheterization may show signs suggestive of PE. Pulmonary embolism is not an indication for Swan-Ganz catheterization, but the patient may receive a catheter as part of the evaluation process. Failure to wedge can indicate complete distal occlusion of a pulmonary artery and indicate PE. Failure to wedge with pulmonary hypertension warrants further investigation such as pulmonary angiogram. Once the Swan-Ganz catheter is in place, angiogram is relatively simple.

A lung scan is a very useful test in the diagnosis of pulmonary embolism. Any patient with a suspected PE should have a ventilation-perfusion ($\dot{V}$-$\dot{Q}$) scan of the lung. A $\dot{V}$-$\dot{Q}$ scan has several possible results. It may be returned as normal, or as indicating low, intermediate, or high probability of pulmonary embolism.

Pulmonary angiogram is the most specific and sensitive test

for pulmonary embolism. However, the test carries significant risks. Morbidity is 4–5% and mortality is 0.2–0.3%. Indications for angiography include indeterminate lung scan, clinically unclear picture, or consideration of thrombolytic therapy or occlusion of vena cava.

Prospective Investigation of Pulmonary Embolism Diagnosis (PIOPED)

The PIOPED was a prospective multicenter study that was designed to evaluate methods of diagnosis for pulmonary embolism. In this study, 931 patients with suspected PE had a $\dot{V}$-$\dot{Q}$ scan performed; 755 of these also had an angiogram performed. The results of the study provide valuable guidance for the diagnosis of PE. The investigators compared the $\dot{V}$-$\dot{Q}$ scan with the pulmonary angiogram (Table 15.2), showing that a negative $\dot{V}$-$\dot{Q}$ scan was very unlikely to be associated with a pulmonary embolism. The scan had a high specificity if it showed high probability for pulmonary embolism, and a high sensitivity if it was not normal (Table 15.3). Other results did not have adequate sensitivity and specificity. Addition of clinical suspicion did not add to the accuracy of the lung scan.

In order to minimize the number of pulmonary angiograms that must be done, an algorithm to evaluate suspected pulmonary embolism has been suggested (Figure 15.1). The workup begins with a chest x-ray, ECG, and arterial blood gases. If after these tests a pulmonary embolism is still suspected, a $\dot{V}$-$\dot{Q}$ scan is performed. The workup then depends on the result of the scan. If the $\dot{V}$-$\dot{Q}$ scan is normal, the chance of a significant pulmonary embolism is low enough not to justify an angiogram or anticoag-

Table 15.2
Comparison of Scan and Angiogram in Diagnosis of Pulmonary Embolism

Scan	Angiogram			No Angiogram
	PE+	PE−	+/−	
High probability	102	14	1	7
Intermediate probability	105	217	9	33
Low probability	39	199	12	62
Normal	5	50	2	74

Table 15.3
Sensitivity and Specificity of Ventilation-Perfusion Scan

Scan	Sensitivity	Specificity
High	41%	97%
High or intermediate	82%	52%
Not normal	98%	10%

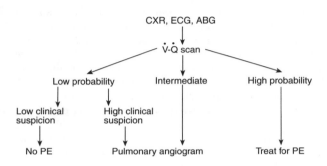

Figure 15.1.   Algorithm for suspected PE.

ulation therapy. If the scan shows a high probability for PE, the
likelihood of pulmonary embolism is high enough to justify anticoagulation therapy without an angiogram. Scans indicating intermediate probability are not predictive enough to form a basis
for therapeutic decisions, and an angiogram is indicated. If the
scan shows low probability and the clinical suspicion of pulmonary embolism is low, no therapy is needed. If the clinical suspicion of pulmonary embolism remains high, then an angiogram
should be performed to confirm the diagnosis.

The initial management of pulmonary embolism is anticoagulation therapy to prevent further thrombus formation and additional emboli. Anticoagulation therapy should be instituted as
described above for deep vein thrombosis.

Thrombolytic therapy may be considered in selected patients. Indications for thrombolytic therapy are obstruction to a
lobe or multiple segments of the lung, or a hemodynamically
compromised patient.

Regimens for thrombolytic therapy include streptokinase,

urokinase, and alteplase (rtPA). Streptokinase is given as 250,000 IU over 30 minutes, then 100,000 IU/hour for 24 hours. Urokinase is given as 4,400 IU/kg (2,000 IU/lb/hour) over 10 minutes, then 4,400 IU/kg/hour (2,000 IU/lb/hour) for 12–14 hours. rtPA is given as 100 mg over 2 hours.

POSTOPERATIVE FEVER

Postoperative fever is usually defined as a temperature of 38°C (100.4°F) or greater on two or more occasions 6 or more hours apart, or a single temperature of 38.5°C (101.3°F) in the postoperative period. Postoperative fever is a sign and not a diagnosis. It can indicate the presence of a serious complication.

Differential Diagnosis

Pneumonia is more common in women who have had a general anesthetic. Other risk factors include extensive abdominal incisions, preexisting restrictive or obstructive lung disease, and preoperative upper respiratory infections. Atelectasis is a consolidation of a lobe or segment and commonly follows a general anesthetic. Atelectasis rarely if ever causes fever in the absence of pneumonia. Pneumonia is usually due to Gram-positive aerobes or Mycoplasmata unless aspiration has occurred, in which case Gram-negative aerobes and anaerobes may be found.

Wound infections may occur in an abdominal wound or vaginal wound (cuff cellulitis). Abdominal wound infections usually result from Gram-positive aerobes from the skin. Obesity, excessive electrocautery use, poor hemostasis, long operative times, immunosuppression, and peripheral vascular disease increase the risk of abdominal wound infection. Vaginal wound infections usually result from vaginal flora and are mixed infections of aerobes and anaerobes. Long procedures, the presence of bacterial vaginosis, and accumulation of blood at the cuff increase the risk of infection. The use of prophylactic antibiotics and the use of vaginal cuff drains reduce the risk of vaginal wound infections.

Intraabdominal infections are usually polymicrobial with a mixed aerobic and anaerobic flora. Bowel injury, long procedures, immunosuppression, and the presence of pelvic inflammatory disease or tubo-ovarian abscesses increase the risk of intraabdominal infection.

Urinary tract infections are associated with catheterization of the urinary bladder and with general anesthesia. They are usually due to Gram-negative aerobes.

Phlebitis is another possible cause of fever, and drug reactions, factitious fevers, and charting errors are less common causes of fever.

Evaluation of Postoperative Fever

The evaluation should begin with a review of the preoperative course, searching for underlying medical conditions placing the patient at increased risk for infection, and proceed with a review of the surgical procedure. The length and type of surgery, and any complications of surgery, should be reviewed. Then the postoperative period should be reviewed for symptoms and signs. Cough, chest pain, or dyspnea can indicate pneumonia. Wound tenderness, erythema, or discharge suggest wound infection. Vaginal discharge or bleeding may indicate a cuff cellulitis or cuff abscess. Lower abdominal pain and ileus are signs of an intraabdominal infection. Dysuria or hematuria are signs of a urinary tract infection. Calf tenderness may indicate phlebitis.

Physical examination is directed toward known causes of fever. Examination of the lungs for bilateral expansion, rales, rhonchi, or rubs is indicated. Any wounds are examined for erythema, induration, or purulent discharge. The abdomen should be examined for tenderness, masses, and bowel sounds. Any drains must be inspected for the character of the drainage. The legs should be inspected for signs of phlebitis. A pelvic and rectal examination to search for masses and cuff cellulitis is performed last.

Laboratory evaluation is directed by the history and physical examination. A complete blood count, urinalysis, urine culture, and blood culture are usually indicated. Chest x-ray is indicated if the history and physical examination indicate a pulmonary problem. Pelvic or abdominal ultrasound scanning can confirm the presence of a cuff or intraabdominal abscess. Abdominal x-rays may show an ileus or a retained sponge or instrument. Air may be retained in the abdomen for several days after abdominal surgery and may not represent perforation of a viscus.

After the initial history, physical examination, and laboratory evaluation, a presumptive diagnosis and plan must be recorded in the chart. Antibiotic therapy is begun on the basis of the presumptive diagnosis. Regimens for antibiotic therapy are shown in Table 15.4.

Table 15.4
Antibiotic Regimens for Postoperative Infections

Type of Infection	Recommended Regimen	Treatment Failures	Penicillin Allergy
Urinary tract infection	First-generation cephalosporin	Based on culture: gentamicin, fluoroquinolones, others	Cephalosporins
Pneumonia	Ampicillin	Ceftriaxone or other third-generation cephalosporin	Ceftriaxone or other third-generation cephalosporin
Pelvic cellulitis	Extended spectrum penicillin or cephalosporin	Clindamycin/gentamicin	Clindamycin/gentamicin
Pelvic abscess	Clindamycin/gentamicin	Surgical drainage	Clindamycin/gentamicin
Wound infection	Extended spectrum penicillin or cephalosporin	Wound debridement	Clindamycin/gentamicin

Antibiotic therapy is continued until the patient is afebrile for 24 to 48 hours. Antibiotic therapy should be administered for 48 to 72 hours before consideration is given of treatment failure unless the patient shows signs of acute clinical deterioration.

POSTOPERATIVE ANEMIA

Postoperative anemia is a common problem. Most surgical procedures are associated with some blood loss, and significant anemia occurs after 0.3–3% of gynecologic procedures. It is critical to determine whether anemia is due to blood loss from surgery or due to ongoing postoperative bleeding. The degree of anemia can be correlated to the drop in hematocrit or hemoglobin levels. Each 500 mL blood loss accounts for approximately a 3% change in the hematocrit level or a drop in hemoglobin of 1 g/dL. Changes in hemoglobin or hematocrit out of proportion to estimated blood loss at surgery may indicate ongoing, hidden blood loss.

Intraperitoneal bleeding that occurs in the first 24 hours is associated with clinical signs of bleeding. It is characterized by drops in blood counts, tachycardia, and abdominal distension. Patients with intraperitoneal bleeding diagnosed in the first 24 hours should usually have reexploration of the abdomen and ligation of the involved vessel. In some cases, interventional radiology may be able to locate the vessel by angiography and occlude the vessel by injection, thus avoiding the need for surgery. Patients who have external bleeding from vaginal or abdominal incisions should be taken to the surgery suite and the vessel isolated and ligated. Delayed intraperitoneal bleeding (more than 24 hours) can be often be managed expectantly. Interventional radiology is also a useful alternative, depending on the degree of blood loss and anemia.

Although it is common practice to check a blood count on the first postoperative day, hemoconcentration in the immediate postoperative period may lead to underestimation of the blood loss. Careful observation of vital signs is the best way to determine excessive blood loss. Patients who have significant blood loss will have tachycardia and postural hypotension. Patients with asymptomatic anemia rarely need transfusion.

Transfusions are indicated for symptomatic anemia. Patients with orthostatic symptoms, including hypotension, tachycardia, and headache, may be transfused with packed red blood cells.

Restoration to a hemoglobin level of 10 g/dL or a hematocrit level of 30% is adequate.

Suggested Readings

Bakiri F, Bendib SE, Maoui R, Bendib A, Benmiloud M. The sella turcica in Sheehan's syndrome: computerized tomographic study in 54 patients. J Endocrinol Invest 1991;14(3):193–196.

Goldhaber SZ. Evolving concepts in thrombolytic therapy for pulmonary embolism. Chest 1992;101(4 Suppl):183S–185S.

Goldhaber SZ. Recent advances in the diagnosis and lytic therapy of pulmonary embolism. Chest 1991;99(4 Suppl):173S–179S.

Goldman MH, Sfedu E, Aboul-Hosn H, Nutt R. Addison's disease presenting in the postpartum state. J Med Soc NJ 1983;80(12):1030–1031.

Hayt DB, Binkert BL. An overview of noninvasive methods of deep vein thrombosis detection. Clin Imaging 1990;14(3):179–197.

Koerner S. Diagnosis and treatment of pulmonary embolism. Cardiol Clin 1991;9(4):761–772.

Lancaster LE. Renal response to shock. Crit Care Nurs Clin North Am 1990;2(2):221–233.

Palevsky HI, Alavi A. A noninvasive strategy for the management of patients suspected of pulmonary embolism. Semin Nucl Med 1991; 21(4):325–331.

Persson AV, Davis RJ, Villavicencio JL. Deep venous thrombosis and pulmonary embolism. Surg Clin North Am 1991;71(6):1195–1209.

The PIOPED Investigators. Value of the ventilation/perfusion scan in acute pulmonary embolism. Results of the Prospective Investigation of Pulmonary Embolism Diagnosis (PIOPED). JAMA 1990 263(20):2753–2759.

Putterman C, Almog Y, Caraco Y, Gross DJ, Ben-Chetrit E. Inappropriate secretion of antidiuretic hormone in Sheehan's syndrome: a rare cause of postpartum hyponatremia. Am J Obstet Gynecol 1991;165:1330–1333.

Rutherford SE, Phelan JP. Deep venous thrombosis and pulmonary embolism in pregnancy. Obstet Gynecol Clin North Am 1991;18(2):345–370.

Sipes SL, Weiner CP. Venous thromboembolic disease in pregnancy. Semin Perinatol 1990;14(2):103–118.

Vaughn TC, Wiebe RH, Hammond CB. Postpartum hypopituitarism and hyperprolactinemia. Am J Obstet Gynecol 1980;137(6):749–751.

Chapter 16

Normal and Abnormal Menses

MENSTRUAL PHYSIOLOGY

Divisions of the Human Menstrual Cycle

The Follicular Phase

The follicular phase begins after menstruation. Initially there is an increase in follicle-stimulating hormone (FSH), which stimulates the growth and maturation of follicles, and a transition from a low to a high luteinizing hormone (LH) pulse frequency. The synthesis and release of LH and FSH are regulated by luteinizing hormone releasing hormone (LH-RH). LH-RH is synthesized in neurons in the hypothalamus, released into the hypophysial portal vessels, and transported by axoplasmic flow to the anterior pituitary gland. Recruitment of follicles occurs during the first 4 to 5 days of the follicular phase, and on days 5 to 7 there is a selection of a dominant follicle. The remaining follicles in the cohort may undergo additional limited growth but will ultimately become atretic. The maturation of a dominant follicle occurs between days 8 and 12. The dominant follicle reaches a mean diameter of 20 mm several days before the LH surge.

The follicle contains theca cells and granulosa cells. Theca cells have LH receptors and respond to LH stimulation by the production of androgens, primarily androstenedione and testosterone. Granulosa cells, which are located inside the follicle, are primarily producers of estrogens.

Ovulatory Phase

Ovulation most often occurs between days 13 and 15. The ovulatory phase begins 2 to 3 days prior to the mid-cycle surge of LH when there is an increase in 17β-estradiol that parallels small increases in progesterone, 17α-hydroxyprogesterone, and inhibin. The increase in progesterone reflects the process of luteinization of granulosa cells following acquisition of LH receptors and the resulting ability of LH to initiate biosynthesis of progesterone and 17α-hydroxyprogesterone. LH and FSH surges begin abruptly and are temporally associated with peak 17β-estradiol levels and the initiation of a rapid rise in progesterone 12 hours earlier. The duration of the LH surge is in the range of 48 hours. Ovulation occurs about 36 hours after the onset of the LH surge.

Luteal Phase

Luteinization (the conversion of granulosa and theca cells to luteal cells with the acquisition of LH receptors) follows ovulation. After luteinization, luteal cells synthesize and secrete large amounts of progesterone and to a lesser extent, estrogens. Following ovulation, there is an increase in the basal body temperature by 0.5–1.0°F. The progesterone metabolite pregnanediol has a thermogenic effect and alters the setting of the thermoregulatory center in the brain. At the time of peak progesterone secretion, there is a 3-day window during which the endometrium is most conducive to implantation. Unless implantation is initiated, luteolysis (death of the corpus luteum) occurs. The corpus luteum needs appropriate LH support (or that of human chorionic gonadotropin (hCG), if pregnancy is established) to continue the secretion of progesterone. Levels of FSH are lowest during the luteal phase, which is due to the combined actions of inhibin and estrogen (acting synergistically with progesterone), which prevents the initiation of folliculogenesis.

Menstrual Phase

As progesterone and inhibin levels fall, there is a rise in FSH levels, which occurs 2 days before the onset of menses. Follicular recruitment for the ensuing cycle is initiated during this time. The process of menstruation is due to declining levels of progesterone and, to a lesser extent, estrogen.

Uterine Changes during the Menstrual Cycle

The uterus is composed of two basic layers; the outer, thick, muscular myometrium, and the inner, thin, glandular tissue, the endometrium. The endometrium responds to estrogen by undergoing rapid mitotic divisions and formation of glandular structures (proliferative endometrium). After ovulation, the corpus luteum produces significant amounts of progesterone, which acts on the endometrium to increase the size of the endometrial glands and to promote the synthesis and secretion of proteins and other factors (secretory endometrium) in preparation for pregnancy and implantation. The secretory endometrium is maintained by the secretion of estrogen and progesterone by the ovary. The decrease in the peripheral levels of these steroids causes degeneration and necrosis of the secretory endometrium, and menses occurs.

Cervical Changes during the Menstrual Cycle

In the follicular phase there is secretion of cervical mucus by the sebaceous glands in the endocervix due to the effect of estrogen. During estrogen dominance, there is an abundant secretion of cervical mucus that has a characteristic "watery" appearance. The elasticity of the cervical mucus is directly dependent upon the presence of estrogen and the absence of progesterone. The measurement of elasticity is referred to as the "spinnbarkeit." Under estrogen dominance, cervical mucus contains a large amount of NaCl, and when a sample of mucus is dried it leaves a distinct "ferning pattern."

When progesterone becomes the dominant hormone, the cervical mucus becomes thick and the ferning pattern disappears. Under progesterone dominance, sperm penetration of the cervical mucus is inhibited (hostile mucus).

Vaginal Changes during the Menstrual Cycle

With a high estrogen background, there is a large amount of glycogen stored in the vaginal epithelium. Substantial changes in vaginal exfoliative cytology occur in different stages of the menstrual cycle, which is a reflection of changing hormone patterns. Under estrogen dominance, superficial cells are predominantly exfoliative. Under progesterone dominance, more intermediate cells are exfoliated.

The Process of Menstruation

Menstruation is always preceded by vasoconstriction of the spiral arteries at the base of the endometrium. This constriction results in endometrial necrosis and damage to the endothelium of the endometrial blood vessels, so that when the arterioles relax, hemorrhage ensues. It is now known that this hemorrhage is due to the release of several local vasodilators, including histamine, bradykinin, prostacyclin, and other prostaglandins.

AMENORRHEA

Primary amenorrhea is defined as the absence of menarche by age 14 with the absence of growth or development of secondary sexual characteristics, or the absence of menarche by age 16 regardless of the presence of normal growth and development and the appearance of secondary sexual characteristics.

Secondary amenorrhea is defined as the absence of menses for a length of time equivalent at least to a total of three of the previous cycle intervals, or six months of amenorrhea in a woman who has been menstruating.

Evaluation of Amenorrhea

The first step in the evaluation of amenorrhea is a careful history, with particular emphasis on psychological dysfunction or emotional stress, family history of apparent genetic anomalies, discussion of nutritional habits and sexual activity. The second step is a physical examination. Abnormal growth and development should be assessed. Evaluation of secondary sex characteristics by the Tanner staging of genitalia and breasts, and any evidence of other endocrine disorders, such as galactorrhea or an enlarged thyroid gland, should be documented. The most important part of the initial physical examination is to document the presence of a normal reproductive tract. Figure 16.1 describes the workup if an abnormality of the uterus or vagina is found.

If no abnormalities are found, proceed to exclude pregnancy, measure thyroid-stimulating hormone (TSH) level and prolactin level, and perform a progestational challenge. If there is a positive withdraw bleed, and normal prolactin and TSH levels are found, then the diagnosis is anovulatory cycles. If the prolactin level is elevated, the diagnosis is hyperprolactinemia. If the TSH level is elevated, the diagnosis is hypothyroidism.

If the diagnosis is not established and no withdraw bleeding occurs, proceed to stimulate the endometrium with an estrogen and progestin cycle. Administer 2.5 mg conjugated estrogen daily for 21 days, with medroxyprogesterone acetate 10 mg daily for the last 5 days. If withdraw bleeding does not occur, then an end organ problem has been diagnosed. Asherman's syndrome

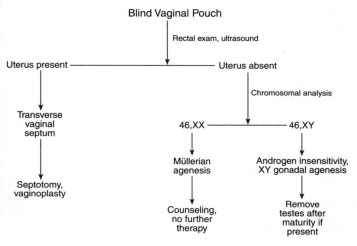

Figure 16.1. Workup of amenorrhea if an abnormality of the uterus or vagina is found.

is the most likely diagnosis and can be confirmed with hysteroscopy or hysterosalpingography.

If withdraw bleeding occurs after stimulation with both estrogen and progestin, proceed to a gonadotropin assay. If the FSH is elevated and the patient is over the age of 30, chromosomal analysis is indicated. If mosaicism with a Y chromosome is found, there is a 25% chance of malignant tumor formation of the ovary. If the gonadotropins are normal or low, proceed to a coronal CT scan to evaluate the sella turcica and suprasellar area for pituitary tumors.

Differential Diagnosis

Classification of Secondary Amenorrhea

Causes of amenorrhea can be divided into four compartments. Compartment I includes disorders of outflow tract or uterus. Compartment II includes disorders of the ovary. Compartment III includes disorders of the anterior pituitary, and compartment IV includes disorders of the central nervous system (hypothalamic factors). Causes of amenorrhea are listed in Table 16.1.

Iatrogenic amenorrhea is caused by surgical removal of

Table 16.1
Causes of Amenorrhea

Compartment I
  Pregnancy
  Intrauterine adhesions
  Disorders of sexual differentiation
    Distal genital tract obstruction
    Müllerian agenesis
  Surgical removal of uterus

Compartment II
  Menopause
  Surgical removal of gonads
  Irradiation of ovaries
  Chemotherapy
  Viral infections
  Chromosomal abnormalities
  Autoimmune disorders
  Enzymatic defects
  Idiopathic (premature ovarian failure)

Compartment III
  Isolated gonadotropin deficiency (Kallmann's syndrome)
  Hypopituitarism
  Hyperprolactinemia

Compartment IV
  Hypothalamic anovulation
    Anorexia nervosa
    Weight loss
    Exercise-associated
    Psychogenic
    Pseudocyesis
    Systemic illnesses
  Inappropriate peripheral feedback
    Functional androgen excess
    Androgen-producing neoplasm
    Liver disease
    Obesity
  Other endocrine disorders
    Thyroid dysfunction
    Adrenal disease

---

uterus, ovaries, or hypothalamus, or by the administration of medications. Estrogen and progestin may cause amenorrhea by effects on the uterus or hypothalamus. Antipsychotic drugs can alter dopamine function in the brain, causing increased prolactin and amenorrhea. Gonadotropin-releasing hormone analogues act on the pituitary to cause amenorrhea.

End organ causes of secondary amenorrhea (compartment I) include uterine adhesions (Asherman's syndrome), which usually is a result of surgical scarring from a dilation and curettage (D & C). Cervical stenosis can result from surgical trauma, infection, or malignancy.

Ovarian causes of secondary amenorrhea (compartment II) include gonadal dysgenesis with limited menstrual function, premature ovarian failure, and resistant ovaries syndrome. Ovarian causes lead to elevated gonadotropin levels associated with low estrogen levels (hypergonadotropic hypogonadism).

Pituitary lesions (compartment III) include destructive pituitary lesions, Sheehan's syndrome, and amenorrhea associated with increased prolactin secretion. Compartment III defects are characterized by low gonadotropin levels and low estrogen levels (hypogonadotropic hypogonadism). In these states, the pituitary will not respond to gonadotropin-releasing hormone (GnRH).

Hypothalamic dysfunctions (compartment IV) include amenorrhea associated with changes in weight, psychogenic amenorrhea, anorexia nervosa, pseudocyesis, amenorrhea caused by environmental changes, secondary amenorrhea of adolescence, amenorrhea associated with thyroid disorders, amenorrhea associated with virilizing disorders, and amenorrhea associated with systemic diseases. These conditions are associated with an abnormality of GnRH release. They result in a hypogonadotropic hypogonadism, and are differentiated from compartment III by the response of the pituitary to GnRH.

Classification of Primary Amenorrhea

Patients who have primary amenorrhea without secondary sex characteristics and have a uterus present have either gonadal failure or a hypothalamic-pituitary disorder. Approximately 50% of gonadal failures are 45,X (Turner's syndrome). Twenty-five percent have 46,X,abnormal X (i.e., short-arm or long-arm deletion). Another 25% have mosaicism. Pure XY gonadal dysgenesis and XY gonadal dysgenesis (Sawyer's syndrome) are rare causes of gonadal failure. These patients have an XY karyotype, a palpable müllerian system, normal female testosterone levels, and lack of sexual development. 17-hydroxylase deficiency (with 46,XX karyotype) is another rare cause of gonadal failure. CNS and hypothalamic-pituitary disorders can be caused by CNS lesions such as brain tumors, by hypothalamic failure secondary to inadequate GnRH release, and by isolated gonadotropin insufficiency.

Patients who have primary amenorrhea with breast development and an absent uterus have either congenital absence of the uterus (Rokitansky-Küster-Hauser syndrome) or androgen insensitivity (testicular feminization). Patients with androgen insensitivity have normal female phenotype and a normal male karyotype (46, XY). They have normal or slightly elevated male blood testosterone levels and have normal-appearing testes in the abdomen. The condition is X-linked recessive and is due to a lack of androgen receptors.

Patients who have primary amenorrhea with no secondary sex characteristics and an absent uterus have either 17,20-desmolase deficiency, agonadism, or 17-hydroxylase deficiency with 46,XY karyotype.

The differential diagnosis for patients with primary amenorrhea with breast development and a uterus present is the same as that for secondary amenorrhea.

Treatment of Amenorrhea

Treatment of amenorrhea depends on the cause and on the patient's desires. Therapy should be directed toward the underlying etiology. If an underlying medical disease is found, it should be treated. If no treatable underlying cause is found, treatment depends on the patient's desire for fertility. If the patient desires pregnancy, ovulation induction is indicated. If the patient does not desire fertility, treatment depends on the patient's estrogen status. Hypoestrogenic patients need estrogen replacement therapy with cyclic progestin therapy (if a uterus is present). Anovulatory patients with elevated or normal estrogen status should have periodic progestin withdrawal to reduce the risk of endometrial carcinoma. Progestin withdrawal can be administered monthly, or every 2 to 3 months to allow the recognition of spontaneous menstruation.

ABNORMAL UTERINE BLEEDING

Normal cycles have an interval of 21–35 days and a duration of 2–7 days. The volume of blood lost varies from 35–150 mL. This represents eight or fewer soaked pads per day, and usually no more than two heavy days. The amount of blood lost during a menstrual cycle can be estimated from the number of pads and tampons used. An average tampon will hold approximately 5 mL blood, and an average pad will hold between 5 and 15 mL blood before it is changed. Changes in the interval or duration of menses are important. Hypermenorrhea (menorrhagia) is excessive bleeding with a normal interval. Polymenorrhea (metrorrhagia) is bleeding that is irregular or too frequent.

Causes of Abnormal Bleeding

Pregnancy complications are common causes of abnormal bleeding. Incomplete or threatened abortion and ectopic pregnancy may present with abnormal bleeding. Intrauterine benign neoplasia (such as polyps or myomas), reproductive tract malignancies, cervicitis, endometritis, salpingitis, endometriosis, adenomyosis, functional cysts, and an IUD may cause abnormal bleeding. Malignancies of the cervix or uterus may present with abnormal bleeding.

Systemic diseases that can cause abnormal bleeding include blood dyscrasias such as thrombocytopenia. In the reproductive-age group, idiopathic thrombocytopenic purpura (ITP) is a common cause of thrombocytopenia. In adolescents, abnormal bleeding associated with thrombocytopenia may result from acute leukemia. Hypothyroidism or hyperthyroidism can cause abnormal bleeding. Liver disease can cause abnormal uterine bleeding (AUB) by interfering with the metabolism of circulating estrogens. Obesity is associated with anovulation and AUB. Diabetes, hypertension, and adrenal disorders can be associated with AUB.

Dysfunctional uterine bleeding is a term used after organic and iatrogenic causes are ruled out. It is predominantly a result of anovulation, but 10–15% of cases of dysfunctional uterine bleeding are associated with ovulatory cycles. If the patient ovulates, the cause of bleeding is usually mechanical and hormonal therapy is unlikely to be helpful. Thus, sampling of the endometrium in the second half of the cycle will help to establish the diagnosis and prognosis.

The key to management of abnormal bleeding is accurate diagnosis. The diagnosis begins with a careful history and physical examination. Pregnancy, thyroid disease, and blood dyscrasias should be excluded. A pelvic examination must be performed whether or not the patient is bleeding. A delay until the patient stops bleeding may lead to a delay in the diagnosis of a pelvic malignancy. A Pap smear should be performed. Sounding of the uterus and endometrial sampling in the second half of the cycle may help to diagnose intrauterine pathology, to exclude endometrial malignancy, or to confirm ovulation. An endometrial biopsy specimen should always be taken if there is a possibility of endometrial hyperplasia or malignancy. Women over the age of 35 who have not been on progestin therapy and women with a history of ten years of anovulation should have a biopsy specimen taken. Hysteroscopy or hysterosalpingography (HSG) should be considered if pelvic examination is normal and ovulation has been documented or the patient is unresponsive to hormonal therapy. Ultrasound examination may help to confirm the presence of fibroids or other pathology.

Treatment of Abnormal Bleeding

Treatment should be directed toward a specific diagnosis. Observation and reassurance is the best therapy in young adolescents with small amounts of irregular bleeding. Oral contraceptives can be used, but they may aggravate an already suppressed hypothalamic-ovarian axis. Hormonal regulation has a cure rate of nearly 90% in anovulatory patients. Cyclic oral contraceptives, cyclic progesterone injection (50–100 mg every 4 weeks), or oral progestins (medroxyprogesterone acetate 5–10 mg/day for 10–14 days) are appropriate therapies. High-dose estrogen followed by progesterone is useful for acute severe bleeding. Estrogen may be given alone or in combination with progestins in the form of oral contraceptives.

Excision of an endometrial polyp or a submucous leiomyoma may be effective in the treatment of abnormal uterine bleeding. Hysterectomy is used only as a last resort. The risks of undergoing hysterectomy are about equal to those of a blood transfusion. Thus, bleeding that is heavy enough to cause moderate anemia, and is not controlled by hormones or other therapies, warrants the consideration of hysterectomy.

DYSMENORRHEA

Dysmenorrhea is defined as painful menstruation. It affects approximately 60 to 70% of menstruating women.

Primary dysmenorrhea is present from adolescence. It is due to excess prostaglandin F2α production by the secretory endometrium, causing smooth muscle stimulation, and is not due to organic causes. Symptoms include lower abdominal cramps, especially during the first 2 days of menses, that may radiate to the back. Nausea, vomiting, diarrhea, fatigue, and headache are associated symptoms. Primary dysmenorrhea usually begins once cycles become ovulatory in the early reproductive years and cycles are regular. Increased intrauterine pressures can be demonstrated. Examination is normal and is performed to rule out secondary causes. No laboratory evaluation is needed. Treatment is with nonsteroidal antiinflammatory medications. Oral contraceptives are also often therapeutic.

Secondary dysmenorrhea is due to an identifiable organic cause. It can be caused by leiomyoma, adenomyosis, polyps, endometriosis, an IUD, or infection. The symptoms depend on the etiology. Symptoms usually begin in the middle-to-later reproductive years (after age 20). Dyspareunia, menorrhagia, and fever may be associated symptoms. The signs are those of the underlying pathology. Pelvic mass, fixed uterus, uterosacral nodularity, or purulent cervical discharge may suggest specific etiologies. Examination is performed to evaluate any uterine enlargement, adnexal masses, and cervical anomalies. Laboratory evaluation is guided by the history and suspicion of any underlying pathology.

Treatment is directed toward etiology. Nonsteroidal antiinflammatory medications or oral contraceptives may be useful regardless of the etiology. Antibiotics are helpful if pelvic inflammatory disease is suspected. GnRH agonists may be used to treat fibroids or endometriosis. Surgical therapy may include laparoscopy or laparotomy to remove adnexal masses. Hysterectomy or oophorectomy is indicated if the dysmenorrhea is severe and can be associated with a defined pathology of the uterus or ovaries.

Suggested Readings

American College of Obstetricians and Gynecologists. Amenorrhea. Technical Bulletin 128. Washington, DC: ACOG, 1989.

American College of Obstetricians and Gynecologists. Dysfunctional uterine bleeding. Technical Bulletin 134. Washington, DC: ACOG, 1989.

American College of Obstetricians and Gynecologists. Dysmenorrhea. Technical Bulletin 68. Washington, DC: ACOG, 1983.

American College of Obstetricians and Gynecologists. Precis V, pp. 368–375. Washington, DC: ACOG, 1994.

Carr BR, Blackwell RE, eds. Textbook of reproductive medicine. Norwalk, CT: Appleton & Lange, 1993.

Yen SCC, Jaffe RB, eds. Reproductive endocrinology. Philadelphia: WB Saunders, 1991.

Chapter 17

Reproductive Endocrinology and Infertility

PUBERTY

Sequence of Events

Puberty is the transition from childhood to adulthood involving physiological and psychological changes. The sequence of events is shown in Figure 17.1. Thelarche (onset of breast development) begins at an average age of 10.5 years. Adrenarche (growth of pubic and axillary hair) begins at an average age of 11.0 years. The growth spurt begins at an average age of 11.5 years, and menarche (onset of menstrual period) begins at an average age of 12.8 years.

Hormonal Events

Levels of estrogen, follicle-stimulating hormone (FSH), and luteinizing hormone (LH) are low prior to puberty. FSH rises first, then LH, then estrogen. Pulses of LH first appear during sleep. Estrogen then increases, causing changes in breasts, bones, uterus, and vagina. Adrenal androgens increase, causing pubic and axillary hair growth. Menarche occurs after the hypothalamic-pituitary-gonadal feedback loop is fully established (Figure 17.2). The average length of puberty is 4 years, with 1.5 to 8 years as a normal range. Ovulatory cycles are usually established after 2 years of menses. Males have pubertal development approximately 1 year later than females. Males may be as much as 2 years behind on growth spurt. Breast and pubic hair changes are staged by the Tanner system.

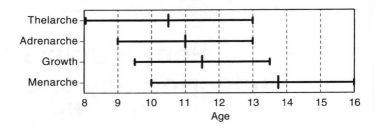

Figure 17.1. Sequence of events of puberty (age ranges are shown as the mean ± 2 standard deviations).

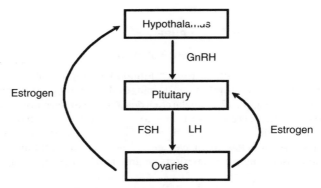

Figure 17.2. Hypothalamic-pituitary-gonadal axis.

Abnormalities of Puberty

Precocious puberty is the onset of pubertal events (secondary sexual development) prior to age 8 in girls and age 9 in boys. These ages are more than 2.5 standard deviations before the mean age. Precocious puberty may be isosexual or heterosexual, true (complete) or pseudo (incomplete). Isosexual precocious puberty is appropriate for genetic and gonadal sex and is the most common type. Heterosexual precocious puberty is inappropriate for genetic sex and includes feminizing of males and virilizing of females. The causes of precocious puberty are listed in Table 17.1.

Idiopathic precocious puberty is due to premature activation of the hypothalamic-pituitary axis. In the female it includes normal menses, ovulation, and the possibility of pregnancy. Idiopathic precocious puberty is the most common type of precocious puberty, accounting for 90% of cases.

Neurogenic causes are usually associated with lesions near the hypothalamus and are usually associated with other signs of CNS dysfunction such as headache and visual disturbance. However, prolonged and repeated observation may be necessary to exclude slowly growing brain tumors. The most common developmental anomalies associated with precocious puberty are microcephaly, aqueductal stenosis, craniostenosis, and tuberous sclerosis. Sturge-Weber syndrome consists of the triad of a flame nevus (cutaneous angioma) over the distribution of the trigeminal nerve; homolateral meningeal angioma with intracranial cal-

Table 17.1
Causes of Precocious Puberty

1. True precocious puberty
   a. Idiopathic
   b. Neurogenic
      (1) Tumors of hypothalamus, pineal gland, cerebral cortex
      (2) Infections—toxoplasmosis, encephalitis, meningitis
      (3) Developmental anomalies
      (4) Trauma
      (5) Sturge-Weber syndrome
   c. McCune-Albright syndrome
   d. Silver-Russell syndrome
   e. Hypothyroidism
2. Pseudoprecocious puberty
   a. Adrenal lesions
      (1) Congenital adrenal hyperplasia
      (2) Cushing's syndrome
      (3) Adrenal tumors
   b. Ovarian tumors
      (1) Granulosa-theca cell tumor
      (2) Luteoma
   c. Exogenous sex hormones
      (1) Estrogens
      (2) Oral contraceptives
      (3) Anabolic steroids
   d. Extrapituitary gonadotropins
      (1) Extrapituitary gonadotropin-secreting tumors
         (*a*) Choriocarcinoma
         (*b*) Teratoma
         (*c*) Hepatoblastoma
         (*d*) Dysgerminoma

cifications; and an angioma of the choroid. McCune-Albright syndrome (polyostotic fibrous dysplasia) consists of café-au-lait spots; fibrous dysplasia; and cysts of the skull and long bones. Forty percent of girls with McCune-Albright syndrome have precocious puberty. Silver's syndrome (also called Silver-Russell or Russell-Silver syndrome) is multiple congenital anomalies with low birth weight; body asymmetry; abnormal jaw; café-au-lait spots; and abnormal fifth digits.

Although most cases of hypothyroidism are associated with delayed puberty, untreated hypothyroidism can lead to precocious puberty. Diminished thyroxine leads to elevated production of thyroid-stimulating hormone (TSH) and an associated increase in production of gonadotropins. Hypothyroidism is the only cause of precocious puberty in which the bone age is retarded.

The most common cause of pseudoprecocious puberty is a functional ovarian tumor, the most common of which are granulosa-theca cell tumors. Exogenous sex hormones may originate from oral contraceptives taken by a child to imitate the mother, estrogen creams, or anabolic steroids used to alter body habitus. Extrapituitary gonadotropins are a rare cause of precocious puberty. The source is usually a gonadotropin-secreting tumor.

Evaluation of Precocious Puberty

The evaluation of precocious puberty begins with a careful history and physical examination. The history includes any medicines taken, including exogenous hormones; neurological symptoms, including headache and visual change; and a history of growth spurts, thelarche, and adrenarche. Physical examination should document height and weight, presence of secondary sex characteristics, any congenital anomalies or body asymmetry, and a total body search for skin lesions such as café-au-lait spots.

Diagnostic tests include measurement of serum estradiol, testosterone, and gonadotropins, and thyroid function tests. Determining the levels of serum dehydroepiandrosterone sulfate (DHEAS) and 17-hydroxyprogesterone (17-OHP) is useful if congenital adrenal hyperplasia (CAH) is suspected. Radiologic tests to rule out CNS tumors should be performed, and a bone age determination should always be performed. Advancement of bone age beyond the 95th percentile documents peripheral sex hormone effect. Gonadal and adrenal tumors can be evaluated by ultrasound or CT scanning.

Treatment of precocious puberty depends on the cause. Surgery is indicated to remove tumors if diagnosed. Hypothyroidism is managed by thyroid replacement. Idiopathic precocious puberty can be treated with gonadotropin-releasing hormone (GnRH) analogues. Girls with menarche prior to age 8, progressive thelarche, and bone age greater than 2 years beyond chronological age should be treated. Monthly injections of GnRH analogues are preferable to daily therapy for most children. Both the child with precocious puberty and her family need extensive counseling. The child is at risk for ridicule and for sexual exploitation.

Delayed Puberty

Delayed puberty is the absence of thelarche by age 13 or menarche by age 15. Constitutional delay is the most common type. These patients have delayed onset of the GnRH pulse generator. Once puberty begins, events proceed along a normal course.

Hypogonadotropic hypogonadism is due to GnRH, FSH, or LH deficiency. Etiologies include CNS tumors or infections, isolated gonadotropin deficiency, constitutional delayed puberty, and anorexia nervosa. Prolactin-producing pituitary adenomas can lead to delayed puberty. Psychotropic drugs such as phenothiazines can lead to elevated prolactin levels and delayed puberty. Primary juvenile hypothyroidism may present with delayed puberty.

Hypergonadotropic hypogonadism is gonadal failure with elevated FSH and LH levels and decreased sex hormone levels. Etiologies include Turner's syndrome and gonadal dysplasia in females, and Klinefelter's syndrome in males.

Diagnostic evaluations of delayed puberty include history and physical examination, with attention to the stigmata of Turner's syndrome and neurological signs. Documentation of normal internal and external genitalia is important. Bone age determination and karyotype may be indicated. Measurement of gonadotropin levels is indicated. If gonadotropin levels are low, a GnRH stimulation test can distinguish pituitary from hypothalamic dysfunction. A CT scan or MRI of the pituitary can determine the presence of pituitary adenomas.

The treatment is based on etiology. Patients with constitutional delay may be treated expectantly. Those with gonadal failure need hormonal therapy. Females need estrogen and progestins and males need testosterone. All patients need counseling for psychological issues.

HIRSUTISM AND VIRILISM

Definitions

Hirsutism is the presence of excessive facial and body hair. It may be present as a normal variant, or it may be due to certain medications or to excessive androgen production in a female. Virilism is the presence of mature masculine somatic characteristics in a female. Virilism may be present at birth or develop later in life. It is a result of excessive androgen.

Biology of Hair Growth

Hair follicles develop at 8 weeks of gestation. The distribution of follicles varies with ethnicity but does not vary by sex. Lanugo hair growth occurs in utero and may be seen in children. Sexual hair responds to sex steroids. Sexual hair grows on the face, lower abdomen, anterior thighs, chest, pubic area, and axillae. Androgens initiate sexual hair growth. Testosterone is the major circulating androgen, but dihydrotestosterone (DHT) is the major nuclear androgen acting on the follicle. 3α-androstanediol is the peripheral tissue metabolite of DHT. 3α-androstanediol glucuronide (3αAG) is utilized as the marker of tissue action. Estrogens retard sexual hair growth, and progestins have minimal effect on hair growth.

Hair grows in phases: anagen is the growing phase; catagen is the phase of rapid involution; and telogen is the quiescent or resting phase. In the resting phase, hair is short and loosely attached. When the anagen phase begins, the epithelial matrix cells around the bulb proliferate and extend downward through the dermis. Continued rapid growth of the matrix cells pushes the hair toward the surface and the hair is shed. The matrix cells keratinize and the catagen phase begins. The column of matrix cells involutes and shrinks, the bulb shrivels, and the telogen phase begins again. Hair length is determined by the length of time the follicle spends in the anagen phase. Scalp hair remains in anagen for up to three years and has a short telogen phase, while arm and body hair has a long telogen phase and a short anagen phase. Occasionally there may be a synchrony of telogen phase in scalp hair. Prolonged high estrogen levels such as occur during a pregnancy can cause a prolongation of anagen in scalp hair. The loss of estrogen that occurs postpartum can lead to a synchrony of telogen phase and an apparent hair loss.

Biology of Virilism

Virilism is always due to excess androgen. Androgens act on testosterone-receptive tissues to lead to the changes associated with virilism, which are listed in Table 17.2. The normal female produces 0.2–0.3 mg testosterone per day. Normally, 50% of circulating testosterone comes from peripheral conversion of androstenedione, with 25% from the ovary and 25% from the adrenal glands. At midcycle, the ovarian contribution increases by 10–15%. About 80% of circulating testosterone is bound to sex hormone–binding globulin. Another 19% is loosely bound to albumin, leaving only 1% free. Androgenicity is dependent on the free fraction of testosterone.

Sources of Androgen

Excess androgen comes from one of three sources—ovarian, adrenal, or exogenous. The sources of circulating androgens in the normal woman are listed in Table 17.3. Ovarian androgen production may be from functional ovarian tissue or from tumors. Androstenedione production is increased with polycystic ovary syndrome, leading to elevated testosterone levels. With excessive stromal tissue, testosterone becomes a significant secretory product of the ovary. Androgenic tumors of the ovary (Table 17.4) are of stromal origin and may produce significant amounts of testosterone.

Adrenal sources of androgen may be due to Cushing's syndrome or to adult congenital adrenal hyperplasia due to incomplete 21-hydroxylase or 11-hydroxylase deficiency. Cushing's syndrome is the persistent overproduction of cortisol. It may be due

Table 17.2
Biologic Effects of Androgen

Hirsutism
Male pattern baldness
Breast atrophy
Striated muscle hypertrophy
Clitoromegaly
Coarsening of vocal cords with deepening of voice
Decreased sex hormone–binding globulin
Increased hematocrit and red blood cell mass

Table 17.3
Source of Circulating Androgens

	Adrenal	Ovary	Peripheral Conversion
Testosterone	25%	25%	50%
Androstenedione	50%	50%	0
DHEA	90%	10%	0
DHEAS	~100%	0	0

Table 17.4
Androgen-Producing Tumors

Sertoli-Leydig cell tumors (arrhenoblastomas)
Hilus cell tumors
Lipoid cell (adrenal rest) tumors
Rarely, granulosa-theca cell tumors

to the oversecretion of adrenocorticotropic hormone (ACTH) (Cushing's disease), ectopic ACTH production by tumors, or an autonomous cortisol-secreting adrenal cortex. Late-onset congenital adrenal hyperplasia is most commonly due to incomplete 21-hydroxylase deficiency. There are three alleles of the gene responsible for 21-hydroxylase production—normal, mild deficiency, and severe deficiency. Classical congenital adrenal hyperplasia occurs in individuals who are homozygous for the severe deficiency. Late-onset disease occurs in individuals who are either homozygous for the mild deficiency, or who carry one mild and one severe deficiency allele. This condition is the most common autosomal recessive disorder, occurring in Ashkenazic Jews (1 in 30), Hispanics (1 in 40), Yugoslavians (Balkan Peninsula) (1 in 50), and Italians (1 in 300).

Exogenous testosterone is often given to women in combination with estrogens by injection or oral forms to treat menopausal disorders. Depot testosterone may have androgenic effects for long periods of time. The workup of hirsutism or virilization should include any injections in the past year. Anabolic steroids may be used illicitly for bodybuilding. Danazol (Danocrine sulfate), which is used for endometriosis therapy, is an androgen.

Evaluation of Hirsutism/Virilism

After the history and physical examination have confirmed hirsutism or virilization and excluded exogenous sources of androgen, attention is turned to the laboratory. Initial laboratory evaluation consists of serum testosterone (normal, 20–80 ng/dL), DHEAS (normal, less than 700 μg/dL), and 17-hydroxyprogesterone (normal, 15–70 ng/dL follicular, 35–290 ng/dL luteal). The workup then proceeds as shown in Figure 17.3.

Measurement of the serum testosterone is the first step in diagnosis. If the serum testosterone is normal, the diagnosis is idiopathic hirsutism. If the serum testosterone is greater than 200 ng/dL, then a tumor is highly likely. If the patient has a palpable adnexal mass, laparotomy or laparoscopy to remove the tumor is indicated. If not, an ultrasound examination may identify a tumor that is not palpable, and if so, removal is indicated.

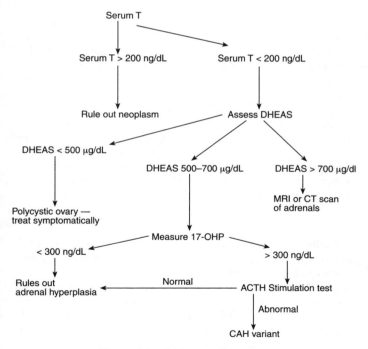

Figure 17.3.   Evaluation of hirsutism.

When the serum testosterone is in an intermediate range (between 80 and 200 ng/dL), then the next step is measurement of the serum DHEAS. If the serum DHEAS is greater than 700 μg/dL, an adrenal tumor is likely and an MRI or CT scan of the adrenal glands is indicated. If the DHEAS is less than 500 μg/dL, then the androgen is of ovarian origin and symptomatic therapy is indicated. If the DHEAS is between 500 and 700 μg/dL, then measurement of the 17-hydroxyprogesterone is the next step. A 17-OHP value of less than 300 ng/dL excludes congenital adrenal hyperplasia. If the value is greater than 300 ng/dL, then an ACTH stimulation test is indicated. If it is normal, then congenital adrenal hyperplasia is excluded and the patient may be treated symptomatically. If it is abnormal, then the diagnosis is congenital adrenal hyperplasia variant.

Therapy

Treatment of hyperandrogenic states is directed toward reduction of circulating androgen. Specific therapy depends on the source of androgen. Ovarian androgen production is usually due to LH stimulation of the stroma. Suppression of LH can be accomplished by oral contraceptive pills. Use of a pill that is high-dose but low in androgen (those containing ethynodiol diacetate) is indicated. If oral contraceptives are contraindicated, medroxyprogesterone acetate can be used. In an older woman who is resistant to hormone therapy, an oophorectomy may be considered. If a functioning ovarian tumor is found, surgical removal is indicated. Adrenal sources of androgen are managed by suppressing adrenal function with glucocorticoid replacement. If an adrenal tumor is found, surgical removal is indicated.

INFERTILITY

Infertility is defined as one year of unprotected intercourse without pregnancy. Approximately 10–15% of the population suffers from infertility. The incidence of infertility has been increasing for the last 40 years. There are many proposed explanations for this increase. Many women defer childbearing to a later age, and fertility declines with increasing age. The increase in sexually transmitted diseases that occurred in the 1970s may have led to increased tubal damage. In addition, there is evidence of an increased concern with infertility—i.e., infertile couples are more likely to seek medical help. All of these factors combine to increase the number of office visits for infertility to over 2,000,000 per year. The causes of infertility are listed in Table 17.5.

Evaluation of the Infertile Couple

The evaluation of the infertile couple is directed toward identifying the cause of infertility. A careful history can help to direct the evaluation, but it is essential to document the sperm count, the presence or absence of ovulation, and the patency of the fallopian tubes prior to beginning any therapy. The menstrual history is essential to assess ovulation. A history of amenorrhea or oligomenorrhea suggests anovulation, and a history of molimina or mittelschmerz suggests ovulation. Abnormal hair growth suggests anovulation secondary to excess androgen. Galactorrhea indicates excess prolactin secretion. Dyspareunia and pelvic pain are symptoms of pelvic infections or endometriosis. Any previous contraception, especially IUD or depot-medroxyprogesterone acetate, should be documented. The sexual history should include frequency of coitus, frequency of penis-in-vagina intercourse, documentation of ejaculation, and any use of lubricants. A history of genital trauma or infection in the male can suggest male factor. Any diethylstilbestrol (DES) exposure in utero of either the male or the female should be documented. In addition to the routine speculum and bimanual pelvic examination, the physical examination must include a breast examination for galactorrhea and a search for hirsutism. An evaluation of estrogen status should be made.

A semen analysis is part of the routine evaluation. A normal

Table 17.5
Causes of Infertility

Tubal disease	25–50%
Anovulation	20–40%
Male factor	40%
Cervical factor	5–10%
Peritoneal factor	5–10%
Uterine/endometrial (e.g., luteal phase defect)	3–10%
Unknown	10%
Combinations	

semen analysis should show a sperm count greater than 20 million/mL, greater than 60% motile, and greater than 60% normal morphology. The normal volume is 3–5 mL. The male should abstain for 48–72 hours prior to giving the specimen. The specimen must not be collected in a condom because this will result in falsely low sperm counts and motility. The specimen can be collected in a clean glass container or in a specimen cup. The specimen must be kept at body temperature and should be analyzed within 2 hours.

Documentation of ovulation by basal body temperature chart (BBT) is also a routine part of the evaluation. The basal body temperature is measured immediately after awakening, before getting out of bed. The temperature should go up 1°F 24 hours after ovulation. The rise in temperature coincides with a rise in progesterone levels to more than 4 ng/mL. A biphasic curve confirms ovulation, although a small proportion of ovulatory women may have a monophasic curve.

Controversy exists over the utility of the postcoital test. This test is performed on the expected day of ovulation. The couple should observe 48 hours of sexual abstinence, then have intercourse. The cervical mucus is examined within 8 hours of intercourse. Evaluation of the postcoital test is described in Table 17.6. Although more than 20 sperm per high power field (HPF) is almost always associated with a normal sperm count, the postcoital test cannot be substituted for a semen analysis.

Hysterosalpingography is used to evaluate tubal patency and the contour of the uterine cavity. It is best performed on day 10 of the cycle. The test is contraindicated in the presence of pelvic infection. The test should be done under image intensification and a minimum number (3–5) of films should be taken. It is best if the patient's gynecologist performs the test, in order to visualize the injection of dye. Hysterosalpingography may itself be ther-

Table 17.6
Evaluation of the Postcoital Test

Factor	Normal	Abnormal
Cervical mucus	thin	thick
Spinnbarkeit	> 8 cm	< 8 cm
Number of sperm	> 5/HPF	< 5/HPF
Ferning	present	absent

apeutic, through a mechanical lavage of the tubes and the dislodging of mucus plugs.

Endometrial biopsy analysis is the most sensitive and specific test for ovulation and for luteal phase defects. The test should be performed 2–3 days before expected menses (day 26). Although taking an endometrial biopsy specimen could interrupt an early pregnancy, the risk is minimal. Use of a 3-mm plastic flexible curette causes minimal pain and bleeding. A luteal phase defect is confirmed if the "lag" between the endometrial biopsy procedure and the subsequent menses is more than 2 days.

Laparoscopy may be used to evaluate suspected anatomic factors and can also be used earlier in the workup if endometriosis is suspected or a history of pelvic pathology or pelvic inflammatory disease is present. Chromotubation with methylene blue may be used to document tubal patency. Laparoscopy provides an opportunity to treat tubal obstruction by lysis of adhesions or other operative procedures.

Treatment of Infertility

Treatment of infertility is directed toward the cause. Nonpatent tubes are frequently due to pelvic inflammatory disease (PID). Each episode of PID increases the risk of infertility. With the first episode of PID, there is a 10–15% risk of infertility; with the second episode, there is a 25% risk, and after the third episode, the risk of infertility is 50%. Lysis of tubal adhesions and tubal reconstruction by laparotomy or laparoscopy may restore tubal patency. Tubal patency, however, does not guarantee successful pregnancy.

Anovulation or oligo-ovulation is a very common cause of infertility. Successful treatment of anovulation depends on the cause. It is essential to rule out underlying endocrine disorders prior to therapy. Women who are morbidly obese frequently have polycystic ovary disease associated with anovulation. These patients have a steady state of elevated LH levels with elevated androgen levels, leading to anovulation. Treatment with clomiphene citrate is indicated as a first step. Women who are very thin (anorexia nervosa, ballet dancers, runners, etc.) will frequently be anovulatory, but there are different mechanisms associated with anovulation in these patients than in obese patients.

Women with exercise-induced anovulation do not have elevated LH levels and elevated androgen levels. Instead, they have elevated plasma β-endorphin levels and a change in the metabolism of estradiol. These women have 16-catechol-estradiol as the primary metabolic product of estradiol. Both β-endorphins and 16-catechol-estradiol interfere with the normal pulsatile release of GnRH and lead to a state of hypogonadotropic hypogonadism. Clomiphene citrate usually does not induce ovulation in these patients, although they do respond to human gonadotropins and human chorionic gonadotropin (hCG).

Women with elevated prolactin levels are often anovulatory. Reduction of the serum prolactin will restore ovulation in these patients. Treatment with bromocriptine is usually successful. Women with hypothyroidism or adrenal abnormalities will often become ovulatory when these abnormalities are corrected.

Therapy for anovulation, then, should be first to seek and to correct any underlying endocrine abnormality. If no endocrine abnormality is present, then ovulation induction is indicated. Clomiphene is begun on the fifth day of the cycle and given for 5 days (days 5–9). The initial dose is 50 mg/day. Ovulation is documented by the use of a basal body temperature chart. If ovulation does not occur in the first cycle of 50 mg/day, the dose is increased to 100 mg/day in the second cycle. If ovulation still does not occur, the dose is increased to 150 mg/day in the third cycle. If ovulation does not occur after 3 or 4 months of treatment at this level, the patient can be considered a clomiphene failure. Although the manufacturer recommends that doses above 150 mg/day not be used, some physicians have reported that pregnancy rates have improved with doses as high as 250 mg/day. If the patient does not ovulate on 150 mg/day of clomiphene, the addition of hCG is indicated. hCG is also indicated if the basal body temperature chart indicates a short luteal phase (less than 11 days). hCG is given as a single intramuscular dose of 5,000–10,000 IU on the seventh day after clomiphene (cycle day 12) or when a follicular diameter greater than 20 mm is documented by ultrasound examination.

Human menopausal gonadotropins (hMG) are supplied as ampules containing 75 or 150 IU each of LH and FSH (Pergonal), and urofollitropin is supplied as an ampule containing 75 IU of purified human FSH (Metrodin). Gonadotropins promote follicle growth by direct stimulation of follicles. They are the treatment of choice for women with hypogonadotropic hypogonadism and are useful in women who do not ovulate with clomiphene therapy. Women with low levels of FSH and estrogen are more likely to respond than those with normal levels.

Safe and successful treatment with human menopausal gonadotropins requires the ability to rapidly measure serum estradiol levels in conjunction with the ability to measure follicular diameter by ultrasound examination. The dose required to induce ovulation varies widely from patient to patient and may vary from cycle to cycle in the same patient. In general, hMG is given as a daily intramuscular injection for 7 to 10 days until a preovulatory follicle is developed. An initial dose of 75–150 IU/day is used. Daily serum estradiol levels are measured. If no response is seen by the fourth day of therapy, the dose of hMG may be increased by 75–150 IU/day. Once the serum estradiol level reaches 100 pg/mL, the daily dose of hMG should be held constant, and daily vaginal ultrasound examination is begun to determine the number and size of follicles.

When the leading follicle is 16–20 mm in diameter, hMG is discontinued and a single intramuscular dose of 5,000–10,000 IU hCG is given to induce ovulation. The hCG is given approximately 24 hours after the last dose of hMG. Follicles grow at a rate of 2–3 mm per day, allowing prediction of the day of ovulation. Ovulation usually occurs 36 hours after the dose of hCG. Subsequent doses of 2500 IU hCG to maintain the corpus luteum are usually given on days 3 and 6 after the ovulatory dose.

Ovarian hyperstimulation and multiple pregnancy are the two most common complications of hMG induction of ovulation. Ovarian hyperstimulation can be avoided if the ovulating dose of hCG is not given. The cycle should be interrupted and hCG not given if the serum estradiol exceeds 2000 pg/mL or if more than three preovulatory follicles are seen. The therapeutic range between normal ovulation and hyperstimulation is very narrow, and hyperstimulation may occur despite careful monitoring.

Ovarian hyperstimulation results in ovarian enlargement, pelvic pain, and weight gain and hemoconcentration due to loss of intravascular fluid into the third space. Classification of ovarian hyperstimulation is shown in Table 17.7. Mild hyperstimulation is relatively common and is managed conservatively. Pelvic and abdominal examination should be avoided. The symptoms will usually resolve in 7 days if no pregnancy occurs, but may persist for weeks if pregnancy occurs.

Moderate hyperstimulation is managed by close observation

Table 17.7
Ovarian Hyperstimulation

Type	Ovarian Size	Weight Gain	Symptoms
Mild	< 5 cm	< 10 lb	Mild pain
Moderate	5–10 cm	> 10 lb	Moderate pain, nausea, vomiting
Severe	> 10 cm	> 10 lb	Ascites, hydrothorax, hemoconcentration, oliguria

of daily weight, hematocrit levels, and abdominal girth. Severe hyperstimulation is uncommon but potentially life-threatening. Hospitalization is usually required. Large fluid shifts from the intravascular space lead to weight gain, ascites, pleural effusion, hypotension, oliguria, electrolyte imbalances, hemoconcentration, and increased coagulopathy. Ovarian hemorrhage can occur and lead to exploratory laparotomy and oophorectomy.

Poor cervical mucus quality can be a barrier to sperm penetration. Low-dose estrogen (micronized estradiol 1 mg) on days 5–13 during the mid-follicular phase may improve the quality of the mucus. Artificial insemination of washed sperm into the uterine cavity may be used to bypass cervical mucus. The use of donor mucus is also a possibility.

A male factor is at least partially responsible for infertility in 30–50% of infertile couples. A variety of conditions can lead to male infertility (Table 17.8). Treatment of male infertility is usually by artificial insemination with donor sperm (AID). Intrauterine artificial insemination with husband sperm (AIH) can be administered for abnormalities of the cervix or mucus, as well as for sperm abnormalities. Very low sperm counts are not amenable to treatment with AIH. Correction of an underlying abnormality, if possible, may restore fertility. Corticosteroids may be of benefit in cases of antisperm antibodies.

There is little doubt that extensive endometriosis causing tubal and ovarian adhesions can be a cause of infertility. Less certain is the role of peritoneal endometriosis that does not involve tubes or ovaries. Many believe that even minimal endometriosis can cause infertility. The mechanism is uncertain, but may possibly be prostaglandin-mediated. Elevated prostaglandin levels could alter tubal function and lead to infertility.

Table 17.8
Causes of Male Infertility

Infections
　Prostatitis, epididymis, mumps
Testicular injury
Varicocele
Heat—increased scrotal temperature can decrease sperm count and
　motility
Drugs
　Marijuana
　Chemotherapy
　Tobacco
　Alcohol—can decrease testosterone, may also decrease libido
Retrograde ejaculation
Hypospadias
Radiation
Congenital
Chromosomal abnormalities
Previous vasectomy
Antisperm antibodies
Sexual dysfunctions

MENOPAUSE

Menopause is the cessation of menstruation. The average age of menopause in the United States is 51 years, with a normal range of 40–60. Due to increasing life expectancy, approximately one-third of women's lives are spent in the postmenopausal years. Menopause may be natural, surgical, or due to other influences such as radiation therapy or chemotherapy. Menopause occurs, on average, 2 years sooner in smokers than nonsmokers.

The climacteric is the process of changing from a reproductive to a nonreproductive state. It occurs over a 3–5-year time span and is sometimes called the perimenopause. Recognition of the climacteric as a process rather than an event is important in effectively managing the problems that women may face during this time. The process of the climacteric is due to oocyte depletion.

The peak number of oocytes is reached at 20 weeks' gestation. The majority of these become atretic by the time of birth. By age 40, they are more difficult to recruit to maturation, leading to anovulation and irregular menses. The remaining follicles secrete less estrogen, causing levels of follicle-stimulating hormone to rise. Lower levels of estrogen lead to the symptoms of the climacteric, which are listed in Table 17.9.

Diagnosis

The diagnosis is made by history, signs, and occasionally by laboratory confirmation. A history of the symptoms listed in Table 17.9 is highly suggestive of the climacteric. Signs include vaginal and vulvar atrophy, pelvic relaxation, and thinning of the hair and skin. Determination of serum FSH levels may be useful in the perimenopausal years if diagnosis is unclear. Levels greater than 40 mIU/mL indicate a postmenopausal state. Measurement of LH levels is rarely indicated. Determination of estrogen levels is usually reserved for evaluating inadequate symptom relief on maximum doses of hormone replacement therapy. Estradiol levels of 40–250 pg/mL are normal, and levels less than 20 pg/mL are menopausal levels. The vaginal maturation index is determined by taking a smear of vaginal mucosa to evaluate the percentage of basal, parabasal, and superficial cells present. An estrogen-dominant environment will have a majority of superficial cells, and a preponderance of parabasal cells indicates a lack of estrogen.

Complications

Osteoporosis is a common complication of untreated menopause. There are over 1 million fractures each year, with two-thirds of them occurring in women. The most common fracture site is the vertebrae, followed by the femur and forearm. Vertebral fractures occur in one-third of women over the age of 65. Hip fractures occur in one-third of women over the age of 90, with a 10–15% mortality rate. Maximum bone density is achieved in the early 30s, with a progressive decline thereafter. The decline ac-

Table 17.9
Symptoms of the Climacteric

Abnormal menstrual cycles—up to 90%
Hot flashes (vasomotor instability)—80%
Emotional lability (not depression)
Vaginal dryness, dyspareunia
Bladder symptoms
Sleep disturbances

celerates at menopause if hormone replacement therapy is not given. The decline in bone mass leads to a height loss of up to 2.5 inches during a woman's lifetime. Risk factors for osteoporosis include Caucasian race, low body fat, short stature, sedentary lifestyle, positive family history, smoking, steroid use, hyperthyroidism, and anticoagulant use.

Cardiovascular disease is the leading cause of death in postmenopausal women. Women have a sharp increase in the risk for cardiovascular disease after the menopause. This risk is associated with a change in serum lipids. At the menopause, women have an increase in total cholesterol and an increase in LDL fraction with a change in the HDL/LDL ratio. Estrogen replacement therapy is associated with a favorable change in the lipid profile and with a decreased risk of cardiovascular disease.

Psychosexual changes are often related to changes in the genital tissue causing discomfort with intercourse. Women who have estrogen deprivation have mood swings, alterations in their ability to concentrate, and decreases in short-term memory. Depression is usually not related to estrogen deprivation, and depression will not respond to estrogen replacement without other therapy.

Endometrial cancer is primarily a disease of postmenopausal women. The risk is increased 3–8 times if estrogen is taken unopposed by progestins with a uterus present. The combination of estrogen and progestins decreases the risk of developing endometrial cancer to less than that of women who take no hormonal therapy. In some women, unopposed estrogen can be safely given if endometrial hyperplasia is excluded. Endometrial cancer develops as a result of endometrial hyperplasia induced by estrogen. This hyperplasia can be detected by annual endometrial biopsy examination or ultrasound measurements of endometrial thickness. An endometrial biopsy analysis should be performed if the endometrial thickness is greater than 5 mm.

Treatment

Hormone replacement therapy is the mainstay of treating menopausal symptoms. Estrogen therapy lowers LDL levels and raises HDL levels, lowers total cholesterol levels, and prevents osteoporosis. It is best to begin estrogen therapy in the first three years of menopause. The following represent alternative regimens of daily doses adequate to prevent osteoporosis and heart disease:

0.625 mg conjugated equine estrogen; 1.0 mg micronized estradiol; 0.05 mg transdermal 17β-estradiol; 1.25 mg estrone sulfate; or 10 μg ethinyl estradiol. All of these regimens appear to be equivalent in their effects. In women who have not had a hysterectomy, cyclic therapy with 10 mg medroxyprogesterone acetate for 12 days each month results in withdraw bleeding in 50% of women and provides protection against endometrial cancer. Continuous therapy with as little as 2.5 mg medroxyprogesterone acetate results in bleeding in approximately 5% of women after 1 year of therapy and in 35% during the first 6 months, while providing protection against endometrial cancer. Contraindications to estrogen therapy are listed in Table 17.10.

Calcium therapy is also useful in preventing osteoporosis. Calcium is given in a dose of 1000 mg/day of elemental calcium if on estrogen, and 1500 mg/day if not on estrogen or if on estrogen doses less than those listed above. Calcium carbonate is usually the best-tolerated form.

Calcitonin prevents bone resorption and is approved by the Food and Drug Administration as a treatment for osteoporosis. It is given as an intramuscular or subcutaneous dose of 100 IU/day. In many patients with osteoporosis, 50 IU/day or even every other day may be adequate to maintain calcium balance. Etidronate is not approved by the FDA for the treatment of osteoporosis, but it prevents bone resorption. It is given in two-week regimens four times a year, as 5–20 mg/kg/day for 14 days every 3 months.

Tamoxifen is a nonsteroidal antiestrogen used as an adjunct therapy for breast cancer. It has estrogenic effects on bone and on the endometrium. Tamoxifen may be useful in alleviating symptoms of menopause in women with a history of breast cancer. It is given in a dose of 10–20 mg orally twice a day. Women on tamoxifen are at increased risk of developing endometrial

Table 17.10
Estrogen Contraindications

Unexplained uterine bleeding
Pregnancy
Active thrombophlebitis
History of thrombophlebitis associated with estrogen
Estrogen-dependent cancers (endometrial, breast)

cancer and should be followed in the same way as women on un-opposed estrogen. It is not known if combination therapy with progestins reduces the risk of endometrial cancer in these women, although it is reasonable to suppose that it does.

Suggested Readings

American College of Obstetricians and Gynecologists. Evaluation and treatment of hirsute women. Technical Bulletin 203. Washington, DC: ACOG, 1995.

American College of Obstetricians and Gynecologists. Hyperandrogenic chronic anovulation. Technical Bulletin 202. Washington, DC: ACOG, 1995.

American College of Obstetricians and Gynecologists. Infertility. Technical Bulietin 125. Washington, DC: ACOG, 1989.

American College of Obstetricians and Gynecologists. Male infertility. Technical Bulletin 142. Washington, DC: ACOG, 1990.

American College of Obstetricians and Gynecologists. Managing the anovulatory state: medical induction of ovulation. Technical Bulletin 197. Washington, DC: ACOG, 1994.

Carr BR, Blackwell RE, eds. Textbook of reproductive medicine. Norwalk, CT: Appleton & Lange, 1993.

Speroff L, Glass RH, Kase NG. Clinical gynecological endocrinology and infertility. 5th ed. Baltimore: Williams & Wilkins, 1994.

Yen SCC, Jaffe RB, eds. Reproductive endocrinology. Philadelphia: WB Saunders, 1991.

Chapter 18

Gynecologic Oncology

VULVAR AND VAGINAL NEOPLASIAS

Condyloma Acuminata

Vulvar condylomata are caused by the human papilloma virus (HPV). The incubation period is usually 2 months but may vary widely. After the first wart appears, there is an expressive period lasting from 6 to 9 months while warts are formed. Immunity begins to develop and a latent period then ensues. The majority of patients will enter a latent period after 6 to 9 months. No new warts are formed during the latent period, and approximately 80% of patients will be in clinical remission.

The diagnosis is usually made by inspection. Biopsy examination is recommended if the warts have an atypical appearance, the course is unusual, or the warts are resistant to therapy.

The conventional therapy has been to apply 25–50% podophyllin. It is now believed that 50–75% trichloroacetic acid or bichloracetic acid is more effective. These therapies should be applied directly to the wart on a weekly basis until the lesions have resolved. Five-percent 5-fluorouracil has been used in a cytotoxic dose, but the side effects are severe and limit its use. It is now primarily used as an adjuvant to laser therapy. Laser vaporization is effective and safe therapy. Laser therapy should be limited to patients in whom outpatient therapy has not been effective. Intralesional interferon is useful in some patients in whom laser ablation has not been successful.

Patients who have condyloma acuminata often ask about the advisability of condom use to prevent spread or recurrence. Patients who are in a monogamous relationship do not need to use condoms because their sexual partner is almost certainly infected and because they will continue to carry the virus even after no warts are clinically visible. Patients who have new partners or multiple partners should use condoms to protect themselves and their partners from acquisition of HPV and other sexually transmitted diseases.

Vulvar Dystrophies

Vulvar dystrophies include a diverse group of syndromes that present with vulvar pruritus. The lesions can be difficult to distinguish on clinical grounds, and biopsy analysis is recommended to establish the diagnosis. Vulvar dystrophies have been divided into three classes by the International Society for the Study of Vulvar and Vaginal Disease (Table 18.1). The classification is based on both gross and histopathologic changes. This simple classification allows a better understanding of vulvar dystrophies and allows comparison of treatment regimens between institutions. If more than one of these lesions coexist, they should all should be reported (e.g., VIN I, lichen sclerosis).

Squamous cell hyperplasias represent 25–50% of vulvar dystrophies. The human papilloma viruses are associated with lesions with atypia, but other lesions are of unknown etiology. Patients with squamous cell hyperplasias tend to be younger than those with lichen sclerosis. The lesions are often elevated, localized, and well-defined. They may be dusky red or may be white. Thickening, excoriations, and fissures result from chronic itching and scratching. The lesions are often unifocal with hyperkeratosis. They are more often associated with dysplasia or carcinoma at diagnosis than is lichen sclerosis. The treatment is with topical corticosteroids. Hydrocortisone 1.0% or betamethasone 0.1%, applied twice daily, are used as initial therapy. Patients who fail to respond to these agents often respond to a more potent agent such as Temovate cream (clobetasol propionate 0.05%). Hyperplastic lesions with atypia are treated by laser ablation of the involved areas.

Table 18.1
Classification of Vulvar Dystrophies

I. Squamous cell hyperplasia
II. Lichen sclerosis
III. Other dermatosis

Lichen sclerosis (LS) can affect any age group. The symptoms are of itching and irritation. The diagnosis may be suspected by inspection but must be confirmed by biopsy examination. In severe cases, the skin has a "parchment" appearance. In early cases, the physical changes can be subtle. The disease is associated with autoimmune phenomena. Approximately 5% of cases have an associated vulvar carcinoma at presentation. Treatment for lichen sclerosis consists of topical testosterone propionate 2% in white petrolatum 2 or 3 times a day. If there is associated itching or a hyperplastic component, a mixture of 3 parts betamethasone 0.1%, seven parts Eurax cream (crotamiton 10%), and testosterone added to make 2% is helpful. Temovate has been reported to be as effective as testosterone and does not have the potential for androgenic side effects.

Vulvar Intraepithelial Neoplasia (VIN)

Vulvar intraepithelial neoplasia is associated with condyloma and HPV. The most common symptom is pruritus. The disease may be unifocal or multifocal, and it is commonly recurrent.

Evaluation requires careful inspection of the entire perineum to include colposcopic evaluation and directed biopsy analyses based upon examination. It is important to evaluate the cervix and vagina for squamous neoplasia due to the high risk of involvement of the entire genital tract.

Treatment of VIN is by laser ablation of lesions. Skinning vulvectomy with split thickness skin grafts has been used, but there have been reports of VIN recurring in the grafts. Skinning vulvectomy is not commonly used today.

Vulvar Carcinoma

Vulvar carcinoma accounts for 3–5% of all female genital cancers. The average age at diagnosis is 65. Associated conditions include hypertension, obesity, and low parity. Women who are immunosuppressed are at increased risk of developing vulvar carcinoma. Squamous cell histology is found in approximately 87% of cases.

A lump, ulcer, or pruritus are the most common clinical manifestations. Two-thirds of women with vulvar cancer have had symptoms for more than 6 months prior to diagnosis. Physician delay in diagnosis is common because vulvar cancer mimics other clinical entities. Any elderly woman with vulvar symptoms should have a careful inspection of the vulva with biopsy examination of any suspicious lesions. The prompt performance of an office biopsy procedure will facilitate the correct diagnosis and subsequent treatment. A punch biopsy specimen from the center of the lesion is the most reliable method for obtaining a pathologic diagnosis.

Grossly, a preinvasive lesion may appear reddish, white, or pigmented and may or may not be slightly raised. Invasive lesions are larger, more indurated, and may be ulcerated. Washing the vulva with a dilute solution of acetic acid (3%) and staining with toluidine blue may help to visualize lesions.

Staging

Vulvar carcinoma is staged clinically. The groin nodes should be carefully evaluated during the physical examination. The staging criteria are shown in Table 18.2.

Treatment

Treatment of vulvar carcinoma is dependent on the stage. Early T1 lesions are first examined by biopsy. If the depth of invasion is less than 1 mm, then the entire lesion is excised locally. If the depth of invasion of the entire specimen is less than 1 mm and the tumor is unifocal with the remainder of the vulva normal, then no node dissection is needed. If the depth of invasion of the entire specimen is more than 1 mm and the tumor is unifocal with the remainder of the vulva normal, then radical local excision is the treatment of choice. The margin of resection is at least 1 cm, and the depth of resection is to the inferior fascia of the urogenital diaphragm.

The risk of groin node metastases is minimal with invasion of less than 1 mm, and node dissection is not needed. Patients with unilateral T1 lesions with greater than 1 mm invasion should have ipsilateral node dissection. Patients with T2 and early T3 lesions without clinically suspicious nodes are treated with radical vulvectomy and bilateral groin node dissection. Patients with clinically suspicious nodes should have individualized therapy. Those with nonfixed and nonulcerated nodes may be treated with radical vulvectomy and bilateral node dissection. Those with fixed or ulcerated nodes may need a course of radiation or chemotherapy prior to surgery.

Table 18.2
FIGO Stage Grouping and TNM (Tumor, Node, Metastasis) Classification for Vulvar Carcinoma (International Federation of Gynecology and Obstetrics, 1988)

TNM Classification	Description
T	Primary tumor
TIS	Preinvasive carcinoma (carcinoma in situ)
T1	Tumor confined to the vulva and/or perineum, 2 cm or less in largest diameter
T2	Tumor confined to the vulva and/or perineum, more than 2 cm in largest diameter
T3	Tumor of any size with (a) adjacent spread to the lower urethra and/or vagina and/or anus, and/or (b) unilateral regional lymph node metastasis
T4	Tumor infiltrating any of the following: upper urethra, bladder mucosa, rectal mucosa, or pelvic bone, and/or bilateral regional lymph node metastases
N	Regional lymph nodes
N0	No node metastasis
N1	Unilateral node metastasis
N2	Bilateral node metastases
M	Distant metastases
M0	No clinical metastases
M1	Pelvic lymph node or other distant metastases
FIGO	**Stage**
I	T1 N0 M0
II	T2 N0 M0
III	T3 N0 M0
	T3 N1 M0
	T1 N1 M0
	T2 N1 M0
IVA	T1 N2 M0
	T2 N2 M0
	T3 N2 M0
	T4 N0/N1/N2, M0
IVB	Any T, any N with M1

CERVIX NEOPLASIA

Epidemiologic studies have concluded that this disease follows a pattern of a sexually transmitted disease. The evidence now implicates the sexually transmitted agent to be the human papilloma virus. The lifetime risk of contracting the virus is 1 in 3 or greater. Yet only 13,000 women are diagnosed with cervical cancer annually. There are cofactors that must assist in the neoplastic process, such as cigarette smoking, presence of oncogenes, and possibly other factors. The median age of occurrence of cervical cancer is 45–50 years, with a range from the late teens to senescence. Risk factors for cervix cancer include early age of first coitus, multiple sexual partners, immune suppression, low socioeconomic status, and lack of Pap smear screening.

The disease begins as a dysplastic process in the squamocolumnar junction. Progression occurs from mild dysplasia to moderate to severe dysplasia and carcinoma in situ over many years. Some patients will have more rapid transformation, and in some patients dysplasia may resolve without treatment.

The average rate of development of invasive cancer is 10–20 years from the first evidence of dysplasia. Invasive cancer is defined by tumor cells breaking through the basement membrane and invading underlying stroma. The tumor then spreads by local invasion. Metastatic spread is via lymphatics to the pelvic lymph nodes. Hematogenous spread is uncommon. Death usually occurs from renal failure secondary to hydronephrosis or hemorrhage from the tumor site.

The Pap smear as a screening test has been extremely successful for the prevention of cervix cancer. Detection of premalignant changes (dysplasia) allows for successful treatment and prevention of cancer. Failures of prevention still occur for several reasons. There are still large populations who are noncompliant with screening guidelines. Healthy women after tubal ligation may not see physicians for screening. Postmenopausal women who see physicians who do not perform pelvic exams for routine care may not be screened. Women with limited access to care may not get adequate screening. Failures of treatment of dysplasia may also be due to a false negative cytology report.

The most common symptom of cervical carcinoma is abnormal vaginal bleeding. Postcoital bleeding is a common symptom. A significant number of women with cervical cancer complain of a malodorous discharge.

Diagnostic Procedures

Colposcopy is a technique for obtaining histologic diagnosis in order to plan treatment. It allows magnified examination of the cervical transformation zone (squamocolumnar junction). Acetic acid is used to highlight hyperkeratotic lesions. The entire transformation zone should be visualized. If it cannot be visualized, the examination is unsatisfactory. Biopsy specimens are taken from the most suspicious areas, and endocervical curettage is performed. Cone biopsy by cold knife, loop excision, or laser excision allow excision of the entire transformation zone as a specimen to be evaluated by a pathologist. A cone biopsy specimen is required when there is an unsatisfactory colposcopic examination, when the endocervical curettage has dysplastic cells present, when the colposcopic appearance is worrisome for invasive cancer without confirmation by biopsy examination, when the biopsy examination shows microinvasive cancer, or when the Pap smear is not explained by the biopsy analysis.

With ablative therapy no tissue is sent for pathologic analysis, as the procedure destroys the transformation zone. Cryotherapy is the most common and least expensive of the ablative therapies. Laser vaporization is more expensive, takes more time, and is no more effective than cryotherapy, although it may allow for less destruction of the endocervical glands. Ablative therapy requires satisfactory colposcopy, a biopsy analysis that explains the Pap smear, an endocervical curettage negative for dysplasia, and no suspicion of cancer.

Staging

Biopsy examination of the cervix is required to make the diagnosis of cervical cancer. A cone biopsy specimen is required to confirm the diagnosis of stage IA. A pelvic examination, physical examination, chest x-ray, and intravenous pyelogram (IVP) are required for staging. Clinical examination is the basis of staging. Cystoscopy and proctoscopy may also be helpful. The stages of cervical cancer are shown in Table 18.3.

Treatment

A subset of stage IA patients with excellent prognostic features (i.e., less than 3 mm of invasion, no lymphatic or vascular invasion, no confluent tongues of tumor on cone biopsy) can be

Table 18.3
FIGO Staging System for Invasive Cervical Cancer (International Federation of Gynecology and Obstetrics)

Stage I	Tumor confined to cervix (extension to the corpus is disregarded)
Stage IA1	Minimal microscopically evident stromal invasion
Stage IA2	Tumor seen on cone biopsy or hysterectomy specimen to be no more than 5 mm deep and 7 mm wide
Stage IB	Tumor larger than Stage IA but confined to the cervix
Stage IIA	Tumor invades vagina but not lower ⅓
Stage IIB	Tumor invades parametria but has not reached pelvic side wall or created hydronephrosis
Stage IIIA	Tumor extends to lower ⅓ of vagina
Stage IIIB	Tumor has extended to pelvic sidewall or there is hydronephrosis
Stage IVA	Spread of tumor to bladder or rectum confirmed by biopsy
Stage IVB	Metastatic spread to distant site (e.g., supraclavicular node or lung)

treated with a simple hysterectomy. Patients with a bad prognosis should have radical hysterectomy and pelvic lymphadenectomy. Stage IB is treated with radical hysterectomy and pelvic lymphadenectomy. Radical hysterectomy is defined as the removal of the uterus with its supporting ligaments (the uterosacral and cardinal ligaments) to obtain good surgical margins around the tumor. It requires dissection of the lower one-third of the ureters down to the bladder and removal of all lymph nodes draining the cervix—the hypogastric, obturator, external iliac, and common iliac nodes. Periaortic nodes may also be removed. Complications of radical hysterectomy include urinary fistula in 1–2% of cases, and bladder dysfunction, including urinary retention, in 20–30% of cases.

Radiation therapy can also be used for stage IB patients, and it is the best choice for all higher stages. External beam radiation therapy or teletherapy is administered as 180 rads or cGy daily Monday through Friday for 5½ weeks until 5040 cGy is reached. Brachytherapy, or intracavitary therapy, consists of a tandem in the cervix and an ovoid in the vaginal fornices. It is generally performed twice, with 2000 cGy given each application. Fewer than 5% of patients experience major complications. Short-term complications include nausea and diarrhea. Long-term complica-

Table 18.4
Five-Year Survival Rates of Cervix Cancer Patients

Stage IA	100%
Stage IB	85%
Stage IIA	70%
Stage IIB	65%
Stage III	30%

Five-year survival for all stages combined is 50%.

tions include radiation cystitis, radiation proctitis, vaginal vault necrosis, and fistulas.

Survival for cervical cancer is related to the stage. Five-year survival rates are shown in Table 18.4. Small cell carcinomas have the poorest outcome, and large cell nonkeratinizing have the best. Approximately 10% of cervical carcinomas are adenocarcinomas, and it appears that stage for stage, adenocarcinomas have similar survival rates.

ENDOMETRIAL NEOPLASIA

Endometrial carcinoma is the fourth most common cancer in females. There are approximately 33,000 new cases annually. It is primarily a disease of postmenopausal women (75%). The average age of onset is 60 years, but 5% of cases occur in females younger than 40 years of age. In 75% of all cases, the tumor is confined to the uterine corpus.

Estrogen exposure is the largest risk factor, and sources of estrogen exposure may be endogenous or exogenous. Women who are more than 30 lbs overweight have a threefold increased risk, and those who are more than 50 lbs overweight have a tenfold increased risk. Late menopause and nulliparity double the risk. Anovulation is a risk factor. Estrogen-secreting tumors increase the risk. Exogenous estrogen in the form of unopposed estrogen replacement treatment can lead to hyperplasia. Simple hyperplasia progresses to cancer in 1% of cases. Complex hyperplasia with atypia progresses to cancer in 29% of cases. Treatment for complex atypical hyperplasia is hysterectomy in patients who have completed childbearing. High-dose progestin therapy with periodic endometrial sampling can be used in selected patients who desire fertility or are not candidates for hysterectomy.

Diagnosis

Ninety percent of patients with endometrial neoplasia have abnormal vaginal discharge, including 80% with abnormal bleeding. Endometrial cells on cervical cytology in a postmenopausal woman should prompt the clinician to perform an endometrial biopsy examination. Histologic assessment can be by fractional dilation & curettage (D & C), although endometrial biopsy as an office procedure is equally sensitive and specific and is safer and less expensive. Hysteroscopy and directed biopsy may be used if the original biopsy is inconclusive.

Transvaginal ultrasound may be of use in the diagnosis. Fewer than 10% of women with postmenopausal bleeding will have endometrial cancer. Endometrial thickness of less than 5 mm is rarely associated with cancer and can potentially spare sampling in 80% of women. Recurrent bleeding after negative evaluation is an indication for hysteroscopy and/or curettage.

Staging

Staging is performed surgically, through total abdominal hysterectomy and bilateral salpingo-oophorectomy (TAH/BSO), pelvic/periaortic lymph node sampling (with specific indications), and peritoneal cytology (Table 18.5). Ideally, the width of the myometrium should be measured along with the width of tumor invasion. Staging also depends on the histopathologic degree of differentiation. Cases should be grouped by the degree of differentiation of the adenocarcinoma. Grade 1 consists of 5% or less of a nonsquamous or nonmorular solid growth pattern. Grade 2 consists of 6–50% of a nonsquamous or nonmorular solid growth pattern. Grade 3 has more than 50% of a nonsquamous or nonmorular solid growth pattern. Notable nuclear atypia, inappropriate for the architectural grade, raises the grade of a grade 1 or grade 2 tumor by 1. In serous adenocarcinomas, clear cell adenocarcinomas, and squamous cell carcinomas, nuclear grading takes precedence. Adenocarcinomas with squamous differentiation are graded according to the nuclear grade of the glandular component. Advanced grade is associated with higher risk of deep myometrial invasion and lymph node involvement (periaortic and pelvic). Endometrioid adenocarcinoma is found in 75–80% of cases. Papillary serous and clear cell histologic types are associated with aggressive biologic behavior.

Table 18.5
FIGO Surgical Staging System for Endometrial Cancer
(International Federation of Gynecology and Obstetrics, 1988)

Stages	Characteristics
IA G123	Tumor limited to endometrium
IB G123	Invasion to < ½ myometrium
IC G123	Invasion to > ½ myometrium
IIA G123	Endocervical glandular involvement only
IIB G123	Cervical stromal invasion
IIIA G123	Tumor invades serosa or adnexa, or positive peritoneal cytology
IIIB G123	Vaginal metastases
IIIC G123	Metastases to pelvic or periaortic lymph nodes
IVA G123	Tumor invasion of bladder and/or bowel mucosa
IVB	Distant metastases including intraabdominal or inguinal lymph nodes

Because endometrial cancer is now surgically staged, procedures previously used for determination of stages are no longer applicable, such as the findings of fractional D & C to differentiate between stage I and stage II. It is appreciated that there may be a small number of patients with endometrial cancer who will be treated primarily with radiation therapy. If that is the case, the clinical staging adopted by the International Federation of Gynecology and Obstetrics (FIGO) in 1971 would still apply, but designation of that staging system would be noted.

Treatment

Treatment of endometrial carcinoma begins with a TAH/BSO and peritoneal cytology. There is disagreement concerning the requirement for lymph node biopsy analysis for all patients with stage I endometrial cancer. Patients with grade 1 or grade 2 tumors and superficial invasion are at low risk for nodal metastases and can be spared the risk of a lymph node biopsy procedure. Selected patients with grade 1 tumors may be treated with vaginal hysterectomy if they are poor candidates for an abdominal approach. If necessary, a frozen section can be performed to guide the decision for lymph node biopsy examination.

Postoperatively, patients are selected for further treatment on the basis of the risk for recurrence. Patients with grade 1 or grade 2 tumors confined to the fundus with superficial invasion are at low risk for recurrence and need no further therapy. Patients with grade 1 or grade 2 tumors that invade the middle third of the myometrium appear to have fewer local recurrences if they receive postoperative radiation therapy, either whole pelvis or intravaginal brachytherapy, although there are no good data to show that radiation therapy increases survival rates in these patients.

Patients with adnexal spread, pelvic node metastases, deep myometrial or cervical invasion, or grade 3 tumors are at high risk for recurrence and should be treated with postoperative radiation therapy. Whole pelvis radiation therapy using 5000 cGy is used unless periaortic nodes are positive, in which case extended field radiation therapy is used.

OVARIAN NEOPLASIA

There are approximately 20,000 new cases and 12,000 deaths from ovarian cancer in the United States every year. Approximately 1 in 70 women will develop ovarian cancer. There is a sharp rise in incidence at age 40 with the peak incidence at age 50–55. The risk increases until age 70, after which it begins to decline. There is a definite difference in risk in different countries, which suggests an environmental or dietary influence. Use of oral contraceptives for as little as three years decreases the risk of developing ovarian cancer.

Diagnosis

No fully effective method of screening to detect ovarian cancer has been discovered. Most patients present with advanced disease. Careful pelvic examination to detect adnexal masses remains the most effective screening technique. Ultrasound examination is useful in helping to identify the origin of a mass but has not been shown to be an effective screening device. Solid or solid-cystic ovarian masses, with internal papules, thick septa, and ascites, are characteristic of malignancy.

When an adnexal mass is found, a determination of serum CA-125 should be made. An elevated level of serum CA-125 is highly predictive of malignancy in postmenopausal women. It has limited value in premenopausal women due to false positives (caused by endometriosis, pregnancy, infection, menses, leiomyoma). Moreover, a normal level of CA-125 does not exclude malignancy. Barium enema is helpful in ruling out bowel malignancy. IVP may rule out a pelvic kidney and establish the course of the ureters.

In reproductive-age women, a cystic mass less than 8 cm in diameter may be managed expectantly with reexamination in 6–8 weeks (after a menstrual cycle). Suppression of gonadotropins with oral contraceptives can be used but does not hasten the resolution of a functional cyst. Seventy percent of adnexal masses smaller than 8 cm will resolve, indicating a functional cyst. Thirty percent of patients will have a persistent or enlarged mass and require operative intervention. A mass larger than 8 cm, or a solid or solid-cystic mass, requires operative intervention. A palpable ovarian mass in a premenarcheal or postmenopausal patient generally requires operative evaluation.

The preoperative evaluation is aimed at excluding other causes of a pelvic mass and preparing the patient for surgery. In addition to pelvic ultrasound examination, IVP, and barium enema, a chest x-ray is performed to check for pleural effusions or metastatic disease. Because breast cancer can metastasize to the ovary, bilateral mammography should be performed.

Tumor markers are useful in the evaluation of ovarian tumors. Different tumor markers are associated with different tumor types (Table 18.6). CA-125 is elevated in more than 80% of patients with epithelial carcinomas but in less than 1% of normal women. Alpha-fetoprotein is found in almost all endodermal sinus tumors and embryonal cell cancers and is useful in following response to therapy. Lactate dehydrogenase (LDH) is potentially useful in the management of dysgerminoma. Preoperative LDH levels are elevated in women with dysgerminoma and fall to normal ranges with therapy. Carcinoembryonic antigen (CEA) levels are not specific for ovarian cancer but are sometimes elevated and, if so, they can be used to follow response to therapy.

Staging

Ovarian cancer is staged surgically. The incision used should allow maximum exposure to the pelvis and allow exposure to the upper abdomen. When the abdomen is entered, the presence or absence of ascites should be noted. Pelvic washings should be obtained in

Table 18.6
Tumor Markers Associated with Ovarian Cancer

Tumor Marker	Type of Ovarian Tumor
CA-125	Nonmucinous epithelial adenocarcinoma
CA-19-9	Mucinous epithelial adenocarcinoma
Alpha-fetoprotein	Endodermal sinus tumor
	Embryonal cell carcinoma
hCG	Embryonal cell carcinoma
	Choriocarcinoma
	Mixed germ cell tumor
Lactate dehydrogenase	Dysgerminoma
Carcinoembryonic antigen	Mucinous epithelial adenocarcinoma

saline from the pericolic gutters, the suprahepatic space, and the pelvis. The diaphragm should be inspected and biopsy specimens or a Pap smear taken. The abdomen should be carefully explored, inspecting the upper abdominal recesses, the liver, the omentum, and the surfaces of the bowel. The retroperitoneal nodes are palpated, and the presence or absence of nodular disease of the pelvis and the size and location of any nodules are noted.

Staging depends on clinical, surgical, histologic, and pathologic findings. The stages of ovarian cancer are outlined in Table 18.7.

Management

Surgery is the initial step in staging and therapy. The tumor is staged and cytoreductive surgery (tumor debulking) is carried out to the greatest degree possible. Stage IA, grade 1 tumors do not require adjuvant therapy, but more advanced and higher grade lesions require further treatment.

Chemotherapy is the most commonly used adjuvant therapy. Cisplatin is the most effective agent against ovarian carcinoma. Taxol (paclitaxel) is a newer agent that has been shown to be effective. Radiotherapy can be administered in the form of intraperitoneal ^{32}P for early-stage disease. Whole abdominal radiotherapy can be considered for more advanced disease.

GESTATIONAL TROPHOBLASTIC DISEASE

Gestational trophoblastic disease includes a spectrum of interrelated disease processes originating from the placenta. Other

Table 18.7
FIGO Staging System for Primary Carcinoma of the Ovary
(International Federation of Gynecology and Obstetrics, 1987)

Stage I	Growth limited to the ovaries
Stage IA	Growth limited to one ovary; no ascites; no tumor on the external surface; capsule intact
Stage IB	Growth limited to both ovaries; no ascites, no tumor on the external surface; capsule intact
Stage IC	Tumor either stage IA or IB, but with tumor on the surface of one or both ovaries; or with capsule ruptured; or with ascites present containing malignant cells; or with positive peritoneal washings
Stage II	Growth involving one or both ovaries with pelvic extension
Stage IIA	Extension and/or metastasis to the uterus and/or tubes
Stage IIB	Extension to other pelvic tissues
Stage IIC	Tumor either stage IIA or IIB, but with tumor on the surface of one or both ovaries; or with capsule ruptured; or with ascites present containing malignant cells; or with positive peritoneal washings
Stage III	Tumor involving one or both ovaries with peritoneal implants outside the pelvis and/or positive retroperitoneal or inguinal nodes; superficial liver metastasis equals stage III; tumor is limited to the true pelvis, but with histologically verified malignant extension to small bowel or omentum
Stage IIIA	Tumor grossly limited to the true pelvis with negative nodes, but with histologically confirmed microscopic seeding of abdominal peritoneal surfaces
Stage IIIB	Tumor of one or both ovaries with histologically confirmed implants of abdominal peritoneal surfaces, none exceeding 2 cm in diameter; nodes negative
Stage IIIC	Abdominal implants greater than 2 cm in diameter and/or positive retroperitoneal or inguinal nodes
Stage IV	Growth involving one or both ovaries with distant metastasis; if pleural effusion is present there must be positive cytologic test results to allot a case to stage IV; parenchymal liver metastasis equals stage IV

terms used to describe this spectrum include gestational tro-phoblastic neoplasia and gestational trophoblastic tumors. The disease spectrum includes complete and partial hydatidiform mole, invasive moles, placental site trophoblastic tumors, and choriocarcinoma. Estimates of the incidence in the United States vary from 1/600 therapeutic abortions to 1/1000–1/2000 pregnancies. Approximately 20% of patients with molar pregnancies develop malignant sequelae or persistent gestational trophoblastic neoplasia (GTN); the majority of these are invasive moles and are not metastatic.

Hydatidiform mole presents with vaginal bleeding, passage of tissue, or abnormal uterine growth during prenatal examinations. The diagnosis is confirmed by ultrasound scanning and by β-hCG titers (beta human chorionic gonadotropin). Complete moles are usually karyotype 46,XX but may be 46,XY. No fetus is present and there is a "snowstorm" pattern on ultrasound examination. Theca lutein cysts are seen in 25% of cases. Post–molar pregnancy GTN occurs in 20% of cases. The high levels of β-hCG can cause hyperthyroidism by stimulating the thyroid gland.

Partial moles are karyotype 69,XXX or 69,XXY. A fetus is often present. The presentation is often of a missed abortion or severe fetal growth retardation. Partial moles may present with severe preeclampsia in the second trimester. Post–molar pregnancy GTN is rare in cases of partial moles but can occur.

Invasive moles are diagnosed when evacuation of a hydatidiform mole does not cause resolution of the β-hCG levels. Placental site trophoblastic tumor usually presents with abnormal bleeding after term delivery and persistently low β-hCG levels.

Treatment

Preoperative evaluation includes a chest x-ray, complete blood count with platelet count, clotting function studies, renal and liver function studies, blood type and antibody screen, and determination of β-hCG levels. Suction D & C is used to evacuate the mole. No therapy is needed for theca lutein cysts. Intravenous oxytocin is begun after evacuation and continued for several hours. Pulmonary complications secondary to deportation of villi to the lungs may occur during the operative or postoperative period. Respiratory distress can also be caused by high output heart failure secondary to anemia, hyperthyroidism, preeclampsia, or fluid overload. Hysterectomy is an alternative to D & C in selected patients.

After evacuation, patients should have weekly determinations of the serum hCG level until it is undetectable. The level should then be checked every 1–2 months for 6–12 months. Oral contraception or other effective contraception is given for 6–12 months. Pregnancy can be allowed after 6–12 months have passed with no recurrence.

The diagnosis of postmolar GTN is made by a β-hCG plateau (less than a 10% decline) or rise (more than 10%) of at least three titers over 14 days. A histologic diagnosis is not necessary. An ultrasound examination of the uterus to exclude a new pregnancy is recommended prior to any therapy. Once the diagnosis is established, immediate evaluation for metastases is mandatory. History and physical examination, complete blood count with platelet count, clotting studies, renal and liver function studies, blood type and antibody screen, and level of baseline β-hCG are determined. Radiologic studies to be performed include chest x-ray, pelvic ultrasound scan, brain CT scan or MRI, and abdominal-pelvic CT scan or MRI of the liver. If the chest x-ray is negative, a chest CT scan should be performed, as up to 40% of those with a negative chest x-ray have a positive CT scan.

Single-agent chemotherapy with methotrexate or actinomycin D is the first line of therapy for patients with a good prognosis. Patients with a poor prognosis are those with any of the following risk factors: duration greater than 4 months, pretherapy β-hCG greater than 40,000 mIU/mL, brain or liver metastases, GTN after term delivery, or prior failed therapy. Patients with a poor prognosis may require some combination of chemotherapy, radiation, and surgery. Initial multiagent chemotherapy with methotrexate, dactinomycin, and an alkylating agent is important. Chemotherapy is continued until three consecutive normal β-hCG levels have been obtained, followed by three additional courses of chemotherapy.

Suggested Readings

American College of Obstetricians and Gynecologists. Cancer of the ovary. Technical Bulletin 141. Washington, DC: ACOG, 1990.

American College of Obstetricians and Gynecologists. Carcinoma of the endometrium. Technical Bulletin 162. Washington, DC: ACOG, 1991.

American College of Obstetricians and Gynecologists. Cervical cytology: evaluation and management of abnormalities. Technical Bulletin 183. Washington, DC: ACOG, 1993.

American College of Obstetricians and Gynecologists. Classification and staging of gynecologic malignancies. Technical Bulletin 155. Washington, DC: ACOG, 1991.

American College of Obstetricians and Gynecologists. Diagnosis and management of invasive cervical carcinomas. Technical Bulletin 138. Washington, DC: ACOG, 1989.

American College of Obstetricians and Gynecologists. Management of gestational trophoblastic disease. Technical Bulletin 178. Washington, DC: ACOG, 1993.

American College of Obstetricians and Gynecologists. Precis V, pp. 297–358. Washington, DC: ACOG, 1994.

American College of Obstetricians and Gynecologists. Vulvar dystrophies. Technical Bulletin 139. Washington, DC: ACOG, 1990.

American College of Obstetricians and Gynecologists. Vulvar cancer. Technical Bulletin 186. Washington, DC: ACOG, 1993.

Chapter 19

Ethics and Legal Issues

ETHICS

Ethics in the broad perspective concerns the distinction between right and wrong and acting accordingly. In medicine, ethics concerns the physician's making decisions that are best for the patient. In obstetrics, where there is concern for two patients, ethical decisions may be more complex and difficult. Ethical dilemmas occur when two or more ethical principles are in conflict. Clear understanding of ethical principles aids in the process of decision making.

Beneficence is the principle of acting in the patient's best interest. It requires that the physician evaluate the patient's clinical problem, outline the various options for treatment to address the problem, and choose the treatment plan that offers the greatest chance of success with the least amount of risk. Autonomy refers to the patient's having the right to make her own decisions. Once the clinical problem has been evaluated and the decision made as to the best plan of management, the physician is obligated to explain the situation and to review each treatment option with the patient, explaining the benefits and risks of each. This process is part of informed consent. The patient's permission is required before embarking on any treatment. The patient has the right to accept or not accept the physician's recommendations.

Nonmaleficence refers to the principle of a physician's not doing harm. A physician has an obligation not to cause harm to patients by treatments administered. Justice refers to the principle that a physician should do what is "just" or "right." This concept holds that there are certain overriding principles that govern human behavior. Justice is essential to the system of ethics known as deontology, in which behavior is governed by adherence to a series of principles or rules that are ranked in order of precedence. For example, an obligation to tell the truth might override an obligation to act in the patient's best interest. The other predominant system of ethics is called the utilitarian system. This system, often referred to in terms of "the greatest good for the greatest number" or as "situational ethics," holds that the course of action that results in the greatest good is the preferred one. Thus any particular "rule" may or may not apply, according to the situation.

All of these principles are always present in the doctor-patient relationship, though one or another of them may be dominant in any given clinical situation. If the doctor prescribes a medicine or a treatment, the mere fact that the patient takes the medicine or undergoes the treatment implies that the patient accepted the physician's beneficence and yielded none of his or her autonomy by undergoing the treatment. It is only when there is conflict in their relationship that ethical concepts are called into play.

An example of conflict is the case of a young married woman who is found to have a stage III squamous carcinoma of the cervix. The physician recommends radiation therapy. The patient refuses because she is afraid of being "burned." In these circumstances, most physicians would decide that beneficence (doing what is best for the patient) would override autonomy (allowing the patient to refuse therapy). Usually such a conflict can be resolved by further discussion with other physicians, members of the patient's family, and other patients who have had radiation therapy. Another example might be the recommendation that a patient undergo an exenteration for recurrent cervical carcinoma. Even though the patient might die from operative complications, the best chance for survival lies with surgery. In this case, the principle of beneficence overrides the principle of nonmaleficence.

The Abortion Conflict

Dr. Daniel Callahan has referred to the abortion conflict as a "chronic public illness." He notes that the conflict has gone beyond a debate to become so polarized that there simply is no middle ground, no room at all for compromise. However the conflict is settled (if it ever is), each physician must develop his or her own method of dealing with the issue of abortion, in terms of the physician's own set of moral beliefs, the practice of medicine, and the needs of the patient. It is not enough for individual physicians to have decided whether they are "pro-choice" or "pro-life," or whether or not they themselves will perform abortions. It is also necessary for each physician to face the issue of how to advise his or her patients when their needs or desires are in conflict with the moral and ethical beliefs of the physician. The major conflict in this context arises when the stated needs of the patient include a legal abortion and the physician is "pro-life."

To apply the principle of beneficence to the doctor-patient relationship, the "pro-life physician" finds himself or herself in a difficult ethical situation. Beneficence and justice may be in conflict. Such a conflict can only be dealt with appropriately in a non-confrontational, nonemotional setting with the doctor-patient relationship maintained on the basis of the beneficence of the physician and the autonomy of the patient. As in other clinical relationships, the physician is to evaluate the clinical situation and make recommendations to the patient, respecting the patient's right to accept or refuse the recommendations. The physician must allow the patient to know the physician's personal beliefs, particularly if those beliefs interfere with a full discussion of treatment options with the patient. Each physician should intellectually consider this situation and decide how he or she is going to manage it, before it arises in a true clinical situation.

The Fetus as a Patient

Until recently the fetus was considered only as a potential heir or person; as such, the fetus was not a citizen and had no "rights" as a citizen, until it was born alive. While in most legal jurisdictions the fetus is not a person or a citizen, recent medical practice treats the fetus as a patient whose best interest is to be considered when making obstetric decisions. Indeed, concern for fetal welfare routinely results in the physician's recommending, and the mother accepting, undergoing the increased risk of cesarean section, even when it is performed solely for fetal indications.

Recent advances in medical science and imaging have enabled the physician to diagnose and directly treat individual fetuses. With the possible exceptions of fetal intraperitoneal or intravascular transfusions or the administration of steroids to the mother to stimulate development of fetal lung maturity, invasive fetal therapy remains experimental. As such, experimental therapy need not be discussed as an option unless the patient continues to insist upon exhausting all possibilities.

LEGAL ISSUES IN OBSTETRICS AND GYNECOLOGY

Malpractice

It is generally held that there must be three elements for malpractice to be present. First, there must be a physician-patient relationship. Second, that relationship must be breached by negligence. Third, damage must result to the patient as a result of the negligence.

A physician-patient relationship exists whenever a patient sees a physician for care. There need not be direct observation or examination of the patient, however, for the relationship to exist. For example, pathologists or radiologists have a physician-patient relationship when they examine a film or a slide. A physician who answers a telephone consultation to an emergency physician may have established a relationship with the patient even though the physician has not seen or examined the patient.

In order for the physician to be negligent, he or she must act in a way that is "below the standard of care." The standard of care is defined as the practice that a reasonably prudent physician would employ in similar circumstances. In order to be beneath the standard of care, a physician must act in a manner that a reasonable and prudent physician would not. Thus the standard of care encompasses a wide range of practices. If a substantial minority of physicians would act in a certain manner, that action is within the standard of care even if the majority of physicians would not act in that manner. The standard of care is often the subject of intense debate among experts in a malpractice trial.

Damages must result from the negligence of a physician in order for malpractice to be present. If practice below the standard of care does not result in damages, no award can be given. For example, if there is evidence of fetal distress and a physician does not act, but the infant has an anomaly not compatible with life and dies in the neonatal period, no award can be given. Damages must result from the negligence of the physician and not from another source. The negligence of the patient or another party may offset the negligence of the physician. For example, if a physician does not perform an evaluation of an abnormal Pap smear and the patient subsequently develops cervical cancer, the physician may be liable. However, if the patient missed subsequent appointments or refused to follow the physician's advice, the patient's negligence may offset the physician's negligence.

Maloccurrence is distinct from malpractice. The practice of medicine is not an exact science. Even with reasonable and prudent care, a patient may have an adverse outcome—a maloccurrence. For example, ureteral injury is a recognized complication of hysterectomy. The presence of a ureteral injury is a maloccurrence but does not mean that malpractice occurred. However, ureteral injury may occur as a result of malpractice if reasonable or prudent care was not given. It is the level of care provided and not the mere presence of an adverse outcome that is necessary for malpractice to occur.

Types of Malpractice Insurance

Most physicians purchase insurance against malpractice claims. Every physician should understand the type and limits of coverage they have purchased. There are two types of malpractice insurance generally available. An "occurrence policy" provides coverage for any event that occurs while the policy is in force. In contrast, a "claims made policy" covers events that occur and ensuing claims that are made while the policy is in force; it does not cover claims made after the policy period for events that occurred during the policy period. For example, assume that a policy has dates of coverage from June 1 until December 31. An event occurs on December 15, leading to a notification of a claim on March 1. Under an occurrence policy, the claim would be covered. Under a claims made policy, the claim would not be covered unless a supplemental policy for future claims (a "tail") had been purchased. It is essential for every house officer to know the type and limits of coverage that they have. Under some jurisdictions, house officers have limited liability or immunity from suit. Under other jurisdictions, house officers are treated as any other physician. Some training programs buy coverage for the house officers. Some of these policies do not provide a "tail" for claims that are made after a house officer leaves a program.

Rights and Obligations of Physicians

All physicians have certain rights and obligations concerning patient care. As with any private individual, physicians have the freedom not to enter into contracts if they do not wish to do so. Thus, physicians need not accept a given patient for care and, in theory at least, do not have to give a reason for the decision. In certain situations, however, physicians may have a legal obligation to care for whoever requests care. For instance, physicians often agree to accept the responsibility to be on call for various services. As a consequence of your hospital or practice affiliation agreements (e.g., emergency room or taking call for another physician who is away), you have agreed to enter into the physician-patient contract for virtually any patient who can reach you. In addition, many physicians are unaware of obligations they may have under antidiscrimination laws and those concerning the handicapped. Generally speaking, these laws prevent physicians from refusing care to patients with any type of handicap, including highly infectious disease (such as AIDS), whether or not the patient has any opportunity to pay for care. A physician may, in most jurisdictions, "fire" a patient without running the risk of an abandonment claim. In order to terminate the physician-patient relationship, the physician must ensure that the patient does not have any immediate life-threatening condition and that the patient has access to another physician for any ongoing condition.

Patient's Rights (Physician's Obligations)

Although a written contract is rarely executed, a contract is implied when a patient seeks the services of a physician and the physician accepts the patient for care. The implied contract usually begins when the patient and the physician meet in a medical setting. In some cases, merely having the patient's name registered for an appointment has satisfied the requirement for a valid contract. Once the relationship is established, the doctor has the duty to provide such care as the ordinarily competent physician would provide under similar circumstances. The physician also has the duty to suggest a referral or consultation when he/she knows, or ought to know, that he/she does not possess the requisite skill or knowledge for proper treatment. It should be pointed out, however, that the physician may limit the therapeutic relationship to include only certain areas of his/her expertise, and to limit his/her availability to certain times or places. However, the physician has the duty either to be available for care of the patient should the need arise, or to provide some other physician of equal skill and training to accept the responsibility for his/her patients when he/she is unavailable, unless other arrangements have been made and are understood by the patient.

Informed Consent

Each patient has the right to be clearly informed as to all of the risks and all of the benefits of any treatment the physician proposes, including the risks and benefits of not having the suggested treatment or of no treatment at all. All adult persons have autonomy—the right to make decisions for themselves as long as those decisions do not harm other persons. When deciding upon a surgical or medical therapy, every patient has the right to refuse such therapy, or to choose an alternative therapy, regardless of the physician's recommendations. However, a physician has the right to refuse to provide medical services if the physician believes it is not in the best interest of the patient. For example, a physician is justified in refusing to perform a cesarean section or hysterectomy, even if the patient requests one, if the physician believes it is not good medical practice.

Different jurisdictions have different standards for adequate informed consent. In some jurisdictions, a reasonable physician standard is used. Under this standard, the physician is required to give the patient the information that a reasonable and prudent physician would provide under similar circumstances. Other jurisdictions use a reasonable patient standard. This standard requires the physician to provide the information that a reasonable and prudent patient would want under similar circumstances. The most stringent requirement is the individual patient standard. Under this standard, the physician must provide the information that the patient would have wanted in order to make a decision, whether or not a reasonable physician or reasonable patient would have needed that information. In any case, for a physician to be guilty of malpractice because of lack of informed consent, it usually must be shown that the physician did not conform to the standard and that the patient would not have undergone the therapy or procedure if such information had been given. It is unclear whether a physician has an obligation to discuss therapies if the physician does not believe they are in the patient's best interest. If the patient requests information about such therapies, the physician is obligated to discuss them. However, in most cases the physician is not required to discuss as options therapies the physician does not believe to be in the best interest of the patient.

Pregnancy

When the patient is pregnant, it is generally accepted that the mother will protect the interest of her fetus, and thus is expected to be able to make decisions about therapy that affect both her and the fetus, e.g., cesarean section. Since the *Roe v. Wade* decision allowing all women the right to abortion during the first trimester of pregnancy, however, some have concluded that the mother may not always act in the best interest of her fetus. Thus, where the decision of the mother seems to conflict with what seems to be the best interest of the fetus, conflict over therapy may arise. These are rare circumstances, and usually arise in an acute situation, e.g., refusal of emergency cesarean section for apparent fetal distress. As such, it may be impossible to find a solution to the conflict.

It is clear, however, that in most states, the fetus is not a citizen and the mother is. Operating upon the mother against her will constitutes battery (negligent use of force by one person against another). Battery is a serious crime—a felony that may be punishable by imprisonment. However, some judges have held that a fetus has rights in these cases, and court orders have been issued to force a woman to undergo cesarean section.

Confidentiality

Physicians must maintain the confidentiality of whatever their patients tell them and whatever diseases or problems the physician discovers or suspects the patient to have. Thus, physicians are prohibited from revealing anything about their patients without specific permission from the patient to do so. In most instances, such permission is assumed when a treating physician discusses the patient's care with another physician who also is caring for, or going to care for or consult on the patient's care with the physician. A general rule to follow is that the patient's personal and medical information may be discussed with another person—usually another physician—when the information shared will be held in confidence by the other person and when it is in the best interest of the patient for the information to be shared. Information may not be shared with insurance carriers or others without the patient's written permission.

Abandonment

Abandonment is the unilateral severance, on the physician's part, of the relationship between the physician and the patient, when continued medical attention is necessary. It is clear that the patient who finds access to the physician denied may feel differently than the physician about whether medical attention continues to be needed. Thus, it is best for the physician who wants to terminate the physician-patient relationship do so in writing, giving the patient adequate time to find another physician (usually a few weeks is reasonable). It may also be helpful to supply a short list of other physicians the physician feels would be capable of providing any care needed.

Fraud

Medical care is based on trust. Physicians are trusted to act in their patient's best interest and to be honest in all dealings relating to medical practice. Fraud (a deception deliberately practiced to obtain unfair or unlawful gain) is unethical. The use of fraudulent claims for reimbursement from patients or insurance companies is unlawful. Deliberate misrepresentation of the efficacy of medical treatment is fraudulent. Since the public usually holds professional practitioners to a higher standard of behavior, physicians must be careful to avoid the slightest hint of fraud, deceit, or lack of honesty.

Sexual Misconduct

The physician-patient relationship between a woman and her gynecologist places the patient in a particularly vulnerable position. By the nature of the relationship, the gynecologist is given permission to touch the breasts and genitals of the patient and to inquire about sexual and other intimate details of the patient's history. The gynecologist is given a great deal of power in this relationship. It is impossible for a patient to enter into a mutually consenting sexual relationship while in the doctor-patient relationship.

According to the AMA report, "Sexual Misconduct in the Practice of Medicine," sexual contact that occurs concurrently with the physician-patient relationship constitutes sexual misconduct. The AMA Council on Ethical and Judicial Affairs provides clear guidelines:

1. Mere mutual consent is rejected as a justification for sexual relationships with patients.
2. Sexual contact or a romantic relationship concurrent with a physician-patient relationship is unethical.

3. Sexual contact or a romantic relationship with a former patient may be unethical under certain circumstances if the potential for misuse of physician power and exploitation of patient emotions derived from the former relationship exists.
4. Education on ethical issues involved in sexual misconduct should be included in all levels of medical training.
5. Physicians have a duty to report offending physicians to disciplinary boards.

It is highly advisable always to have a chaperone present during a pelvic or breast examination, irrespective of the physician's gender. A chaperone can provide benefits to both the patient and the provider. Chaperones provide reassurance to the patient and can also serve as a witness to events occurring in the room if later questions should arise. The presence of a third person in the room may prove embarrassing to the patient if sensitive issues are discussed, and a patient's request that the chaperone leave should be honored. However, it is preferable, if possible, to allow the patient to dress completely and to hold such discussions in a consultation room rather than in an examination room.

Suggested Readings

American College of Obstetricians and Gynecologists. Coping with the stress of malpractice litigation. Committee Opinion 150. Washington, DC: ACOG, 1994.

American College of Obstetricians and Gynecologists. Ethical decision-making in obstetrics and gynecology. Technical Bulletin 136. Washington, DC: ACOG, 1989.

American College of Obstetricians and Gynecologists. Professional liability: a resident's survival kit. Washington, DC: ACOG, 1989.

American College of Obstetricians and Gynecologists. Sexual misconduct in the practice of obstetrics and gynecology: ethical considerations. Committee Opinion 144. Washington, DC: ACOG, 1994.

Association of Professors of Gynecology and Obstetrics. Exploring issues in obstetric and gynecologic medical ethics. Washington, DC: APGO, 1991.

Chervenak FA, McCollough LB, eds. Ethical dilemmas in obstetrics. Clin Obstet Gynecol 1992;35:707–853.

Papper S. Doing right: everyday medical ethics. Boston: Little, Brown, 1983.

Index

Note: Page numbers followed by a "t" denote tables; those followed by "f" denote figures.